W9-BEX-248

Change Your Smile

Change Your Smile

Third Edition

RONALD E. GOLDSTEIN, DDS

Clinical Professor of Oral Rehabilitation
Medical College of Georgia School of Dentistry, Augusta

Adjunct Clinical Professor of Prosthodontics
Boston University Henry M. Goldman School of Dental Medicine

Adjunct Professor of Restorative Dentistry
The University of Texas Health Science Center at San Antonio

Visiting Professor of Oral and Maxillofacial Imaging and Continuing Education
University of Southern California School of Dentistry, Los Angeles

Contributors

LOUIS BELINFANTE, DDS

Chief of Oral and Maxillofacial Surgery
Emory Adventist Hospital
Smyrna, Georgia

Former Special Lecturer in Esthetic Dentistry
Emory University School of Dentistry
Atlanta, Georgia

FOAD NAHAI, MD

Professor of Surgery
Emory University School of Medicine
Atlanta, Georgia

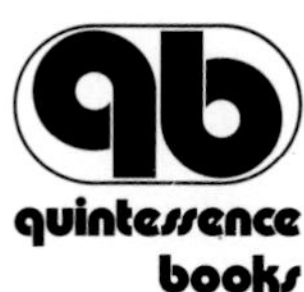

Quintessence Publishing Co, Inc
Chicago, Berlin, London, Tokyo, São Paulo, Moscow, Prague, and Warsaw

Library of Congress Cataloging-In-Publication Data

Goldstein, Ronald E.
Change your smile / Ronald E. Goldstein ; contributors, Louis Belinfante, Foad Nahai. —3rd ed.
p. cm.
Includes bibliographic references and index.
ISBN 0-86715-291-5
1. Dentistry—Aesthetics. 2. Prosthodontics. I. Belinfante, Louis.
II. Nahai, Foad, 1943– . III. Title.
RK54.G63 1996
617.6'05—dc20 96-9359
CIP

Illustrations by Christine Young.
Illustrations in Chapter 5 by Fredrick Perssons, courtesy of Nobel Biocare.

Photographs on pages 39, 68, 100, 104, 120, 126, 151, 177, 178, 179, 180, 220, and 231 were originally published in: Ronald E. Goldstein: *Esthetics in Dentistry*. Philadelphia: J. B. Lippincott, 1976.

Published by Quintessence Publishing Co, Inc
551 N. Kimberly Dr.
Carol Stream, IL 60188

Editor: Patricia Bereck Weikersheimer
Design Manager: Jennifer Sabella
Printed in Hong Kong.

Dedication

This book is dedicated to the memory of a dentist who was the ultimate dental-patient consumer advocate. Aside from being a perfectionist and committed to excellence, he was a protector of patients' best interests.

His love of dentistry and his concern for people fueled his passion for helping others. His life and example served to inspire all who knew him. He helped me. He inspired me.

This book is dedicated, then, in loving memory, to my father, Dr. Irving H. Goldstein.

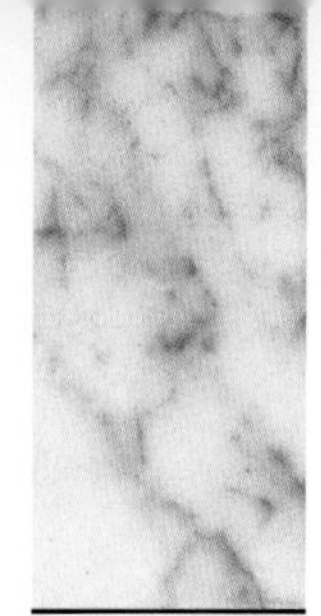

CONTENTS

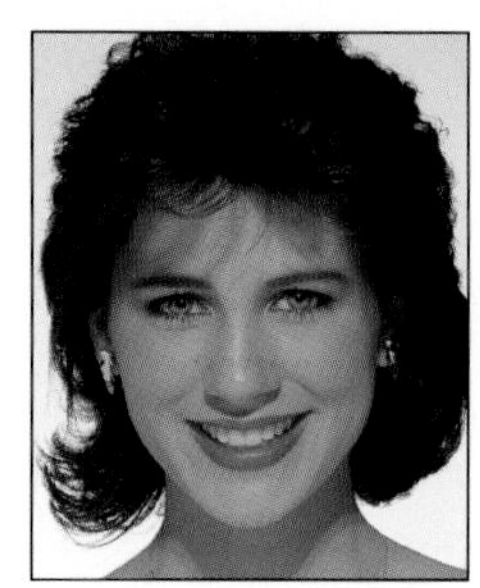

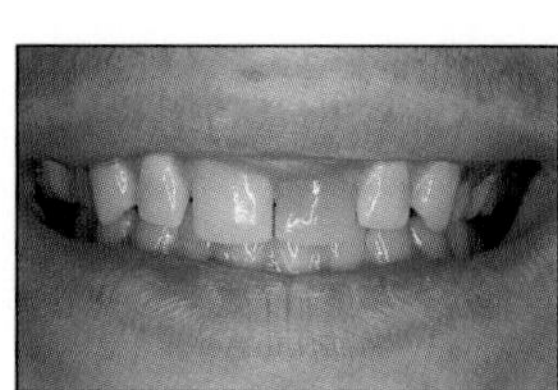

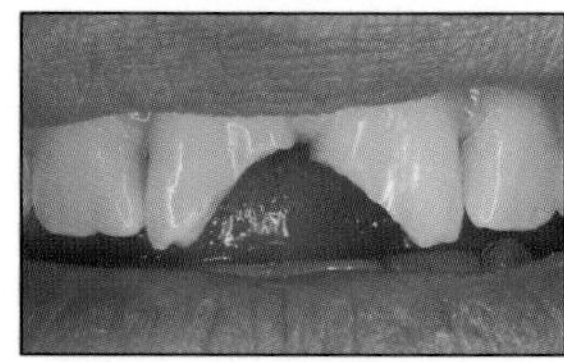

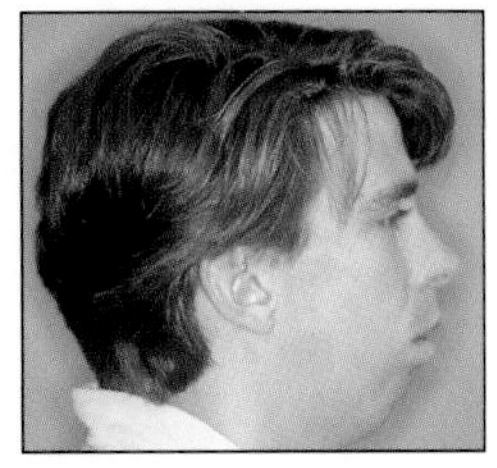

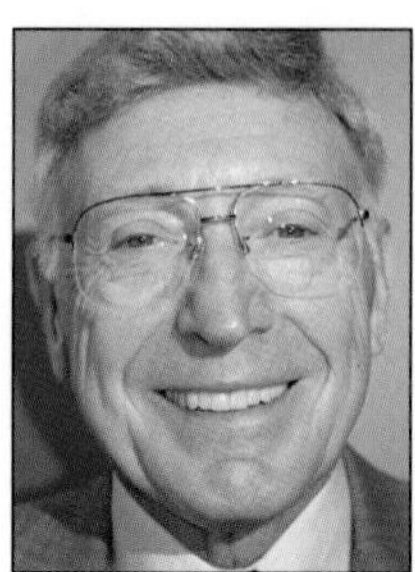

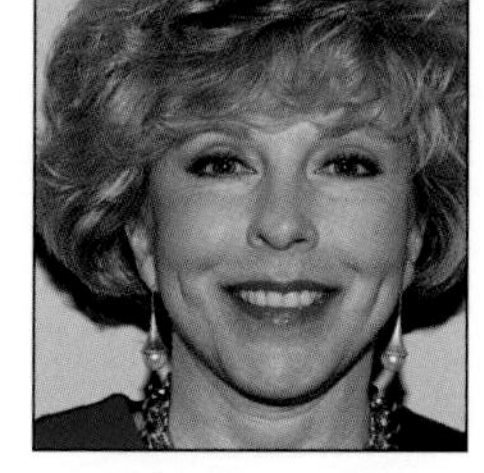

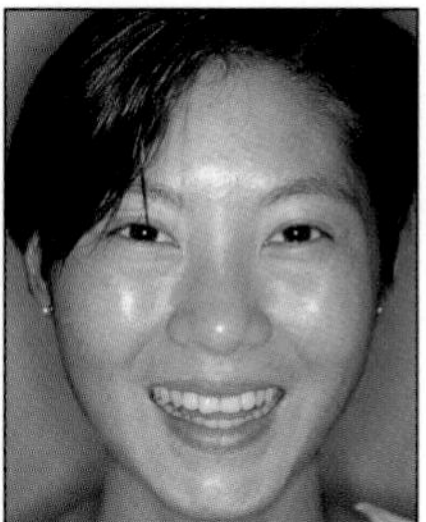

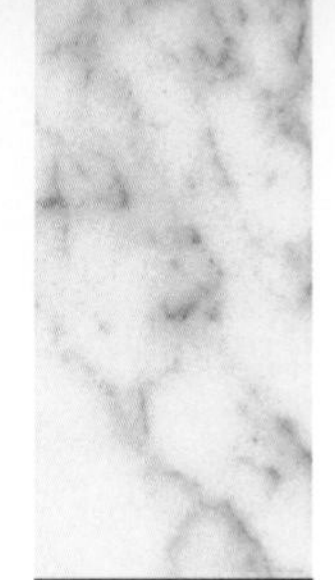

FOREWORD

This book is the ultimate sees all, knows all, tells all about cosmetic dentistry. No stone is unturned, no tooth is unfixed. The author, my dear friend and cosmetic dentist, Dr. Ronald Goldstein, has covered every facet of cosmetic dentistry, whether it be repairing, straightening, reshaping—you name it. He shows how every type problem can be corrected.

I am a firm believer in smiles—beautiful smiles. A smile is a curve that sets everything straight.

I have been through many of the procedures Dr. Goldstein describes in this definitive tome. I have worn the little plastic slip-on teeth which in my town we call "Hollywood splints." Then I had late-in-life orthodontia and my teeth were finally straight. But by then they had become etched, chipped, ribbed and stained.

Then came that lucky day when I met Dr. Goldstein as he and I disembarked the Concorde from Paris, where he had enlightened European dentists about new procedures. While a customs officer ruffled through my suitcase, I made a date with Dr. Goldstein to have my teeth bonded. The rest is history. Here I am in my late 70s with the most radiant smile I've ever had. I enjoy being on the cutting edge of progress and I truly believe you can have a better life through cosmetic care.

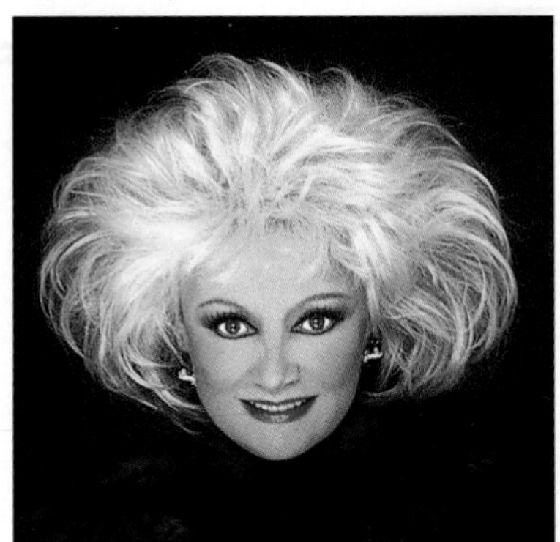

Phyllis Diller

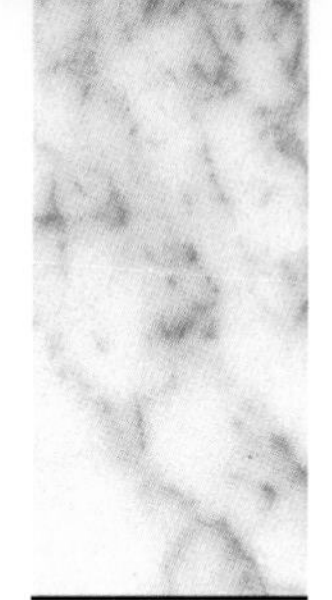

PREFACE

Some years ago I picked up a *Psychology Today* survey on body image. The consensus of the thousands of respondents fascinated me. One of the things they most wanted to change was their smiles! I wondered how many of them realized how much a smile can be transformed by cosmetic dentistry. It was then I decided to write *Change Your Smile.*

First published in 1984, the book is now in its third edition. It has been translated into six languages, helping millions of people throughout the world obtain the smile they have dreamed about. This new version has been rewritten and updated with new photographs and illustrations, and new tips on how to save money and time and prevent failure. This third edition brings you into the new world of esthetic dentistry, where high-tech makes it possible for you to virtually see how your new smile will look. *Change Your Smile* is designed to assure you that you do not have to go through life with a smile you do not like. Life is too short!

In thirty-eight years of practicing cosmetic dentistry, I have seen how more attractive smiles have dramatically improved my patients' self-images. They feel better and smile more. But what about your smile? Do you have an underbite or overbite? Unhealthy gums? Fractured teeth? Signs of simple aging? You can feel better about your smile, and yourself too—regardless of your age, your budget or the extent of your problem.

The pages that follow are filled with examples of the characteristics you might like to change in your smile. Shown are the ranges of possible solutions. You will learn the benefits and potential limitations of various treatments, their costs, and how long results will last. After you have read the book, you will know what to discuss with your dentist before you have invested your time and money.

I began writing *Change Your Smile* believing that the better educated we are about our goals and needs, the more expertly we will exercise the right to get the results we want. My hope is that reading this book will give you the tools you need to communicate with your dentist to do just that. After all, it is your smile.

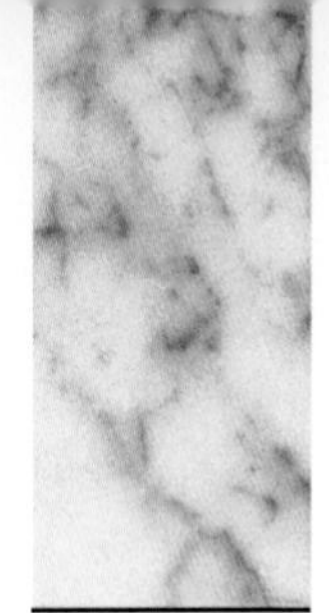

ACKNOWLEDGMENTS

So many people have helped to make *Change Your Smile* possible. Most of them were acknowledged in the two previous editions, but certain individuals deserve recognition for making this third edition possible.

First and foremost is my partner, David Garber, who helped in every way by reading and rewriting many areas of the manuscript and who produces such excellent dentistry. I am very grateful for the help and good counsel of my mentor, Charles Pincus, of blessed memory, whom I miss dearly. I owe a great deal of appreciation to my sons, Cary and Ken, and my daughter, Cathy Schwartz, who provide me with instant advice and who also produce great dental treatment. I also want to thank my extended family—my associates Maurice Salama and Angie Gribble have been so helpful whenever I have called upon them.

So many other people helped me create the various esthetic results of this book that it would take too long to enumerate them. Nevertheless, this edition was aided with the talent and valuable technical skills of ceramist Pinhas Adar, Fausto Catena, and our long-standing dental technician, Mark Hamilton.

This new edition was improved by the splendid editorial talent of Fran Goldstein (no relation). Thanks also go to Susan Hodgson, and especially to my administrative assistant, Kelly Sadowski, who handled the bulk of details necessary to bring this book to fruition.

A great deal of thanks goes to my entire office staff, and especially to the talented dental assistants who have helped me over the years. I am indebted to: our office manager, Teresa Anderson, dental assistants, Regina Baird, Kelly Binner, Debbie Michalec, and Denise Robinson, and particularly for the unusual dedication and many talents of Charlene Bennett. At various times I have been privileged to use the secretarial abilities of Candace Paetzhold, Cynthia Clement, and for many years, Margie Smith. Our hygiene team has been of much help to me as well as to the patients. I would particularly like to thank Cindy Brooks, Paula Stewart, Kim Nimmons, Gail Heyman, and especially our double-teaming hygienist/computer imaging specialist, Barbara Wagner.

Communication has always been at the core of what this book is about, so I thank our treatment coordinators, Diane Wright and Carla Williams, who went to great lengths interpreting this book's philosophy to patients.

Finally, I am indebted to many other individuals who helped with suggestions and especially in proofing the new edition: Rick, Amy, and Jody Goldstein, Katie, Jennie, and Steve Schwartz, and my wife Judy whose good judgment continues to make this a better book.

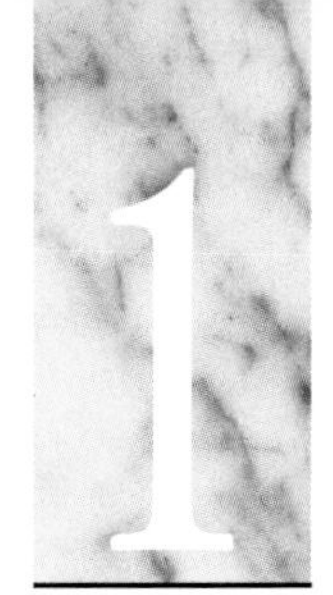

FACING IT

Like it or not, we live in a beauty-conscious society. In fact, since the turn of the century the American advertising community has pushed the idea that "beautiful is better." This is particularly true in the entertainment industry where actors, actresses and models meet and perform before millions of admiring fans each year.

Not all of the "beautiful people" were born that way, however. Many have helped nature along by taking advantage of plastic surgery, as well as cosmetic dentistry. Melanie Griffith, Cher, Jane Fonda and Phyllis Diller, to name just a few, have all openly displayed the results of their cosmetic surgery to the world.

Fortunately, such self-improvement is no longer the exclusive domain of the rich and famous. Nor is it considered a sign of self-indulgence or vanity. Quite the contrary, taking steps to improve your appearance today is considered an investment in your health and well-being, and it is as socially acceptable as it is personally gratifying.

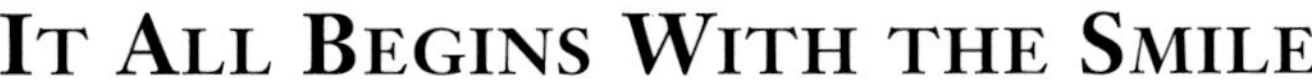

IT ALL BEGINS WITH THE SMILE

In our modern competitive society, a pleasing appearance often means the difference between success and failure in both our personal and professional lives. And

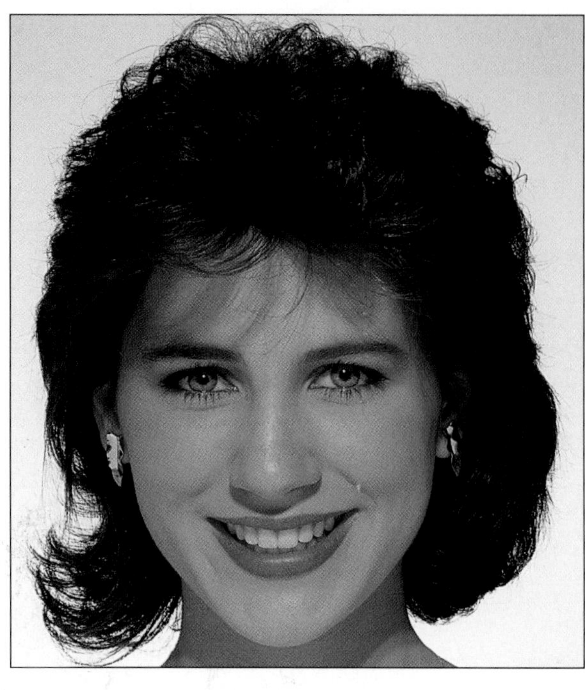

IMPROVED SMILE IN ONE APPOINTMENT

A simple one-hour cosmetic contouring appointment was all it took to give this young woman a new, improved smile.

because the mouth is one of the focal points of the face, it should come as no surprise that the smile plays a major role in how we perceive ourselves, as well as in the impressions we make on the people around us.

If you feel good about your smile, you are much more likely to flash it on others in a pleasing and perhaps even disarming manner. A charming smile can open doors and knock down barriers that stand between you and a fuller, richer life.

If, on the other hand, you are dissatisfied with your smile, you may suffer from low self-esteem that causes you to hold back when you should be embracing life. Even if your teeth are practically textbook perfect, if in your mind's eye a slightly chipped or crooked incisor is a facial deformity, that perception will influence both your self-image and the way you interact with others.

A CHARMING SMILE CAN OPEN DOORS AND KNOCK DOWN BARRIERS THAT STAND BETWEEN YOU AND A FULLER, RICHER LIFE

Malformed teeth or gums can suggest that you're different in a negative way. If you're a hermit or a confirmed social eccentric, this may not be a problem. But for most people, unflattering smiles cause undue embarrassment and distress.

In more than thirty-five years of practicing dentistry, I've never seen two mouths that were exactly alike. It stands to reason then that yours is also unique. And so is the way you feel about it.

Are *you* ready for a new smile? The fact that you picked up this book suggests that you are at least interested in what cosmetic dentistry has to offer. Perhaps you've wondered whether straighter, more even teeth might help you feel more confident in your professional life, or if a whiter, brighter smile might boost a flagging social life.

If you're not completely happy with your smile, perhaps it's time to get a new one! The following self-analysis will help you make that determination.

Are You a Candidate for Cosmetic Dentistry?

Why change your smile? If you're happy with it, don't! But ask yourself the following questions:

Yes	No	
❑	❑	1. Are you self-confident about smiling?
❑	❑	2. Do you ever put your hand over your mouth when you smile?
❑	❑	3. Do you photograph better from one side of your face?
❑	❑	4. Is there someone you believe has a better smile than you?
❑	❑	5. Do you look at magazines and wish you had a smile as pretty as the models'?
❑	❑	6. When you read a fashion magazine, are your eyes drawn to the model's smile?
❑	❑	7. When you look at your smile in the mirror, do you see any defects in your teeth or gums?
❑	❑	8. Do you wish your teeth were whiter?
❑	❑	9. Are you satisfied with the way your gums look?
❑	❑	10. Do you show too many or too few teeth when you smile?
❑	❑	11. Do you show too much or too little gum when you smile?
❑	❑	12. Are your teeth too long or too short?
❑	❑	13. Are your teeth too wide or too narrow?
❑	❑	14. Are your teeth too square or too round?
❑	❑	15. Do you like the way your teeth are shaped?

If you answered "no" to every question except 1, 9 and 15, you are content with your smile.

It's as Old as the Pyramids

We are not the only people to place a high premium on the smile. In fact, throughout history many of the civilizations noted for achievements in other areas also demonstrated an interest in cosmetic and restorative dentistry.

For example, two false teeth encircled with gold wire believed to have been designed as substitutes for missing molars were discovered years ago in the ancient Egyptian cemetery of El Gigel. On another continent, four thousand-year-old references mention the Japanese custom of tooth staining called *ohaguro*, a practice that resulted in a set of dark brown or black teeth, which recent studies suggest may have been designed to prevent decay. At the height of the Mayan civilization, a system of dental decoration involved filing the teeth into intricate shapes or decorating them with jadeite inlays.

Although times have changed, human nature has not. Just as our predecessors sought solutions to their esthetic and restorative dental problems, so do we. Fortunately, modern dentistry not only provides us with better materials and technology, but ensures that today's procedures are performed with minimal discomfort and maximum safety.

Beginning the Journey

Esthetic or cosmetic dentistry strives to merge function and beauty with the values and individual needs of every patient. Esthetic dentistry involves a certain attitude, as well as artistic ability and technical competence.

Time and expense are two factors that you must consider when seeking cosmetic dental treatment. Although it may be tempting to opt for shortcuts and "bargains," remember the old saying, "You get what you pay for." The best esthetic dentistry requires a highly personalized approach, and thus is not typically offered at discount prices, nor covered by insurance.

THE BEST ESTHETIC DENTISTRY REQUIRES A HIGHLY PERSONALIZED APPROACH, AND THUS IS NOT TYPICALLY OFFERED AT DISCOUNT PRICES, NOR COVERED BY INSURANCE

Also remember to keep the lines of communication open with your dentist. Let him or her know what you want and expect from the beginning. And make sure that you understand all of the available treatment options before making any decisions.

Helping you determine how to improve your smile, and how to look and feel better about yourself, are the goals of this book. The chapters that follow discuss specific problems related to the teeth and gums and provide a variety of solutions. The best place to begin, however, is with a close examination of your facial proportions.

Facial Proportions: Perfect Isn't Always Better

Every day your face is assessed countless times by everyone you meet, regardless of whether you are a model, actor, construction worker or department-store clerk. *And all too often—whether you realize it or not—you are accepted or rejected because of your facial appearance alone.*

Do you have a beautiful or handsome face? Modesty notwithstanding, if you said "yes," you're in the minority. Most people can find fault with their faces because there is no such thing as a perfectly symmetrical one.

That's not all bad, however. Recent studies indicate that most people actually *prefer* facial asymmetry to symmetry. In other words, within limits, the most appealing face is one with some sort of imbalance.

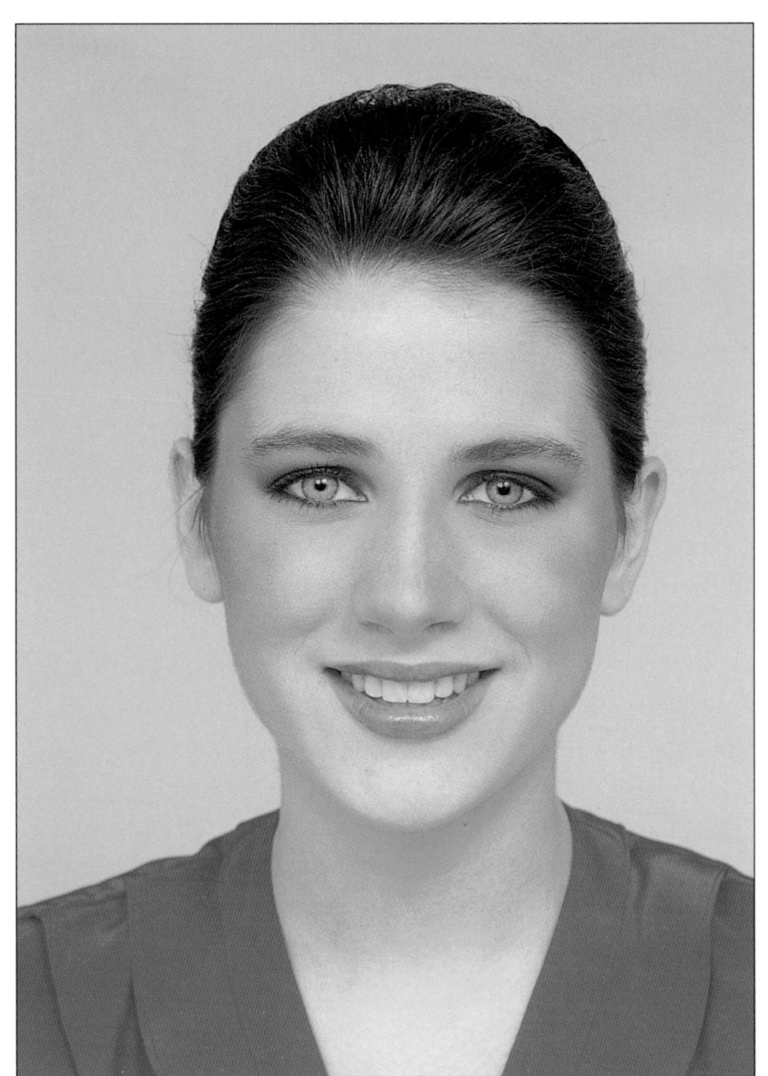

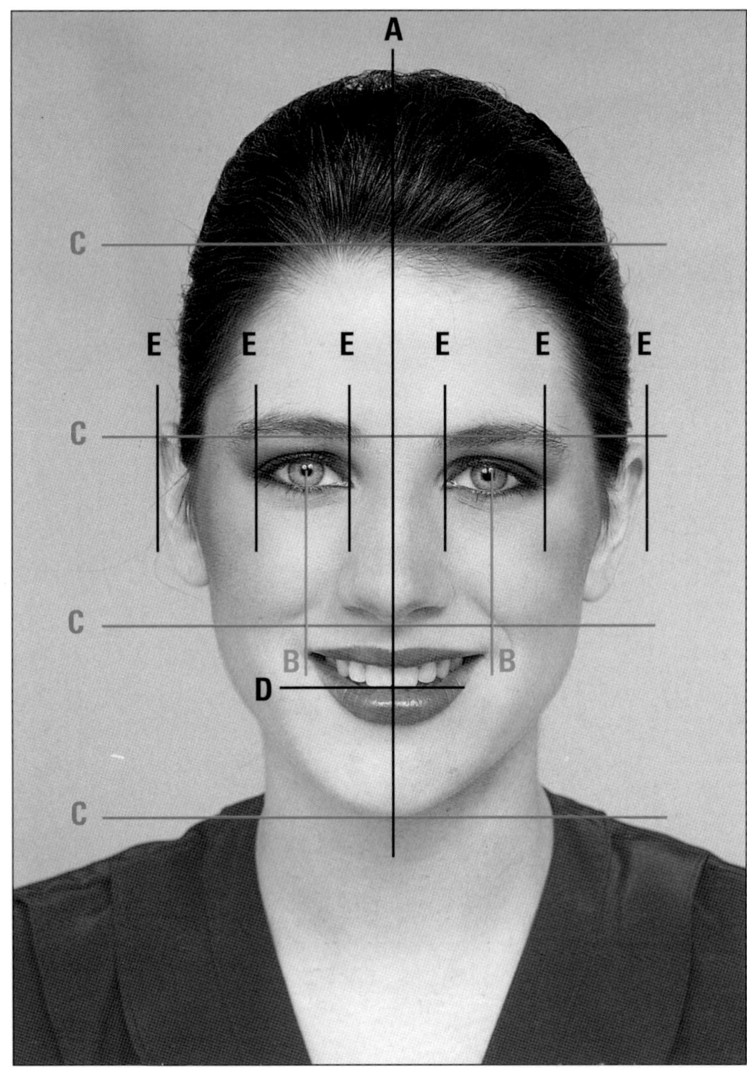

FACIAL PROPORTIONS

This model was chosen as a "perfect face" to measure because it is almost perfectly proportioned. When inspecting your face, make sure your hair is back so you can see your complete facial outline. From the front view, the face can be vertically divided into halves as seen by line A, which is the midline. Vertical lines can then be drawn from the pupil of the eye to the corners of the mouth (line B).

The face can also be horizontally divided into thirds as seen by line C. The lower third of the face can be further subdivided into: $^{1}/_{3}$ distance from the base of the nose to where the lips meet (line D); $^{2}/_{3}$ from where the lips meet the bottom of the chin. Many oral surgeons use this formula when developing a treatment plan. This face also meets the ancient Greek criteria of the perfect face width, which is five times the width of the width of one eye (line E).

The dilemma lies in determining where you need improvement. Many people erroneously believe that all of their facial defects reside in their smile when, in fact, their problems lie elsewhere. In these cases, plastic or oral surgery, rather than dental treatment, may be necessary.

Still other people who *do* have deformities of the teeth and gums may seek the help of a dentist, yet fail to obtain the proper treatment. For example, you may think, "If only my two front teeth were capped, my smile would look great," when in reality, such treatment might create a *less* appealing smile by making your two front teeth "stand out" while other problems go uncorrected.

If you're like most people, you probably don't see what's in the back part of your mouth. But observers see it every day when you speak or laugh. That's why it's important to evaluate *every part that shows*, not just those that are most apparent. And while it's not necessary to correct every esthetic eyesore at once, it is important to know the components of a beautiful smile so that you can discuss your particular problems with your dentist and develop a treatment plan that meets your long-term goals.

IT'S IMPORTANT TO EVALUATE EVERY PART OF YOUR MOUTH THAT SHOWS

If you're not happy with your smile, or if you are curious about the possibilities of changing it, take the test on p. 8. One purpose of this test is to make you aware that a smile consists not only of the front four or six teeth, but of *all* of the teeth and gum tissues that show when the lips are in a smiling position.

Although you are ultimately your own best critic, such an analysis can provide you with objective parameters upon which to base your cosmetic dentistry decisions.

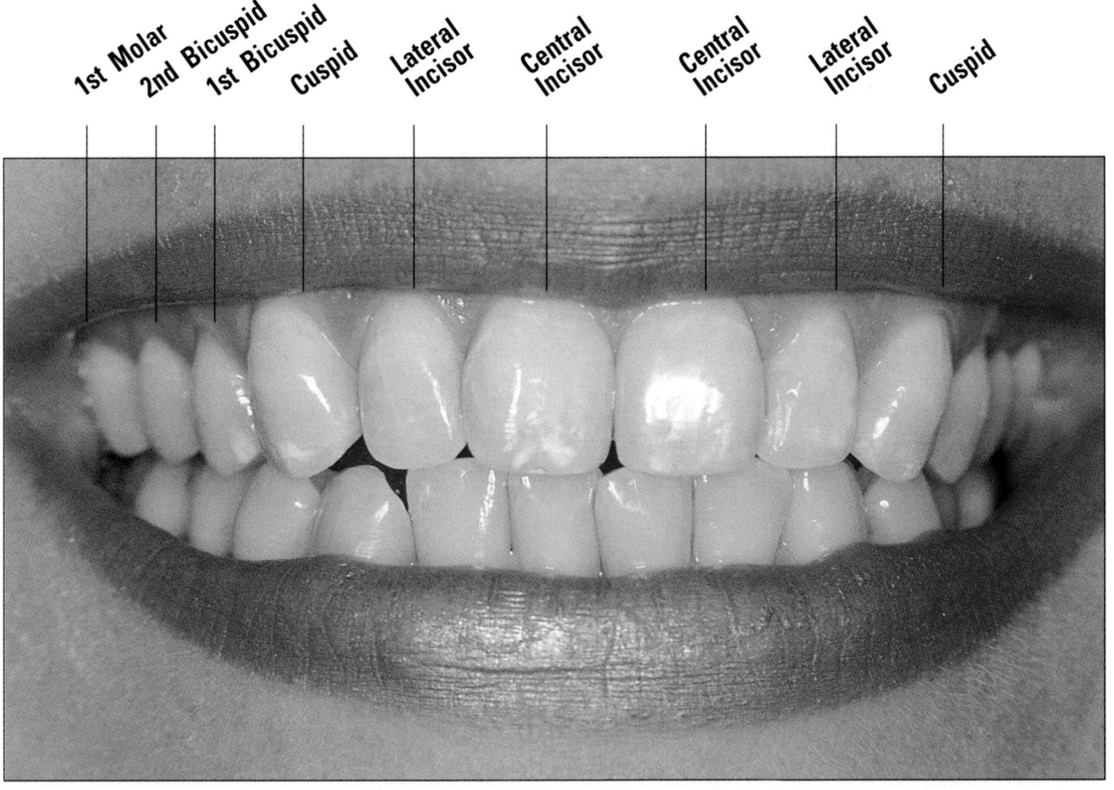

This woman has a wide enough smileline so you can see all the way back to her first molars. Try to learn the names of the teeth because they will be referred to throughout this book.

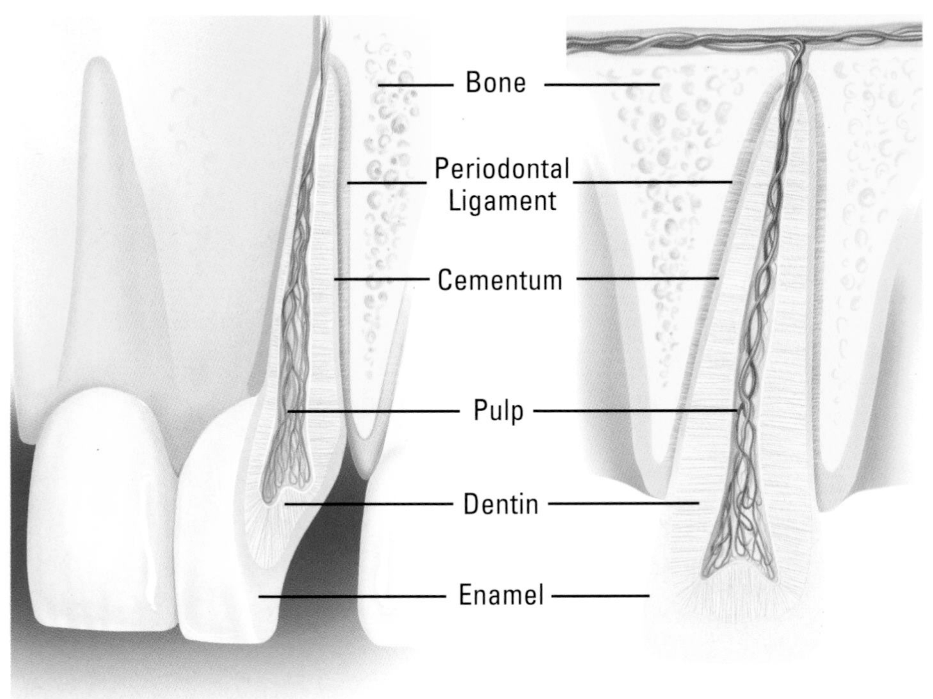

This cross section shows the basic parts of an upper front tooth. The translucency seen on the biting edge can be due to thinness of the enamel in that area. During the aging process, the size of the pulp chamber is reduced. This is one reason that the teeth of older people may be less sensitive.

Now You're Ready to Analyze Your Smile

If you've determined you are a candidate for cosmetic dentistry, it's now time to get down to specifics. Perform this smile analysis in front of a close-up mirror and in good light.

Smile Analysis

Yes **No** **Teeth**

❑ ❑ 1. In a slight smile, with teeth parted, do the tips of your teeth show?
❑ ❑ 2. Are your two upper front teeth slightly longer than the adjacent teeth?
❑ ❑ 3. Are your two upper front teeth too long?
❑ ❑ 4. Are your two upper front teeth too wide?
❑ ❑ 5. Are your upper six front teeth even in length?
❑ ❑ 6. Do you have a space between your front teeth?
❑ ❑ 7. Do your front teeth protrude or stick out?
❑ ❑ 8. Are your front teeth crowded or overlapping?
❑ ❑ 9. When you smile broadly, are your teeth all one color?
❑ ❑ 10. Do your teeth have white or brown stains?
❑ ❑ 11. If your front teeth contain tooth-colored fillings, do they match the shade of your teeth?
❑ ❑ 12. Is one of your front teeth darker than the others?
❑ ❑ 13. Are your lower six front teeth straight?
❑ ❑ 14. Are your lower six front teeth even in appearance?
❑ ❑ 15. In a full smile, the back teeth normally show. Are your back teeth free of stains and discolorations from unsightly restorations?
❑ ❑ 16. Do the necks of your teeth indicate erosion, a ditched-in "V," that either can be seen or felt with your fingernail?
❑ ❑ 17. When you smile broadly, does your top lip rise above the necks of your teeth so that your gums show?
❑ ❑ 18. Do your restorations—fillings, laminates and crowns—look natural?

Gums

❑ ❑ 19. Are your gums pink and "knife-edged," or are they red and swollen?
❑ ❑ 20. Have your gums receded from the necks of the teeth?
❑ ❑ 21. Does the curvature of your gum around each tooth create a half-moon shape?

Breath

❑ ❑ 22. Is your mouth free from decay or gum disease that can cause bad breath?

If you could alter your smile, what would you most like to change? ____________________

____

Facing It

What Your Smile Reveals

Teeth

1. *In a slight smile with teeth parted, do the tips of your teeth show?*

When you smile slightly or when you speak, the edges of the front teeth should show slightly. If your upper teeth have been worn too much or if you have a low lipline, you may appear as if you have no teeth and forgot to wear your dentures. In these cases, composite resin bonding or crowning can eliminate the problem. However, your dentist should study your bite (the way your teeth meet) carefully before performing any lengthening procedure.

Before

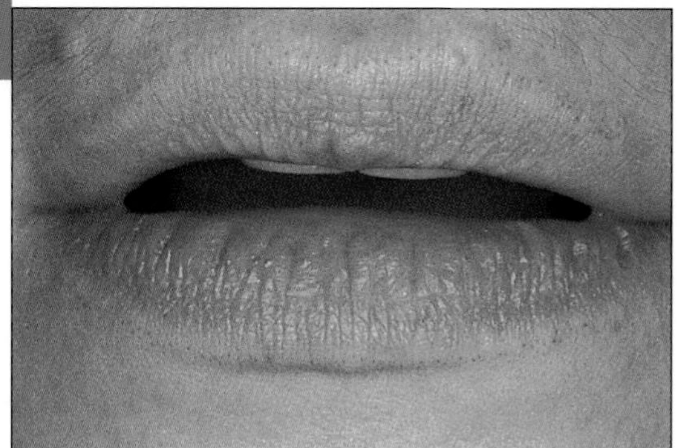

Low lipline

This thirty-eight-year-old businesswoman was concerned with her low lipline, which made her appear as if she had no teeth.

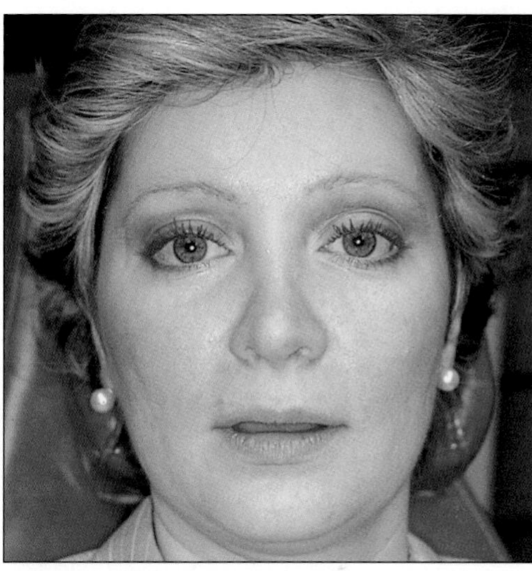

Before treatment.

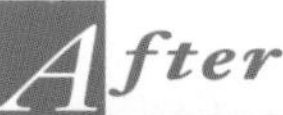

After

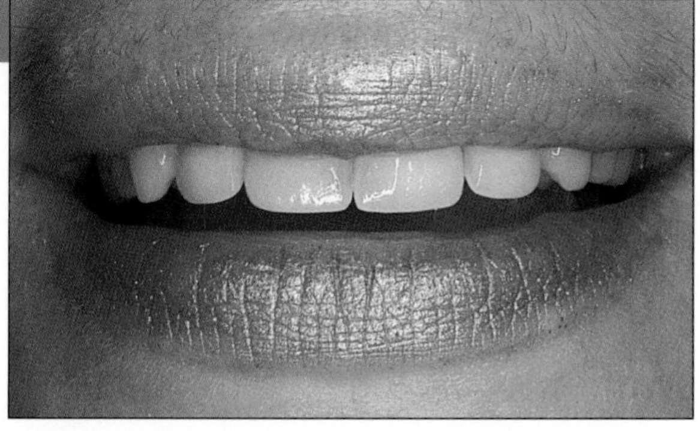

Orthodontics plus full crowns

Orthodontic treatment improved the bite (the way the teeth meet) so the front teeth could be lengthened. After orthodontic treatment, full crowns were placed on the upper front teeth to improve this woman's smileline.

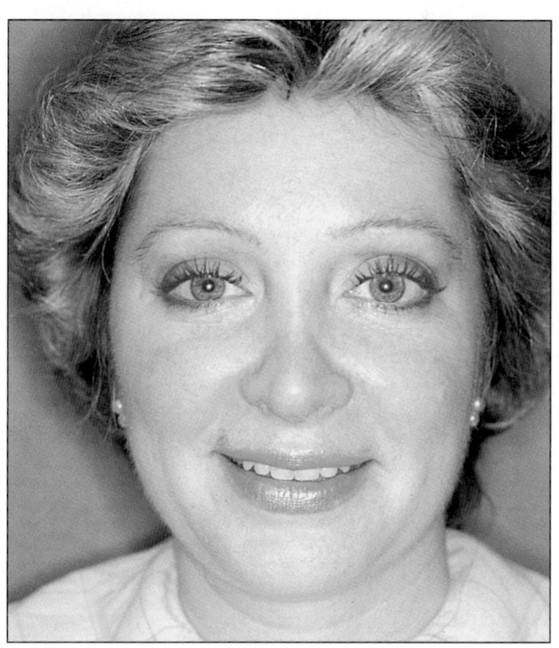

After treatment.

2. *Are your two upper front teeth slightly longer than the adjacent teeth?*

If they are, you probably have a youthful smile. Typically, the upper six front permanent teeth appear with the two central incisors slightly longer than the two adjacent teeth or lateral incisors. The cuspids or "eyeteeth" support the corners of the mouth and should be approximately the same length as the central incisors. A smileline is created by drawing an imaginary line from the biting edges of the back teeth around to the front teeth. This smileline is perceived by others as being youthful if the line is curved downward with the central incisors being the lowest part of the curve, or aged if the line is flat.

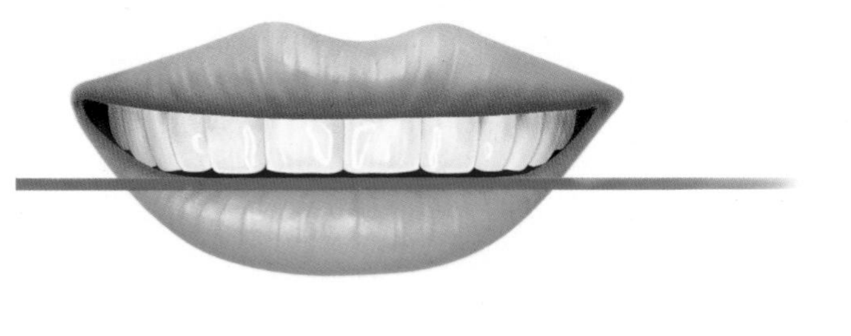

Older smileline

An older-appearing smileline is one in which the front teeth have been so worn that the teeth appear straight across.

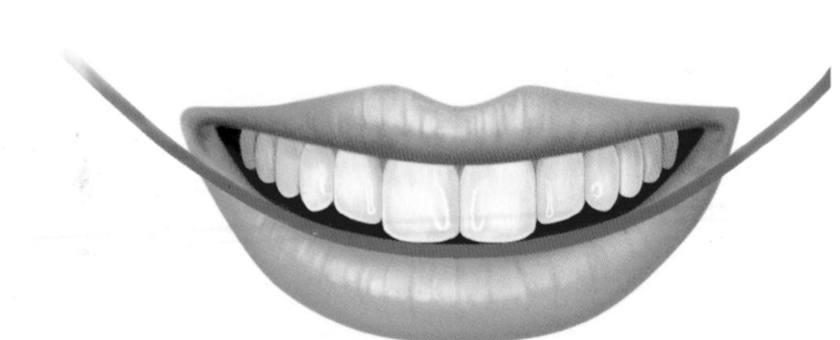

Youthful smileline

In the more youthful smileline, the front teeth are longer and help create a line that comes slightly downward in the middle and up at the corners.

If your teeth have already worn, you may be able to change your smileline by having the worn teeth rebuilt with composite resin bonding, laminates or full crowns. An alternative treatment is cosmetic contouring.

3. *Do your two upper front teeth appear to be too long?*

Sometimes the lateral incisors are too short or the central incisors are too long, producing a "bunny look." In such cases, it is possible either to lengthen the lateral incisors with composite resin bonding or porcelain laminates, or to reshape the central incisors with cosmetic contouring.

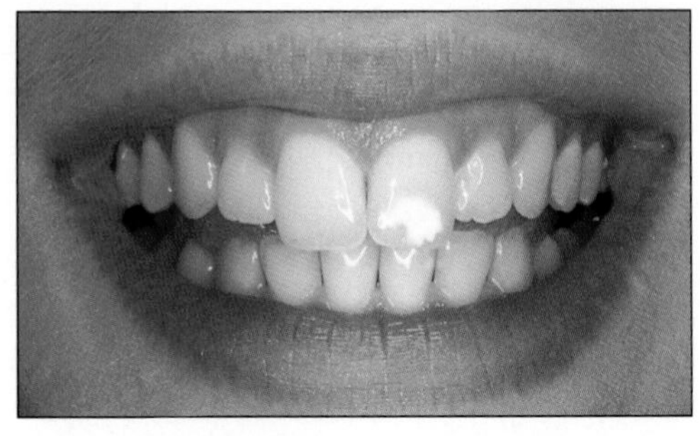

Too-long front teeth

This 15-year-old had very long teeth, which creates a "bunny" look to this otherwise perfect smile (see p. 51).

4. *Are your two front teeth too wide?*

Front teeth that are too wide can make your face appear fatter. Either orthodontics or restorative dentistry can help make the teeth look more proportionate. Orthodontically repositioning the teeth so they are closer together is usually the ideal treatment. However, it is often possible to correct the problem by altering the disproportion with restorative dentistry, which sometimes includes treating more than the two front teeth.

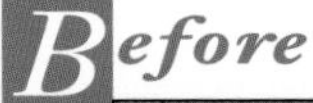

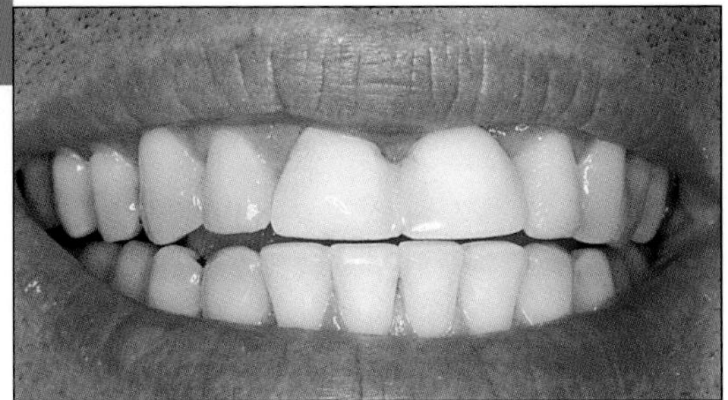

Too-wide Front Teeth

This dentist was unhappy with his smile, particularly with his two front teeth, which he felt were too wide.

After

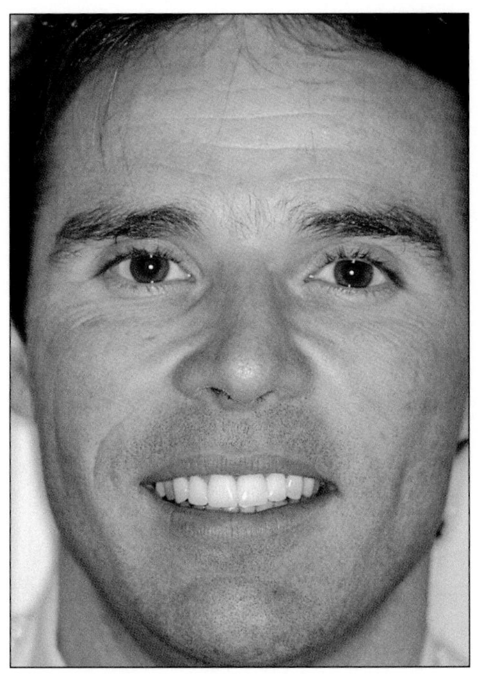

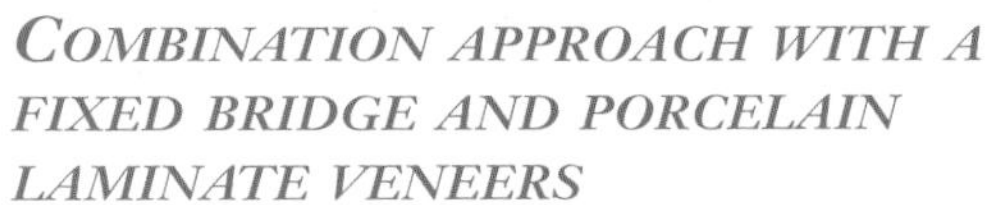
Combination Approach with a Fixed Bridge and Porcelain Laminate Veneers

An all-ceramic anterior bridge and a porcelain laminate veneer on the right lateral incisor corrected the problem, giving this patient the smile he had always wanted.

5. *Are your upper six front teeth even in length?*

Examine your teeth to see if the edges are flat as one tooth touches another, or if there are slight spaces and curves between the teeth. Teeth that are perfectly even may be the result of bruxism, or extreme wear from abnormal grinding. A smile is much more interesting—as well as youthful looking—when the central incisors are slightly longer than the adjacent teeth. This creates delicate shadows and individuality among the teeth and appears more natural.

TOO-EVEN TEETH

Teeth that are too even across the front are usually the result of wear. Normally, the two front teeth (central incisors) erupt slightly longer than the adjacent lateral incisors. Symptoms such as jaw, ear, neck or back soreness may indicate a bite or facial joint (TMJ) problem (see p. 239).

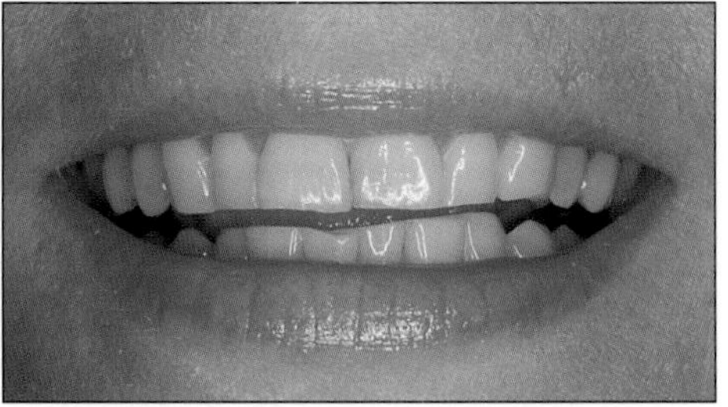

6. *Do you have a space between your front teeth?*

If you have a diastema or space between your front teeth, have it checked, particularly if it hasn't always been there. Such spaces can grow larger, indicating a physical problem such as gum disease or a bad habit such as tongue thrusting. If no problems exist and you like the look, enjoy your trademark smile. If, on the other hand, you don't like the space, it can be closed with either fixed or removable orthodontic appliances, or bonding or laminating procedures, depending on its size.

Before

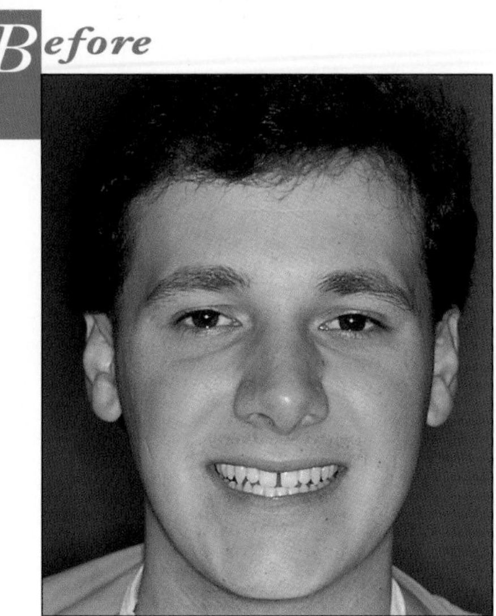

SPACE BETWEEN FRONT TEETH

A space between the two front teeth can be distracting, causing the viewer to look from your eyes to your mouth.

After

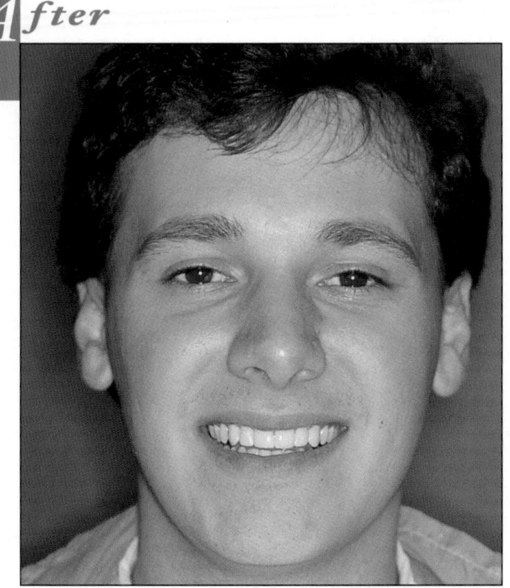

COSMETIC CONTOURING AND BONDING

The teeth were first cosmetically contoured so the new shapes would blend in better with each other. Closing such spaces allows people to see your entire face rather than focusing on distracting parts of it.

7. *Do your front teeth protrude or stick out?*

Protruded teeth can cause facial deformity, not just an unappealing smile. Although some people choose to have the teeth removed, that's usually not the best solution. Instead, the problem should be corrected by having the teeth repositioned orthodontically. The results not only look more natural, but it's a less-expensive solution.

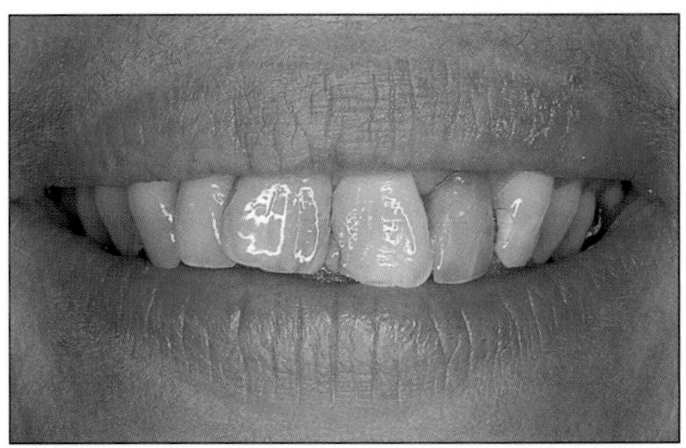

Protruding, discolored, and crowded teeth. Treatment for this lady consisted of tooth repositioning and crowning the front teeth (see p. 168).

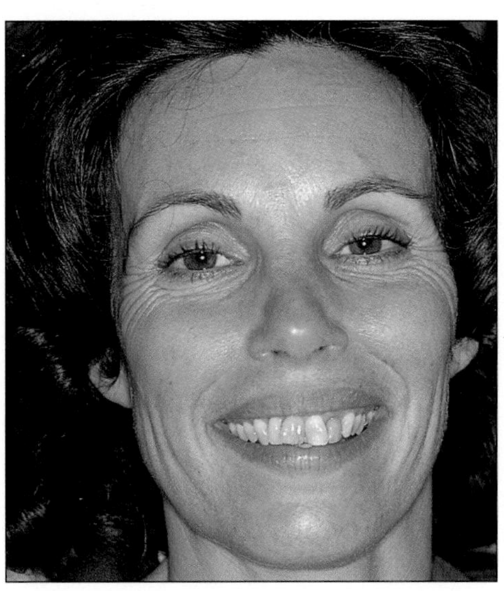

8. *Are your front teeth crowded or overlapping?*

Crowded or overlapping teeth can detract from an otherwise attractive smile. Moreover, crooked teeth are difficult to clean, increasing the likelihood of gum disease or even tooth loss. Again, the best solution is usually to straighten the teeth with orthodontic appliances, because that preserves the natural tooth structure and ensures that the teeth are in proportion to the smile.

ADULT ORTHODONTICS

Adult orthodontics makes up approximately 40 percent of most dentist's practices. Because today's braces are easier to place and less noticeable than ever, more adults are opting to correct dental problems.

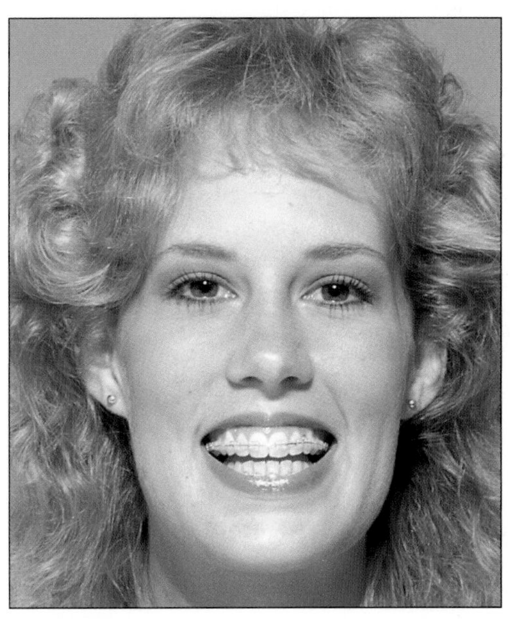

9. *When you smile broadly, are your teeth all one color?*

Multicolored or stained teeth, especially those that are dark brown or gray, may indicate damage from use of the antibiotic tetracycline or minocycline (see p. 40). If the stains are not too dark, it is possible to return the teeth to their natural color or to make them appear lighter through bleaching. Darker stains can be treated with composite resin bonding, laminate veneers or crowns.

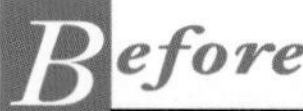

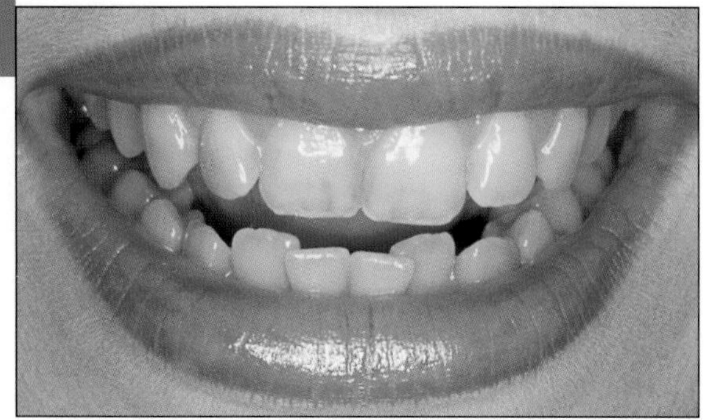

TETRACYCLINE-STAINED AND CROWDED TEETH

This 20-year-old student wanted to have the color of her teeth improved, especially for a statewide competition of the Miss America Pageant.

After

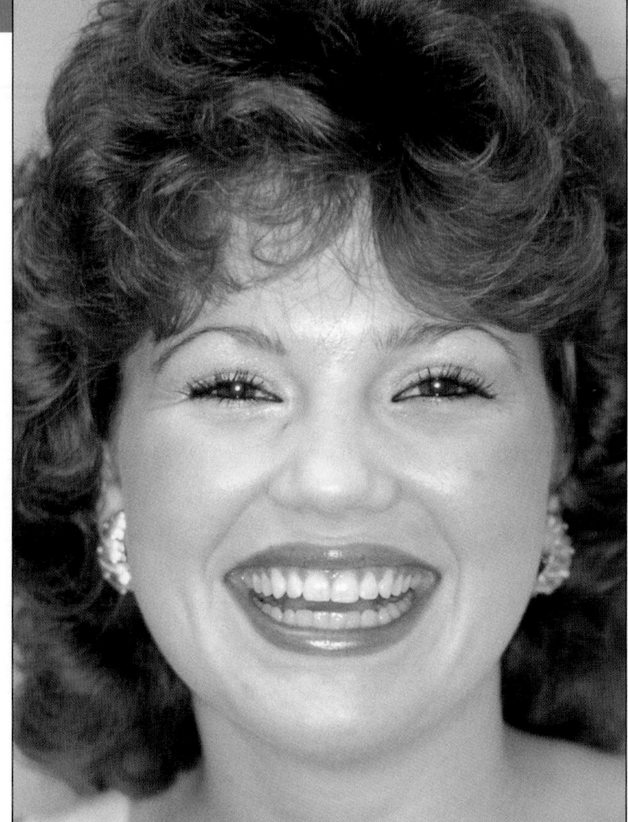

BLEACHING AND REPOSITIONING

A series of nine bleaching appointments, plus slightly repositioning her front teeth orthodontically, made for a much-improved smile in only two months.

10. *Do your teeth have white or brown stains?*

White stains, called "headlights" by some, are actually areas of enamel that are less calcified than others. These distracting spots can be cosmetically contoured or treated with microabrasion or bleaching to make them less noticeable. Alternatively, they can be masked with composite resin bonding or porcelain laminates. Brown stains on a single tooth or on multiple teeth may also be the result of diminished calcification. These stains can usually be treated with the same techniques as above.

Before

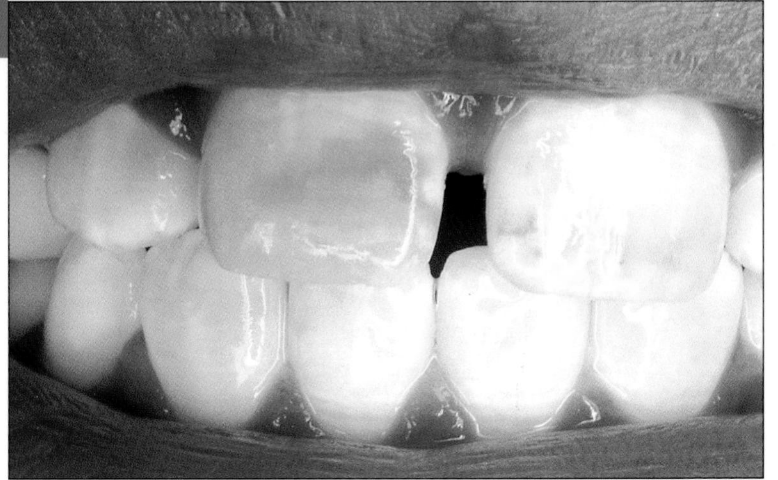

DARK STAINS

This 11-year-old-boy hated to smile because he was kidded by his friends about his dark front teeth. It was believed that the child was given too much of a particular prescription drug, which caused the stain.

After

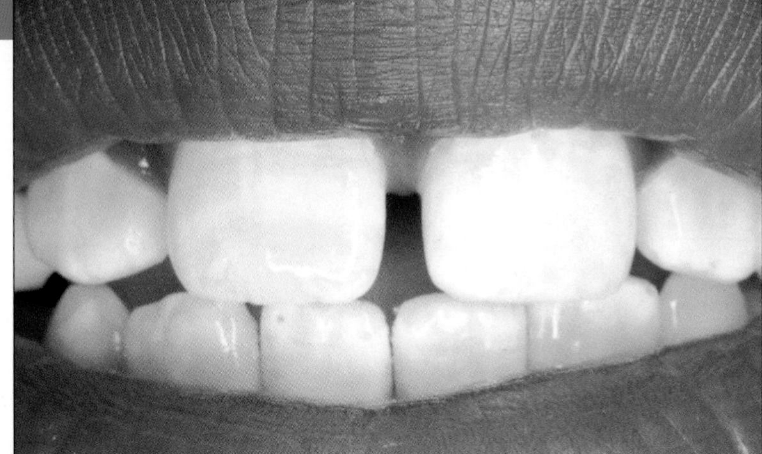

BLEACHING

After one bleaching treatment, the stains nearly disappeared. Stains of this type, however, often require several bleaching treatment sessions.

11. *If your front teeth contain tooth-colored fillings, do they match your teeth?*

Tooth-colored fillings in the front teeth that matched perfectly when they were placed may not look as good after a few years. Certain foods can stain these fillings, as can habits such as smoking and drinking coffee and tea. You may need more frequent professional cleanings with a prophy jet (which uses a high powered-abrasive with baking soda) or replacement. Bonding, laminating or crowning may eventually be necessary to restore the teeth and change their shapes for a more attractive smile.

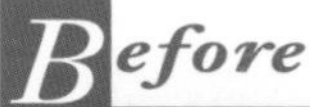

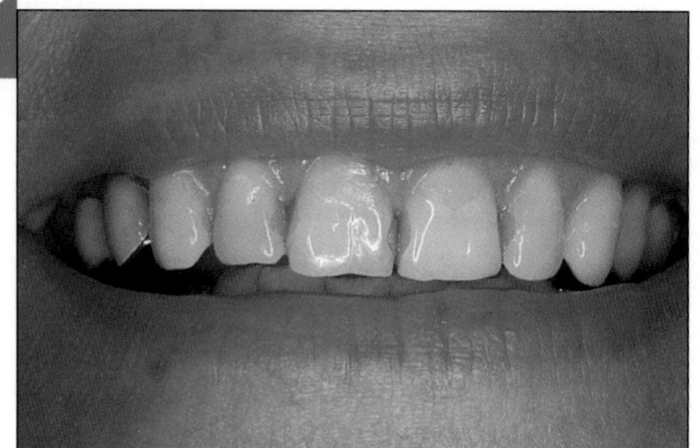

DISCOLORED FILLINGS

This 41-year-old woman was dissatisfied with her fillings, which discolored too rapidly. When front teeth have as many large fillings as these, the larger surface area is susceptible to stain each time they are replaced. Although crowning may be the final solution, an alternative to the full crown is bonding with composite resin.

After

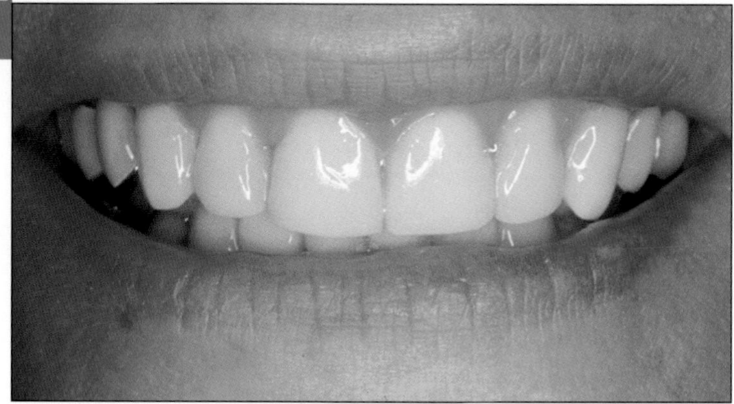

REPLACED DISCOLORED FILLINGS

All twelve upper and lower front teeth were bonded. Bonding teeth that have such large fillings may involve covering the entire front tooth surface. If the teeth were merely refilled, it would only take a short time before the junction of the filling and tooth became a site for new discoloration. The teeth were also cosmetically contoured for a more attractive smile.

12. *Is one of your front teeth darker than the others?*

If one of your teeth is darker than the others, it may indicate that the nerve inside is injured, damaged or dead. In such cases, the nerve may require treatment in order to save the tooth. Afterward, the dark tooth often can be lightened with bleaching procedures or the darkness masked with composite resin bonding or laminating. Sometimes, however, treatment includes the placement of a metal post inside the tooth for reinforcement, followed by a crown or "cap."

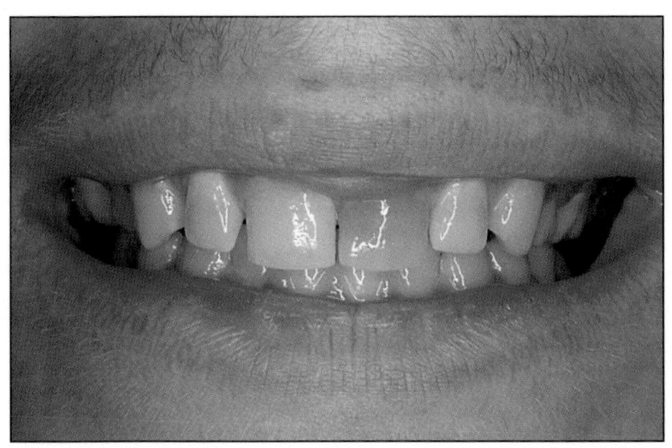

INJURED FRONT TOOTH

If one of your front teeth is much darker than its counterpart, the nerve (pulp tissue) in the tooth is injured. Untreated, the tooth can continue to darken (see p. 46).

13. *Are your lower six front teeth straight?*

If your lower six front teeth are crooked, it is best to have them repositioned or straightened by an orthodontist. However, for those people who refuse such long-term treatment, cosmetic contouring can usually make the teeth appear much straighter than they are.

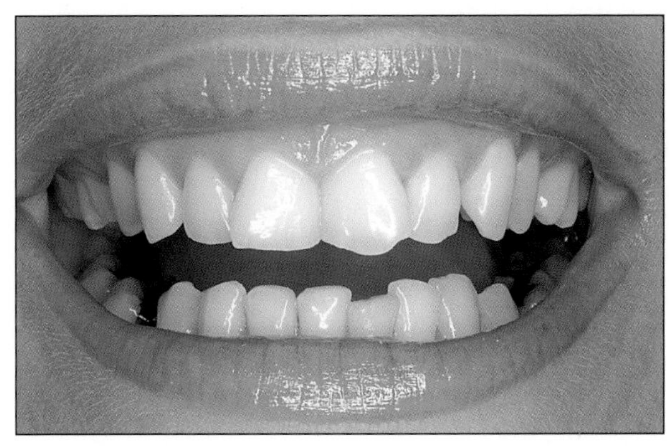

OVERLAPPING AND CROWDED FRONT TEETH

This 29-year-old model and actress had overlapping, crowded front teeth. She was concerned about being restricted from posing for close-up photographs, but ruled out orthodontics because she wanted immediate results. She was also reluctant to reduce the teeth for crowning (see p. 151).

14. *Are your lower six front teeth even in appearance?*

Uneven lower teeth, with one or more teeth longer than the others, can be a distraction when you speak. Through cosmetic contouring, the teeth can often be reshaped to appear even.

Before

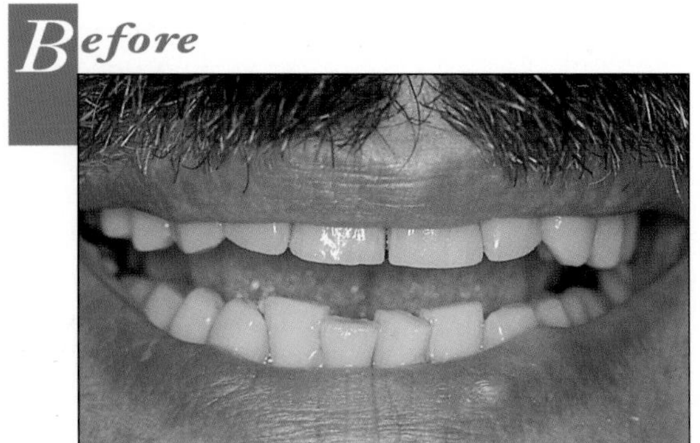

CROWDED LOWER TEETH

These lower teeth looked like fangs when this 42-year-old businessman talked or smiled.

After

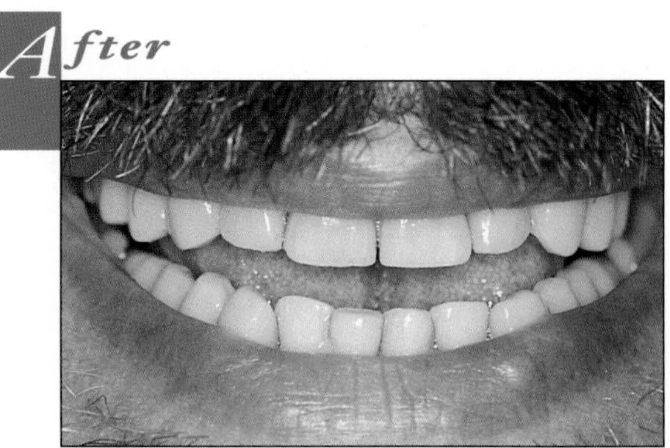

COSMETIC CONTOURING

In a single cosmetic contouring session, the teeth were reshaped, which helped make them appear much straighter.

15. *Are your back teeth free of stains and discolorations from unsightly restorations?*

A discolored back tooth caused by a defective filling can spoil an otherwise attractive smile. Moreover, the discolored tooth may indicate decay or leakage from an old silver filling that needs to be replaced. Have it checked by your dentist. If fillings are replaced, be sure a technique that returns the tooth to its normal color is used.

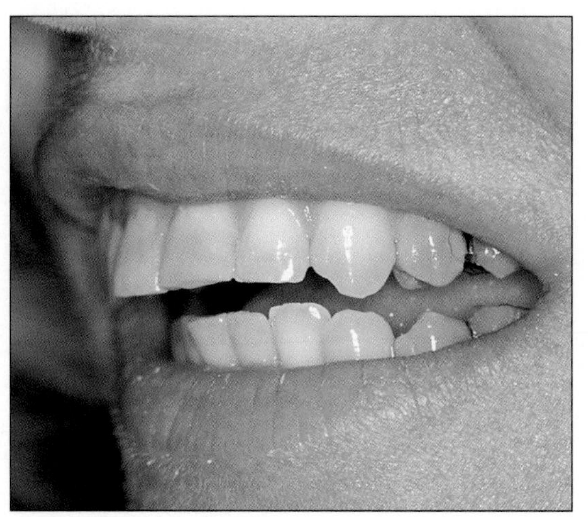

DISCOLORED BACK TEETH

A discolored side tooth can be an unwanted distraction when smiling. One common cause of such discoloration is a faulty silver filling. These silver (amalgam) restorations can later corrode, and the mercury can leak into the inner walls of the tooth, changing its color. Treatment may be replacement of the filling with a protective liner or one of the newer tooth-colored posterior composite-resin filling materials (see p. 77).

16. *Do the necks of your teeth indicate erosion, a ditched-in "V," that can be seen or felt with your fingernail?*

These deformities can progress rapidly, resulting in tooth discoloration and sensitivity. However, they usually can be corrected easily and esthetically with composite resin bonding. The primary advantage, however, is that such tooth repair prevents further erosion and possible damage to the nerve.

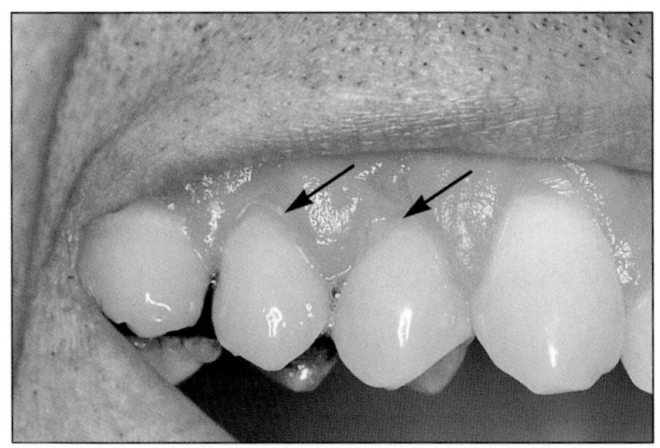

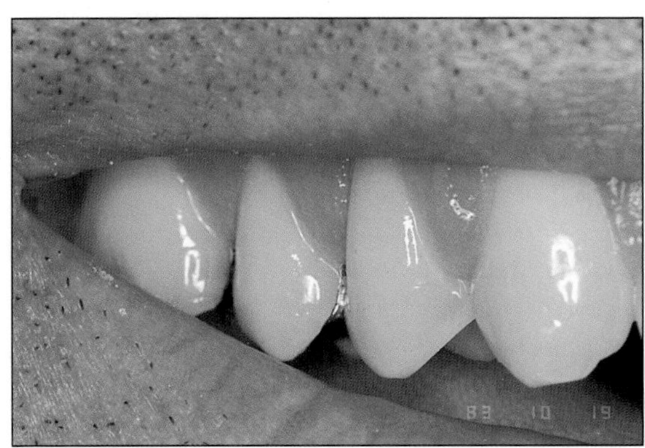

ERODING TEETH WITH GUM RECESSION

If your gum tissue recedes, the roots of your teeth can become exposed, as shown above left. If this happens, the softer root covering or cementum can easily be destroyed by improper brushing. This 42-year-old lawyer had erosion (or "ditching out") around the necks of his upper bicuspids. This type of defect should either be treated with a tissue graft (see p. 222) or bonded with composite resin as the photo on the right depicts.

17. *When you smile broadly, does your top lip rise above the necks of your teeth so that your gums show?*

If your teeth and gum tissue show on a full smile, you probably have a high lipline, or short upper lip (see p. 23, liplines). If so, make sure your gums stay healthy because they are always on display. You should also avoid crowning or capping your front teeth, if possible. The gumline around a cap can eventually recede and reveal a telltale line that shows that the tooth is not really your own. So, if you have a choice, try to have the tooth bonded with composite resin in case of fracture or other deformity.

18. *Do your restorations—fillings, laminates and crowns—look natural?*

Most people want their restorations to look natural. This requires not only technical expertise, but artistry on the part of both the dentist and the laboratory technician. How much of a perfectionist are you? Using a scale from "1" through "10," rate yourself. If you're a "5," an ordinary technician can probably satisfy you. If, on the other hand, you are a "9" or a "10," make sure your dentist uses a top-notch or "master" ceramist.

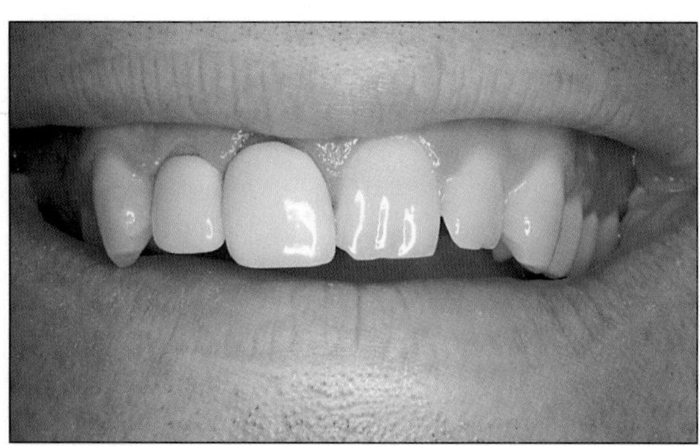

UNNATURAL-LOOKING CROWNS

Unnaturalness in this smile is revealed by the dark line around the two right front crowned teeth. Also, the shapes of the crowned teeth are inconsistent with the adjacent teeth. Finally, the porcelain is so opaque (lacking translucence) that it does not blend in with the color, or even texture, of the adjacent teeth. Since this young man was a model, his smile was of the utmost importance. Due to the unnaturalness of his smile, it limited the work he could do.

Gums

19. *Are your gums pink and "knife-edged," or are they red and swollen?*

Gums should be pink and well-defined, not red and puffy. Dark or red gum tissue around teeth or restorations may indicate periodontal disease, an allergic reaction or an ill-fitting restoration. To protect your gum tissue, be sure to brush and floss properly and maintain a well-balanced diet. An extra cleaning appointment during the year also may go a long way toward helping you maintain healthy gums.

INFLAMED GUM TISSUE

This patient's high lipline reveals an otherwise attractive set of teeth. The smile, however, is ruined by red, swollen and puffy gums. This is typical of patients with gum disease. The puffy gums are caused by bacterial plaque. Proper oral care can restore this smile to its original beauty.

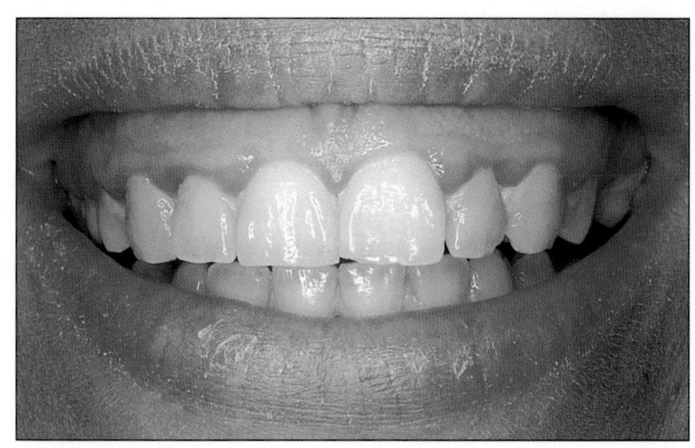

20. *Have your gums receded from the necks of the teeth?*

If your gums are receding or clefting (forming tiny "ditches"), don't ignore it! This type of problem typically grows worse, eventually exposing the roots of the teeth, which, in turn, erode quickly and cause even more damage. Your dentist may refer you to a periodontist, a specialist in treating gum disorders, for treatment. Frequently, bad brushing habits are the culprit.

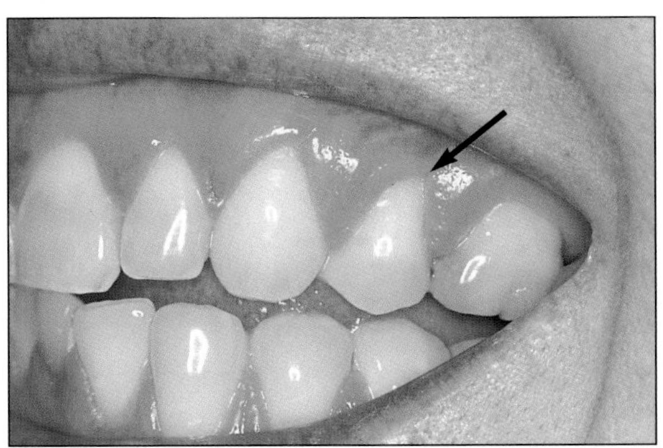

GUM RECESSION

This 30-year-old woman has a potential problem with gum recession. Note the beginning clefts at the neck of the bicuspid (see p. 222).

21. *Does the curvature of your gum around each tooth create a half-moon shape?*

The gum contour should never be flat unless a bone deformity or overgrowth of tissue is the cause. If your gum contour is flat instead of curved, your teeth may appear too short. Periodontal surgery, which typically is required to correct this condition, should be performed before any other type of cosmetic treatment is initiated. Note the attractive curvature pictured on p. 217.

INSUFFICIENT GUM CONTOUR

A flat gum contour, not nearly as attractive as curved (half-moon shaped) gums, can be the result of gum (periodontal) disease. However, the contour can usually be made to look much healthier and more attractive with periodontal treatment.

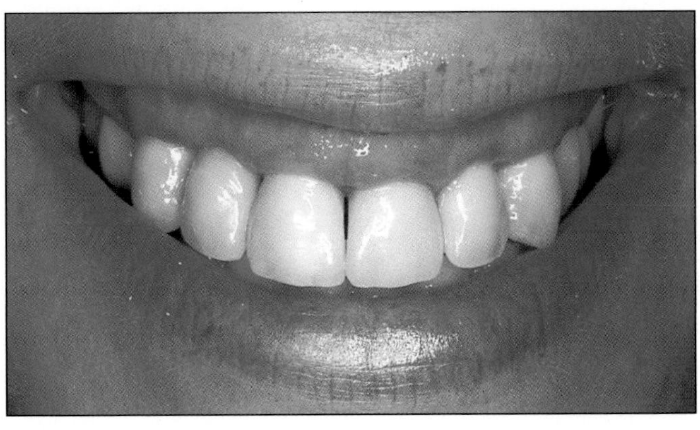

Breath

22. *Is your mouth free of decay or gum disease that can cause bad breath?*
No one always has pleasant breath. However, if you consistently experience bad breath—even with regular brushing and flossing—see your dentist. Unpleasant breath can indicate tooth decay, gum disease or systemic illness.

If after responding to the preceding questions you believe that you can benefit from cosmetic dentistry, the next step involves discussing your wants and needs, as well as possible treatment alternatives, with your dentist.

Questions to Ask Your Cosmetic Dentist

1. What are my cosmetic options?
2. What will the final result look like?
3. How long will my restorations last?
4. What type of maintenance is required?
5. How closely will the restoration(s) match my natural teeth?
6. Will I have to change my eating habits?
7. How well will the restorations wear?
8. What guarantees do I have?
9. What are my payment options?

Liplines Determine Gum Exposure

There are three types of liplines: high, medium and low. A high lipline exposes a lot of gum tissue above the front teeth. A medium lipline reveals up to—but does not include—the upper gumline of the front teeth. A low lipline doesn't reveal the gum tissue at all.

The difference in these liplines can influence the type of restoration that you and your dentist choose to improve your smile. For example, for a person with a high lipline, extra attention must be given to the health of the gums and how they meet the teeth, particularly when a crown restoration is being considered (see p. 27).

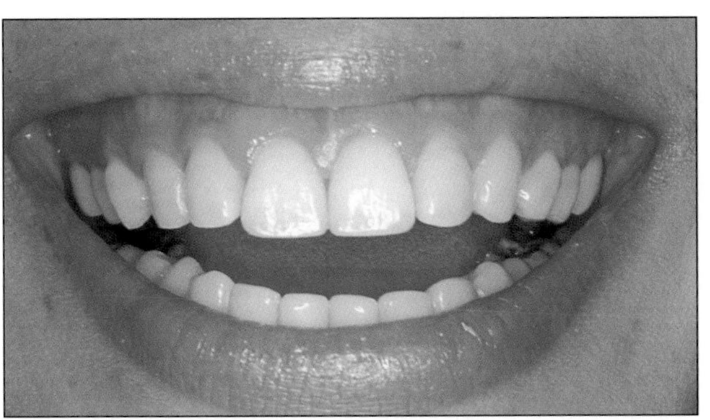

High lip line

Beautiful teeth help create a beautiful smile. This patient has a high lipline, one in which the gum tissue is exposed when she smiles. Notice the nice contour of her healthy gums.

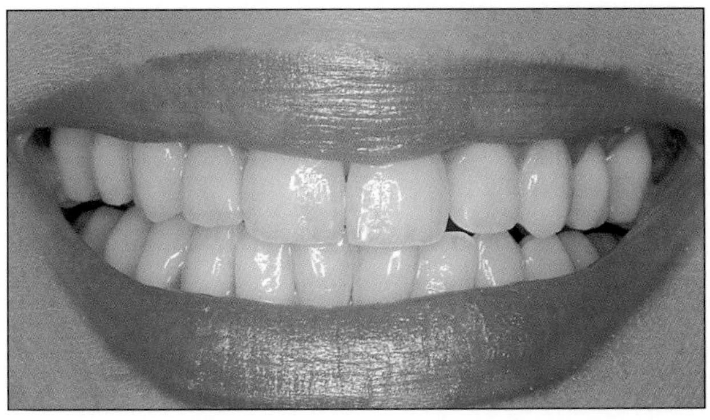

Medium lip line

This attractive smile is a good example of a medium lipline, or one that shows up to, but does not include, the upper gumline of the front teeth. It also shows that the two front teeth (central incisors) are slightly longer and wider than the two adjacent lateral incisors. The cuspids, or canines, are more pointed and are about the same length as the central incisors. The tissue fills in the spaces between the teeth nicely and frames their beautiful contour.

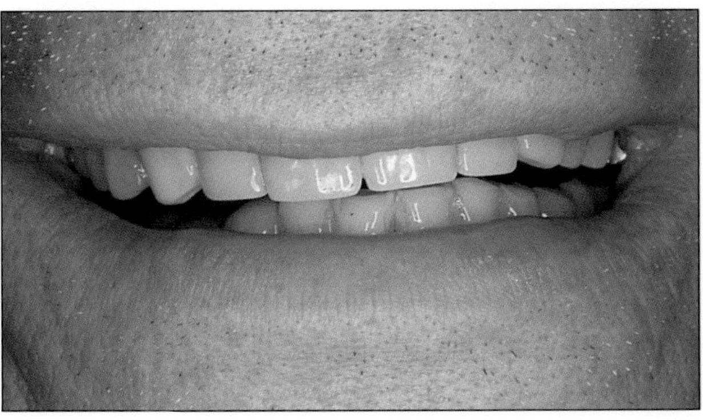

Low lip line

This man has a low lipline, one in which no gum tissue shows when he is smiling. With this type of lipline, tooth wear can eventually make the person appear as if he or she has no front teeth.

For a person with a medium lipline, there is only a moderate degree of difficulty in crown restoration because the gums are rarely exposed. Finally, in a person with a low lipline, no esthetic problem exists between crown and gumline.

Lipline shape also influences the type of crown chosen. Some porcelain crowns, for example, are fused to metal, and the metal may show around the gumline (see p. 73). If you have a low lipline, the metal will never be visible to others. If you have a high lipline, however, you'll want a crown that is designed in such a way that the metal is never exposed.

The lipline can be cosmetically modified by lengthening or shortening the teeth. When gum disease occurs, the lipline may be changed drastically because the loss of gum tissue actually changes the amount of tooth that is exposed.

Below is a simple quiz designed to give you insight into the type of lipline you have. Ask yourself the following questions:

What Type of Lipline Do I Have?

1. When I smile, do more of my upper or lower teeth show?
2. How much of my lower teeth show?
3. When I smile broadly, how much of my upper gums show?
   - Can I see upper teeth, but not the gums surrounding the teeth? (This indicates a low lipline.)
   - Can I see only the tips of the gum tissue between the teeth? (This indicates a medium lipline.)
   - Can I see a lot of the gum above the upper teeth? (This indicates a high lipline.)
4. How many teeth are revealed with my widest smile?

The lips play a leading role in how your face looks. They control many expressions and influence attractiveness. The relative position of your teeth in the arch of your mouth determines your lip position. Thus, any change in the type, size, position or vertical or horizontal overlap of your teeth may change your facial appearance. An extreme example is the person who can't close his or her lips over the teeth because of severe protrusion.

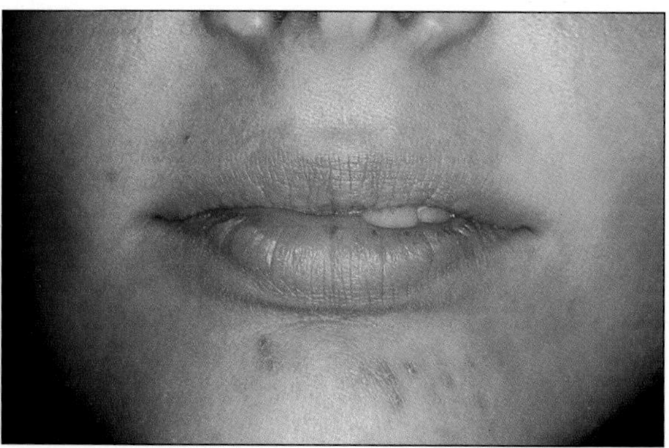

Severe protrusion

The protrusion of two of this woman's front teeth is so great that she cannot close her lips over her teeth. The protrusion also causes her lips to pucker out and makes the lower part of her face look collapsed.

Tooth position can also affect the appearance of the cheeks. The relative fullness of the cheeks is determined not only by the thickness of the tissue itself, but by the position of the teeth or restorations. For example, some people with dentures look as if their lips and cheeks have collapsed. This is due to poor placement of the denture, which, in turn, leads to an inadequate fit.

Smilelines Determine Tooth Exposure

The length of the upper lip also affects the esthetics of the smile. Basically, people display their teeth when smiling in one of four ways: They show only upper teeth; they show only lower teeth; they show both upper and lower teeth; or they show neither upper nor lower teeth. When enhancing esthetics, it is important to preserve the natural smile as much as possible.

The appearance of your entire face can be affected by your lip position. For example, your lower lip can determine the relative prominence of your chin. If your lower lip protrudes, the prominence of the chin is diminished. If your lower lip recedes, the prominence of the chin is enhanced. Likewise, your upper lip can determine the relative prominence of your nose. You may have acquired abnormal lip mannerisms when speaking or smiling in an attempt to hide unsightly teeth or because the back teeth do not provide adequate support.

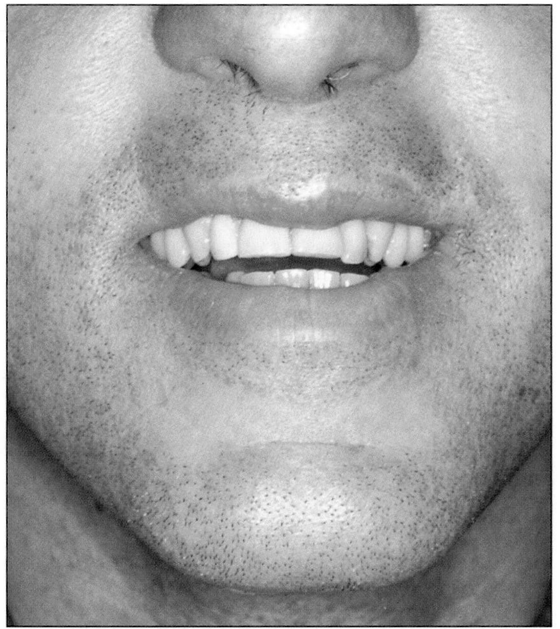

Lower protrusion

This sports and television star had a "bulldog" (or protruding) chin complicated by upper teeth that were inside the lower teeth. There was also severe erosion at the necks of the upper teeth (see p. 182).

The midline of your face (an invisible line from the forehead to the chin) and its relationship to the midline of your teeth also affect the esthetics of your smile. Ideally, the midline of the teeth should follow the midline of the face. However, facial features may "slant" one way or the other, making it difficult to determine the true midline in the teeth. In some cases, an off-center midline can be acceptable and may even enhance the illusion of the natural shape. In other cases, off-center midlines can be corrected through various restorative techniques.

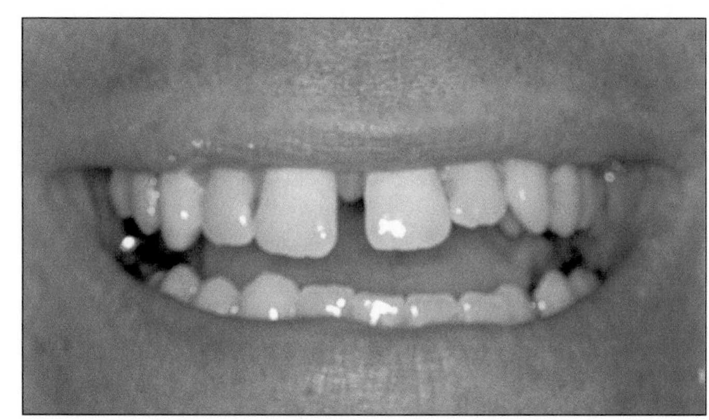

Midline deviation

The space between this man's front teeth calls attention to what is called a midline deviation. Ideally the midline of the face should coincide with the midline of the teeth. Correction for this patient appears on p. 110.

Before

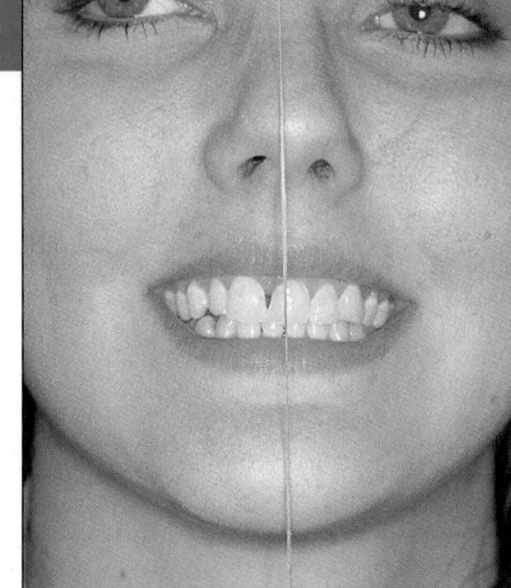

Off-center midline

This young woman had a severely deviated midline. She declined orthodontic treatment, preferring an "instant result."

After

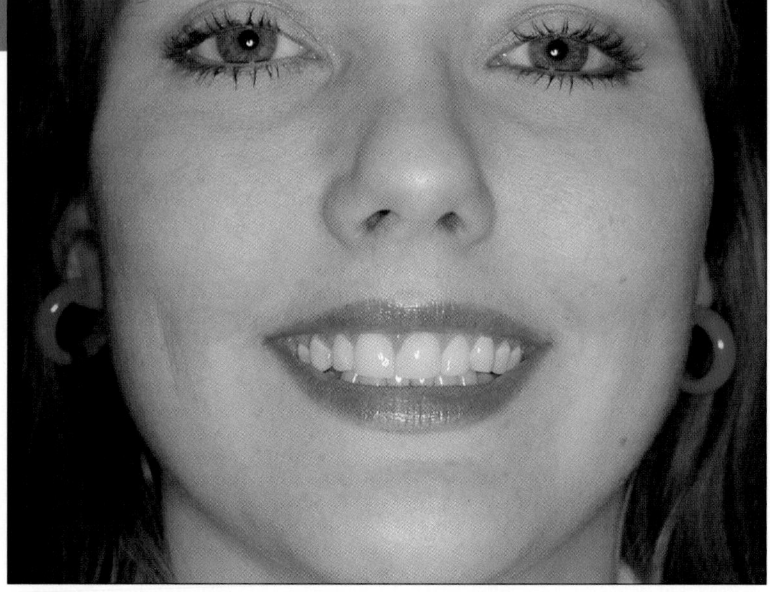

Direct composite resin bonding

An effective compromise result was obtained through direct composite resin bonding. Although the dental midline still does not match the facial midline, the smile is now more pleasing.

The Right Smile for You

Does your smile project the type of image you want?

Both men and women spend time, money and effort to project sex appeal. But you can have a super body, a sexy hairstyle and designer clothes and still fall short of a great image because your smile isn't attractive. Even if it's not a turn-off to you, it might be a turn-off to others!

First, consider the shape of your teeth. Although there's no anthropological basis for masculinity or femininity, square teeth are considered more masculine, and rounded teeth more feminine.

If you aren't happy with the image your teeth project, your cosmetic dentist can reshape them to give you a whole new look. And that look is up to you. There are no rules. Some women want a delicate and more rounded shape to their teeth; some prefer a bold, athletic look. Likewise, many men desire an angular "masculine" smile, while others want a softer appearance.

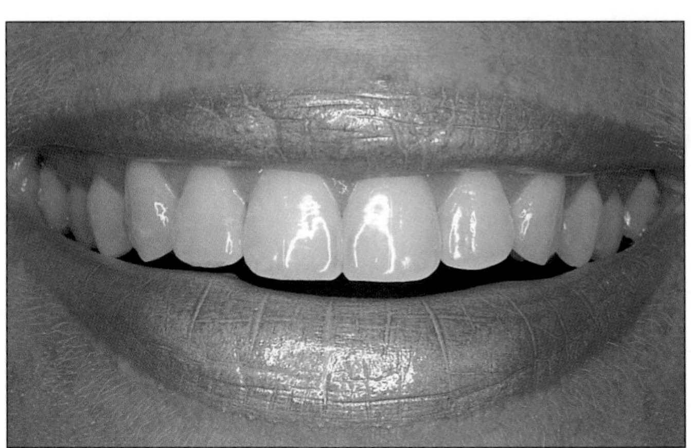

Feminine type smile

There is no anthropological basis for masculinity or femininity in teeth. However, we tend to think of teeth that are nicely curved as softening the smile and we perceive this as a more feminine look. Note, also, the slight openings at the biting edges between the teeth. These are called *incisal embrasures* and help make the teeth look distinct instead of joined together.

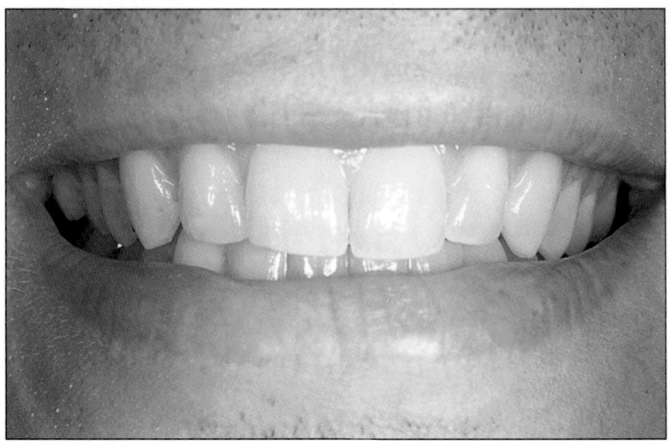

Masculine type smile

This is a fine example of a masculine smile with a medium lipline. The teeth are more angular, and the central incisors provide a bolder or stronger look in relation to the lateral incisors. They are squarer, less rounded, and slightly more textured than in the above photograph. A more youthful smileline is created when the central incisors are slightly longer than the lateral incisors. The teeth are all one color, but the canines or cuspids are usually slightly darker than the other teeth due to the thickness of the teeth.

Before

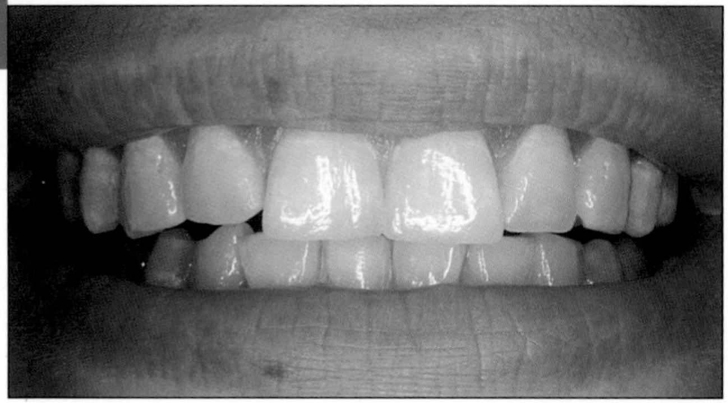

After

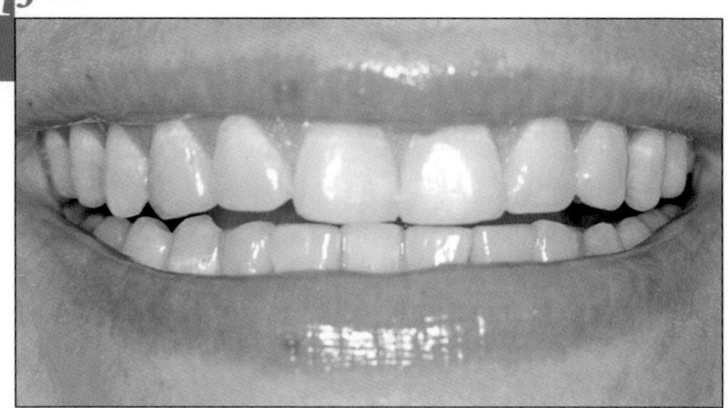

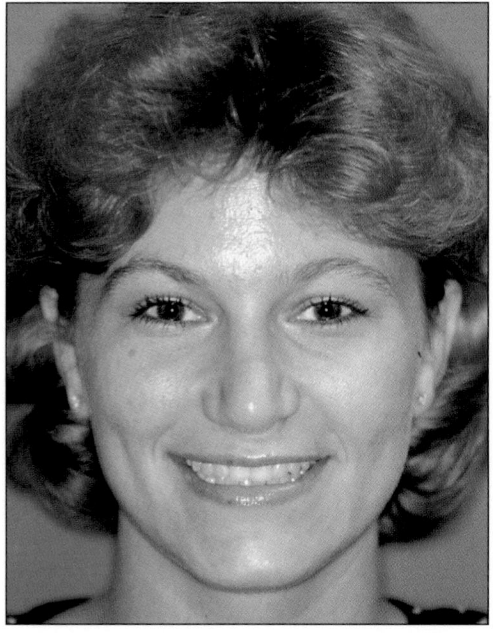

One appointment to a more feminine smile

Here is how a simple cosmetic contouring can change a smile with a "masculine" appearance to one that has a softer and more "feminine" look.

Before

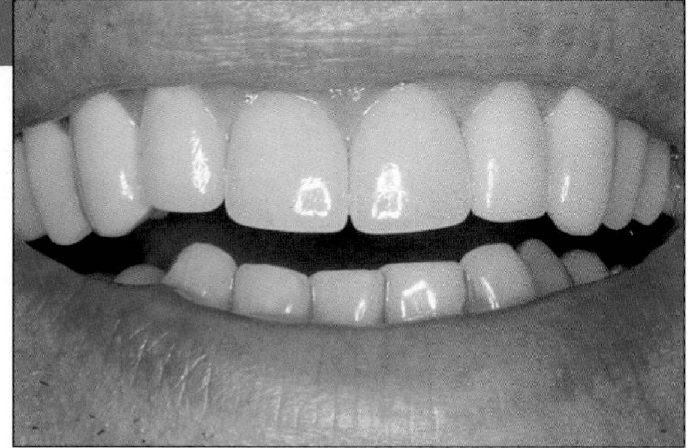

Teeth shape does make a difference

Although this 50-year-old dentist had recently had his teeth crowned, both he and his family were displeased with the final result.

After

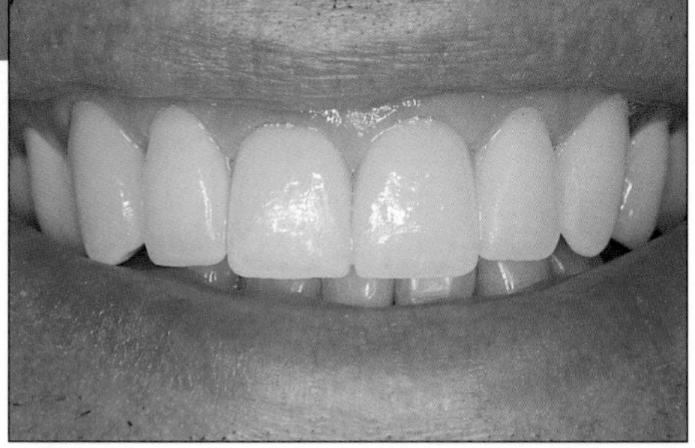

New crowns

The dentist's teeth were recrowned with more "masculine" appearing shapes and a lighter color. Both the dentist and his family were pleased with his new smile.

Your height is also a factor. Keep in mind that people don't always view you directly from the front. What do you look like from an angle? Problems that are practically invisible from one perspective may become prominent from others. New technology, such as computer imaging and extraoral video cameras can demonstrate a view of any angle or perspective from which you may be viewed by others.

Regardless of your height, make sure you analyze your smile from the angles at which most people view you. Holding a mirror straight in front of you if you are extremely short or tall does little to give you the perspective from which most others see you. Obviously, when you face another person in a seated position, everything is equalized.

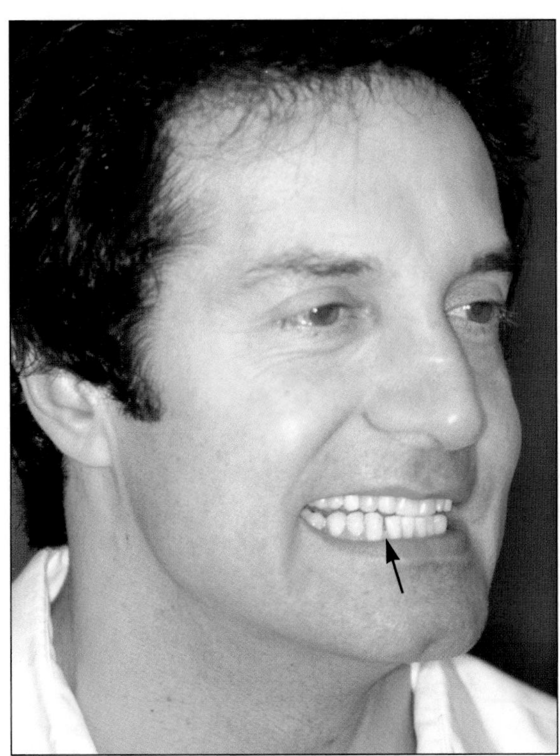

SPACES BETWEEN TEETH

Even a small space can be a detriment to someone in a profession such as acting or modeling, because such people are seen and photographed from different views and angles. This well-known actor had a space between his lower teeth and had worn down the biting edges of his front teeth.

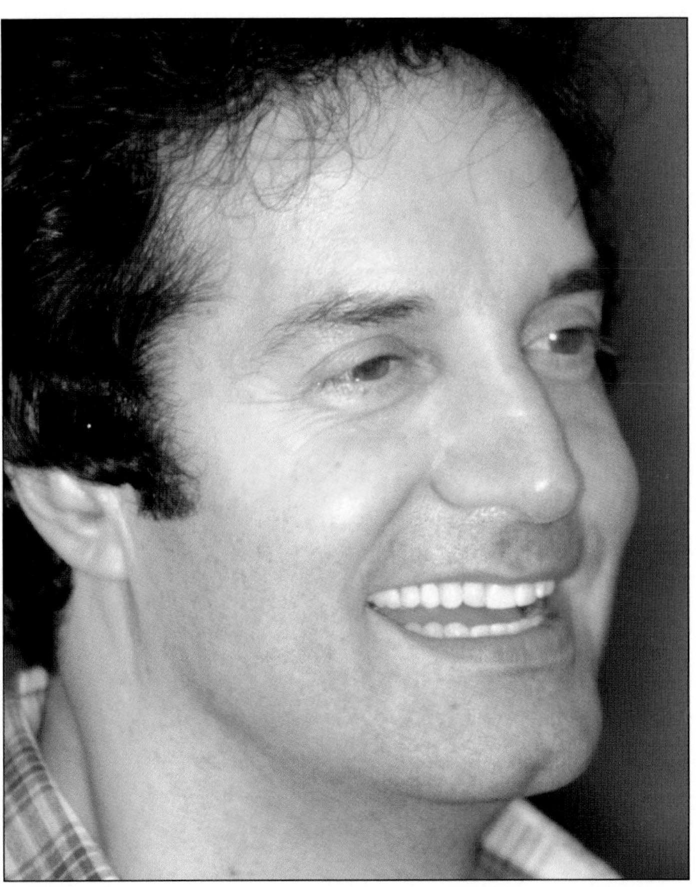

BONDING AND COSMETIC CONTOURING

Only one appointment was needed to close the space as well as recontour the upper and lower teeth to help create a more attractive smile. Television can overemphasize a space, making it look much larger than it is.

If You're Short

If you're short, most people look at you from above. Therefore, pay particular attention to your lower teeth. If they are crooked, consider orthodontic repositioning. If orthodontics is out of the question, then consider cosmetic contouring, bonding or laminating as a compromise.

In shorter people, the very tops or biting edges of the lower front teeth are also quite visible. If the dentin has become exposed due to an erosion of the enamel, the result can be brown or orange-brown areas of discoloration that not only spoil an otherwise attractive smile, but make you look older than you are (see illustration below and on p. 179). However, this problem usually can be solved quickly and easily with composite resin bonding.

Finally, if you are having your lower teeth crowned or having a bridge inserted, consider a restoration in which the metal is masked completely. Be sure to advise your dentist of your preferences before treatment begins. If he or she has to overbuild the metal later in order to hide it, your teeth will look bulky and gum irritation may result. Moreover, if the dentist has to revise the treatment plan simply because you failed to express your wishes, you may be charged extra for it.

If You're Tall

If you're tall and have slightly flared upper front incisors, your teeth will look much shorter because of the angle at which the shorter viewer sees them. Likewise, upper front teeth that are slightly indented will look longer.

Because the upper gumline is usually not as visible in the tall person as the lower gumline is in the shorter person, the esthetic problems encountered and the approaches taken to solve them are often quite different.

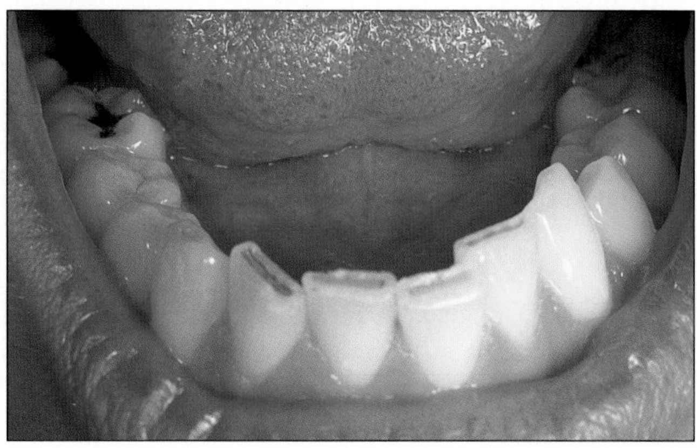

Incisal erosion

Bruxism, or grinding of the front teeth, caused loss of enamel on the biting edges of this 28-year-old woman's teeth. As the underlying, softer dentin becomes exposed, it becomes susceptible to stains from tobacco and certain foods. One form of treatment for these stains is composite resin bonding (see p. 179).

Choosing a Cosmetic Dentist

For the sake of convenience, most people choose to visit a neighborhood dentist. When seeking a cosmetic dentist, however, don't let location alone be a deciding factor. For instance, would you prefer a dentist who uses the most up-to-date, high-tech diagnostic and treatment equipment? Will your esthetic problem require computer imaging to allow you to see just how your smile will appear after treatment?

The following suggestions can help you make an appropriate choice:

- **Contact your local or state dental society.** Most dental societies have listings of members' specialties. A phone call will typically produce the names of those dentists whose practices are well prepared in both philosophy and training for cosmetic dental treatment.
- **Contact your local or state dental school.** Most dental schools have departments that focus on various aspects of esthetic dentistry, and increasing numbers of schools teach courses in esthetic dentistry.
- **Contact your local dental specialists.** These include orthodontists, oral surgeons, endodontists and periodontists. These specialists, who are familiar with the dentists in their communities, often can provide recommendations and referrals. Most specialists have certain dentists they typically refer to, so make it clear that you wish to see the very best in cosmetic dentistry . . . someone the specialist would choose to see for his or her own esthetic dental care.
- **Contact professionals in related fields.** These include plastic surgeons, cosmetologists, and modeling or theatrical agencies. Ask who they would see for cosmetic dental treatment. They often know the best people in the business.
- **Ask a friend.** Although other sources typically are better, if you know someone who has completed cosmetic dental treatment and is satisfied with the results, ask for a recommendation.
- **Contact the American Academy of Esthetic Dentistry (AAED) and the American Academy of Cosmetic Dentistry (AACE).** They can provide names of member dentists in your area, as well as information on cosmetic dental procedures. Write the AAED at 500 N. Michigan Avenue, Suite 1920, Chicago, IL 60611, or call (800) 993-2626. Write the AACD at 270 Corporate Drive, Madison, WI 53714, or call (800) 543-9220.

Also be sure to ask if the dentist to whom you have been referred has a copy of this book. If he or she does, chances are the dentist practices the techniques discussed.

Is This Where I'm Supposed to Be?

Your own dentist may be the best person to see for your cosmetic dental treatment, but you may not know it! A patient who had been coming to me for more than 25 years once asked who I would recommend for her esthetic dentistry. She had no idea that I was qualified for the job. Obviously, I had neglected to let her know that I shared her esthetic concerns.

However, if you are unsure of your dentist's abilities in the area of restorative and cosmetic dentistry, consider asking him or her for a referral.

The Next Step Is Up to You

The following tips can help you find the right dentist for your cosmetic treatment.

• Ask for a consultation. Expect to pay a separate fee for the dentist's time, as well as additional fees for X-rays, computer imaging, models and records.

• Outline your expectations. Preparing a "wish list" before your first meeting with the dentist is often helpful.

• Bring photographs. If you want to have your teeth restored to a previous condition, bring your dentist some photographs that show what you used to look like. Or, if you're hoping to change your smile, be ready with suggestions about how you'd like to look after treatment is completed.

• **Ask to see photographs of patients with similar conditions the dentist has treated.** Most dentists, especially those who practice cosmetic dentistry, like to show the results of their treatment with "before" and "after" photos.

• Get a second opinion. Don't be reluctant to seek more than one opinion, particularly if you're not convinced that the dentist can fill your needs.

• **Don't shop for bargains.** Bargains can be deceptive. Instead, look for a dentist who will spend the time it takes to give you what you want. Otherwise, you may end up spending twice the money and time on make-over treatment.

• **Try wax-ups.** With a wax-up, your dentist applies wax either to a cast mold made from your teeth or directly to your mouth to give you some idea of how the final treatment result will look.

• **Ask for computer imaging.** If you're a perfectionist, you'll want to see what your smile can look like with various treatment alternatives before treatment begins. Many dentists who perform a great deal of cosmetic dentistry either have their own computer imaging system or have access to one.

• **Ask for a referral.** Don't be reluctant to ask for a referral if you aren't fully confident in the dentist's ability to satisfy your needs. If you are a perfectionist, explain this before treatment begins. Your dentist will probably appreciate your candor, and it may help him or her decide whether or not to undertake your esthetic treatment! As in any profession, some dentists are willing to expend more time and effort to satisfy patients' needs than others.

Before

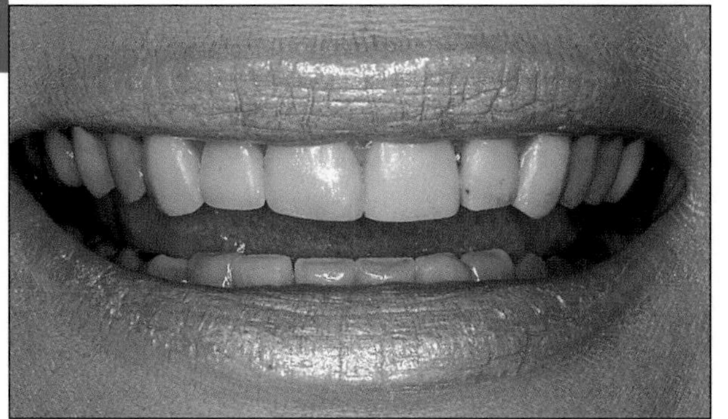

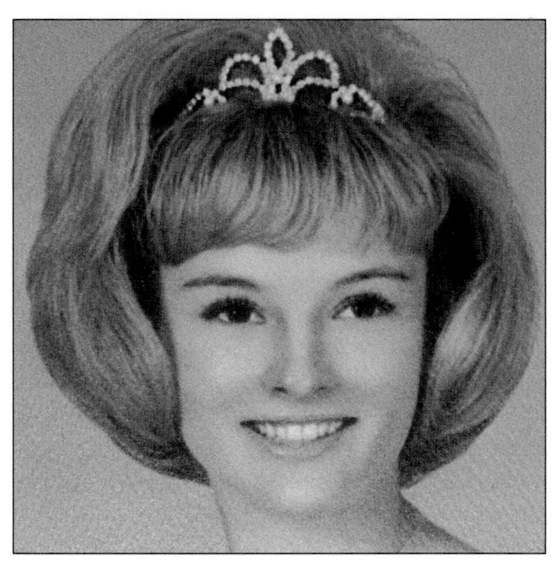

BULKY TEETH

This former beauty queen was unhappy with her smile. She wanted to recapture the look she had when she was younger.

After

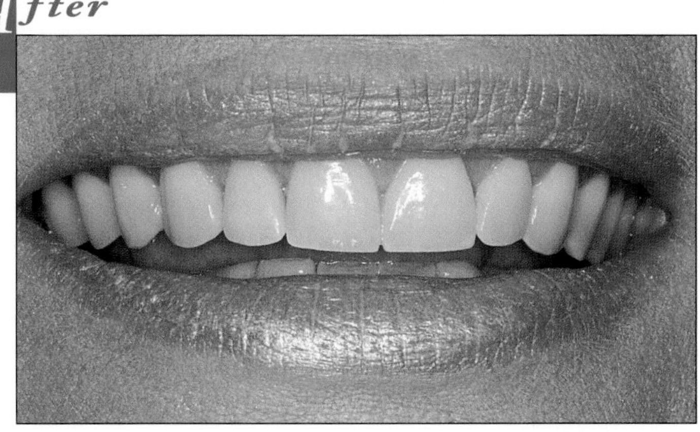

PORCELAIN LAMINATE VENEERS

The patient brought several photos to her initial appointment. Computer imaging also gave her an idea of the results she could expect. Now her smile and her entire face look more youthful.

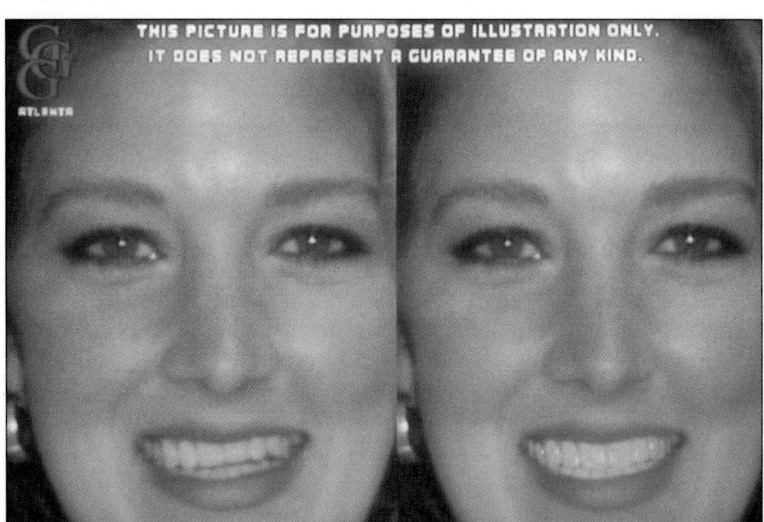

Computer imaging is a good way to visualize how your proposed new smile will look in relation to your face (see p. 190).

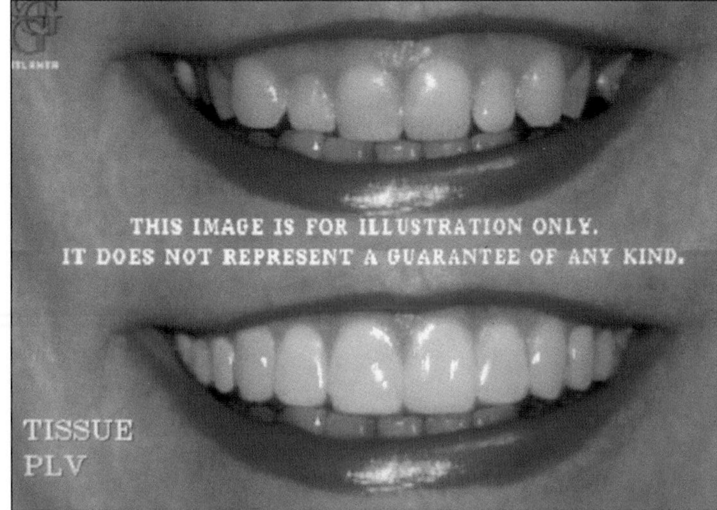

Computer imaging can also help you see close-up the potential changes in your smile.

- **Be aware of your problems and their potential treatment alternatives.** Read this book! The more knowledgeable you are, the better.
- **Show up for your appointment early.** You'll need time to complete forms and relax. The more relaxed you are, the easier it will be for you to communicate, a critical component of esthetic dentistry.
- **Bring any X-rays or models you have had made.** It will save you time and money if new X-rays and models don't have to be made.
- **Be frank about money problems.** You won't be "penny wise and pound foolish" if you discuss what can be done within your budget. Also, bring dental insurance booklets and forms to the appointment. **Although insurance typically doesn't pay for cosmetic treatment per se, the restorative portions of your treatment, such as crowns or bridges, may be covered.**

What About Fees?

Cosmetic dentistry is as much an art as it is a science. And just as the fee for a world-renowned artist or photographer is higher than that of a local artist, so it is with dentistry.

When looking for a cosmetic dentist, first take into account the dentist's skill and experience level. Has he or she been practicing for only two or three years? Or does that person have 15 or 20 years' experience?

Evaluate the dentist's artistic skills too. Ask to see photos of patients who have undergone treatment similar to what you are considering. And then study them! But don't just look at color. The chart on pp. 70-71 will give you an idea of what to look for.

Also find out how much time the dentist is willing to spend on your treatment. A "budget" price may result in a dentist who's in a hurry to finish. Make sure that the fee reflects an adequate amount of time to satisfy your emotional as well as your physical needs.

MATCH YOUR NEED FOR PERFECTION AND A BELIEVABLY NATURAL RESULT WITH WHAT YOU ARE WILLING TO PAY

Finally, keep in mind that cosmetic dentistry is a team effort. The skill of the dentist's support staff—the hygienist, the dental assistant and especially the technician who may be fabricating your restorations—is critical. Making a tooth look natural isn't easy. That's why some world-class ceramists charge more to make a crown than many dentists charge for the entire procedure!

The bottom line: Don't base your decision solely on price. Instead, match your need for perfection and a believably natural result with what you are willing to pay. As is so often the case, you usually get what you pay for!

Paying for Cosmetic Dentistry

Once you decide on cosmetic dental treatment, you can arrange the best payment method with your dentist. **Your insurance program may cover some aspects of treatment, but rarely is cosmetic improvement included.** However, if you have a good dental insurance program, chances are you have partial coverage for some cosmetic procedures. If your treatment can't be justified for health reasons, don't ask your dentist to falsify records so that you can receive insurance reimbursement.

In addition, many insurance companies have restrictions. For example, they may pay only up to a specified amount for a crown. Most policies are designed to emphasize preventive dentistry, so make maximum use of this by having as many cleanings and X-rays as are necessary at the insurance carrier's expense.

If you're using insurance, begin your treatment by submitting an estimate with the proposed treatment and related costs outlined for your carrier. Once this estimate is approved, you can begin treatment with a clear idea of your financial responsibilities.

Also expect to pay in advance. Whether or not you have dental insurance, your dentist will probably ask you to pay in advance, particularly if he or she devotes most of the practice time to cosmetic work. This is a customary practice long established by plastic and reconstructive surgeons. If cash flow is a problem, try to set up the treatment in stages so that you can pay as it progresses. If, for example, you need a crown right away, consider wearing an acrylic temporary until you have the money to pay for the final restoration. Another alternative is to arrange a customized payment plan with your dentist.

Communication Is the Key

The secret to getting exactly the new smile that you want lies in total communication. Learn as much as you can about esthetic dental procedures, as well as the names and parts of your teeth. Then determine what you need and want, and convey this message clearly to your dentist. You want to make sure your "dream smile" is attainable in reality!

THE SECRET TO GETTING THE NEW SMILE THAT YOU WANT LIES IN TOTAL COMMUNICATION

If you want to improve your smile, you'll find that the following chapters give you a comprehensive overview of exactly what to expect.

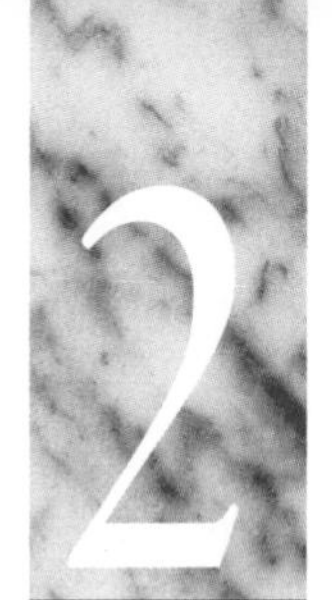

Getting Rid of Stains

If your teeth are stained or discolored, chances are you've gone to some lengths to achieve a whiter, brighter smile. Perhaps you've experimented with the variety of toothpastes on the market today, many of which offer special ingredients guaranteed to give you not only a dazzling smile, but sex appeal as well! Maybe you've purchased some of the home bleaching kits sold in drugstores and supermarkets. Or, in an attempt to draw attention away from your teeth, you may have cultivated a year-round tan or accentuated your hairstyle or clothing.

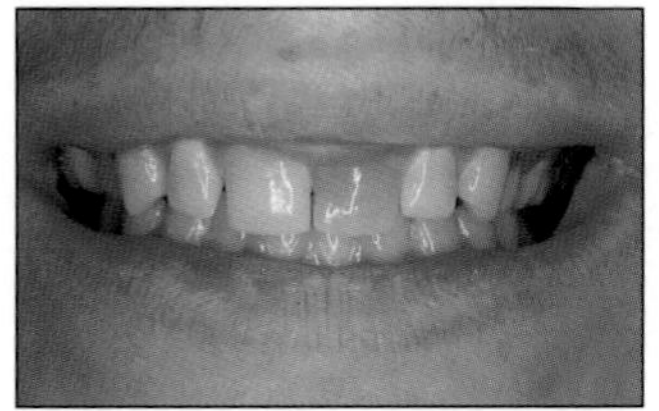

Unfortunately, these efforts ultimately fall short. Most over-the-counter products disappoint consumers because they fail to provide more than a temporary removal of surface deposits on the teeth. And measures taken to camouflage or de-emphasize the smile do little or nothing to lessen the feelings of vulnerability and inadequacy that many people with discolored teeth experience daily.

Today, however, there is no need to suffer from social embarrassment or psychological trauma because of stained or discolored teeth. Suitable cosmetic dental treatment can provide both predictable and positive long-term results.

This chapter describes the most common tooth stains and their methods of treatment.

Why Teeth Stain

There are basically three types of stains or discolorations: surface stains, soft deposits, and stains that are actually part of the basic tooth structure.

Surface stains occur primarily between teeth and on the surfaces of crooked teeth. Typically dark brown, these stains are caused by strong discoloring agents such as coffee, tea and tobacco. These discolorations usually can be managed with daily oral hygiene combined with regular visits to your dentist for professional cleanings.

Before

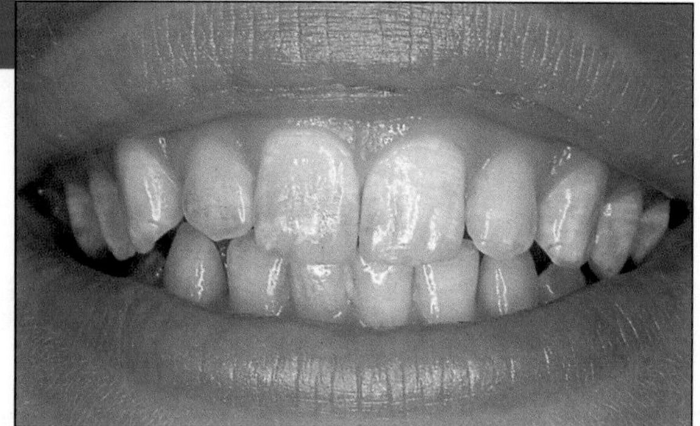

Stained teeth

This young lady was so concerned about her unattractive smile that she sometimes avoided smiling.

After

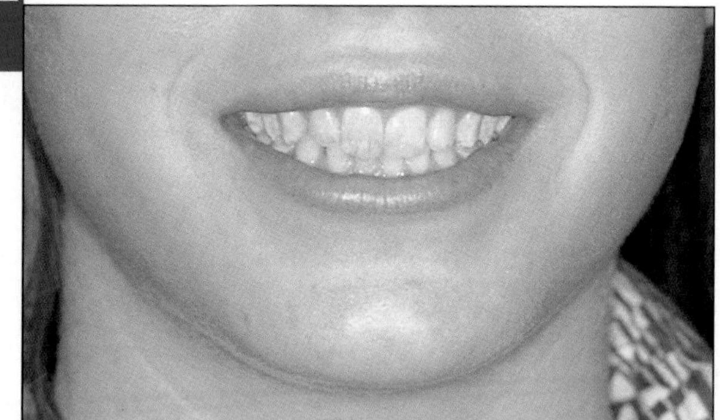

Much of the stain was removed by polishing the teeth with an extra-coarse cleaning paste. Additional stain could be removed with either bleaching or one of the other masking procedures.

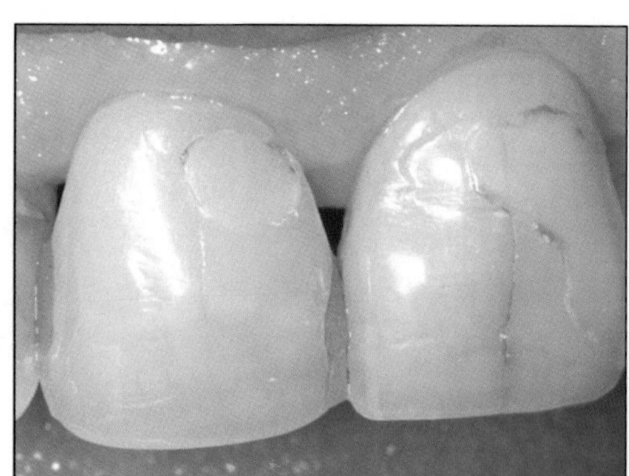

Microcracks

Microcracks, which can be caused by chewing on ice or other hard objects, can stain over time from food and tobacco. **Don't chew ice!**

One type of surface stain, however, is not so easily removed. These stains actually get "trapped" in the tooth's structure because of *microcracks*, tiny fractures in the tooth's enamel usually caused by chewing on ice or other hard objects. Microcracks are so small that they generally go unnoticed until they become stained, often from food or tobacco. The solution requires a more aggressive treatment than professional cleanings alone, typically bleaching or bonding.

A second class of stains is caused by *plaque*, a sticky film that builds up on the teeth over time, or *tartar (calculus)*, a cement-like substance that forms when plaque is not removed. Often bacterial in origin, these stains may be the by-product of ineffective oral hygiene. They appear as dark areas around the gumline, most often on the lower front teeth. They typically disappear after a thorough dental scaling and polishing.

Before

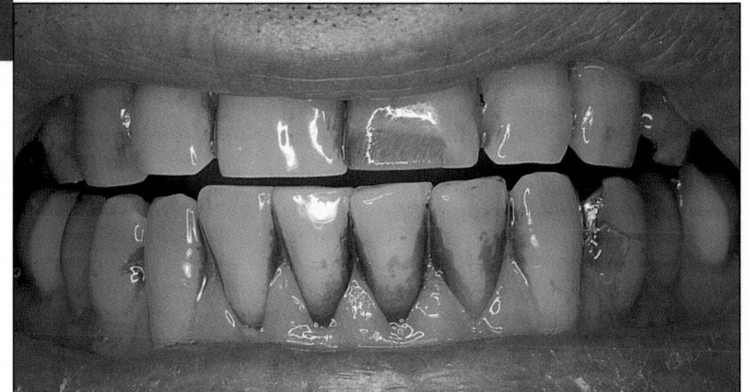

COFFEE STAIN

This 63-year-old internationally known executive was embarrassed about his stained teeth. He drank about eight cups of coffee per day, which was determined to be the cause of the staining. Even though he had frequent cleanings, the stains rapidly returned due to the amount of coffee he drank.

After

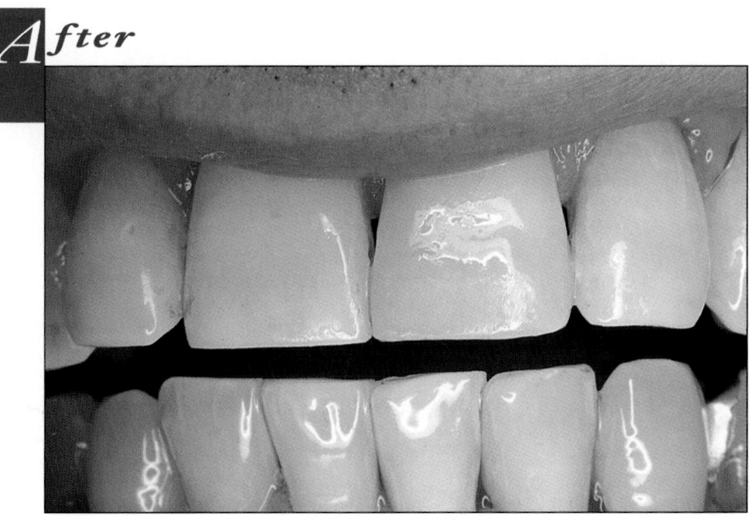

TEETH CLEANING AND BONDING

The first step in treating stained teeth is a professional cleaning to see how much stain will be removed. In this patient, the discolored and worn filling in the left central incisor was then replaced through composite resin bonding. The patient was advised to avoid coffee consumption to protect the esthetic life of the newly bonded restoration as well as his natural teeth. Following this dietary change, the stains have been much less noticeable between his more frequently scheduled cleaning appointments.

The third category of stains encompasses those that are actually part of the tooth's structure. These discolorations include white splotches on the enamel surface and bands of brownish-gray across the teeth. They may be due to faulty hardening of the tooth before birth or the interruption of normal enamel formation by medications or disease. *Tetracycline stains*, which appear as unsightly yellow, dark brown or blue-gray discolorations, often develop in people who were treated with the antibiotic tetracycline before the age of eight or in those people whose mothers took the drug while pregnant. Although it is now known that even mild dosages of tetracycline can cause permanent tooth damage, children were once given the drug routinely. Today its use is restricted in children under eight years of age and in pregnant women. Further research now indicates that the antibiotic minocycline may cause staining in the teeth of adults.

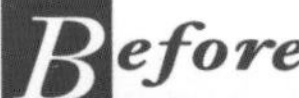

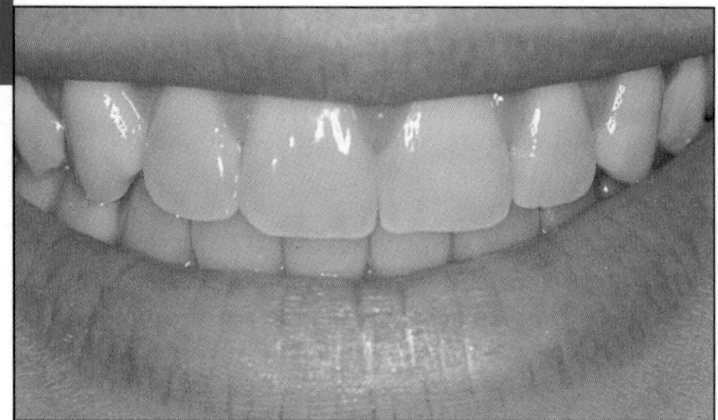

TETRACYCLINE STAINS

This 18-year-old student was unhappy with her darkly stained gray-brown teeth. Although it is usually more difficult to obtain a good result by bleaching teeth of this color, bleaching was nevertheless attempted.

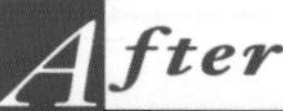

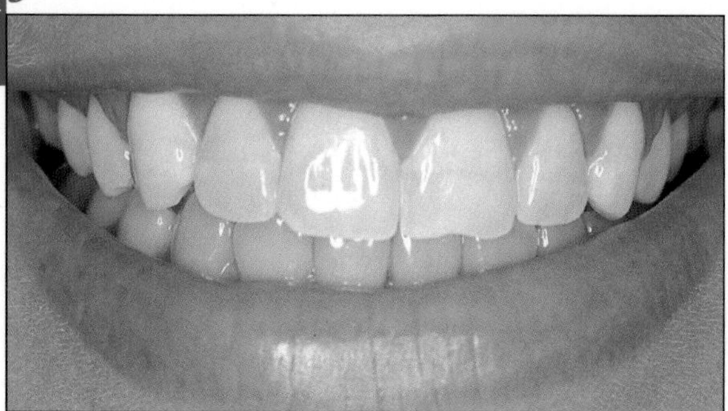

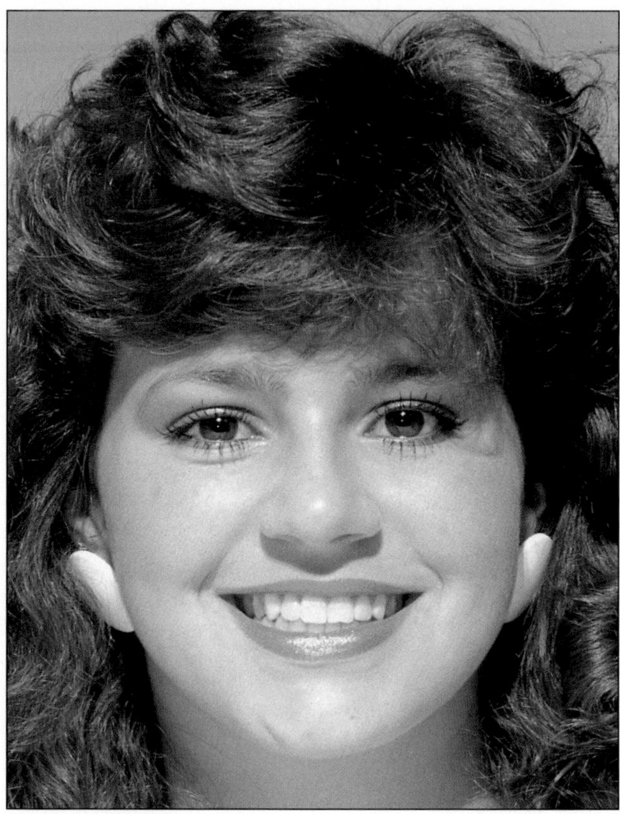

IN-OFFICE BLEACHING

Gray- or brown-stained teeth usually do not respond as well to bleaching as do yellow teeth; however, after eight in-office treatments, this patient's ten upper teeth were successfully bleached. An additional in-office bleaching "touch-up" treatment should be scheduled every one and a half to two years unless matrix (at-home) bleaching is used. This patient's problem proved that it is sometimes wise to attempt bleaching to see just how well the teeth respond.

Finally, stain can be caused by advanced decay or old or defective silver fillings. Both problems can cause the teeth to appear brown or gray and can make a person look older than his or her years.

Many patients, in an attempt to eliminate these unsightly stains, scrub their teeth vigorously with harsh abrasives and cleansers. Unfortunately, these stains are "locked in," and overzealous brushing usually does nothing more than destroy the teeth's enamel surfaces and abrade delicate gum tissue.

Before

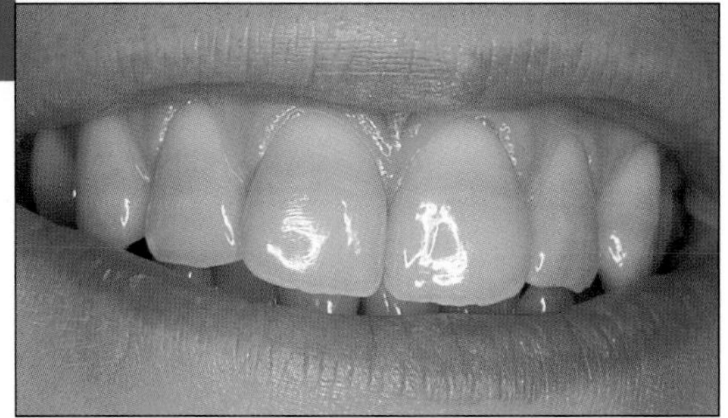

TETRACYCLINE STAINS

This 16-year-old had darkly stained teeth as a result of having taken the antibiotic tetracycline as a child. Such stains can result if the antibiotic is taken by the mother during the final six months of pregnancy and/or by the child up to eight years of age. The teeth remain perfectly healthy, but they become discolored. Notice the ribbon effect or band of darker color in the upper third of the teeth.

After

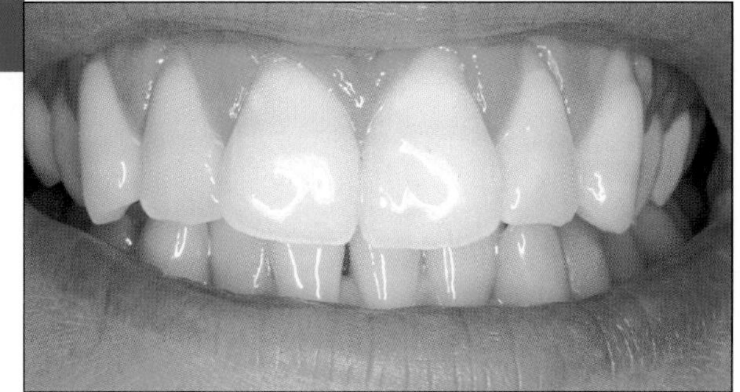

IN-OFFICE BLEACHING

Following multiple in-office bleaching treatments, the teeth are much lighter. The best treatment is to combine in-office with "matrix" or "at home" nightguard bleaching. A prettier smile through bleaching is possible about 75 percent of the time.

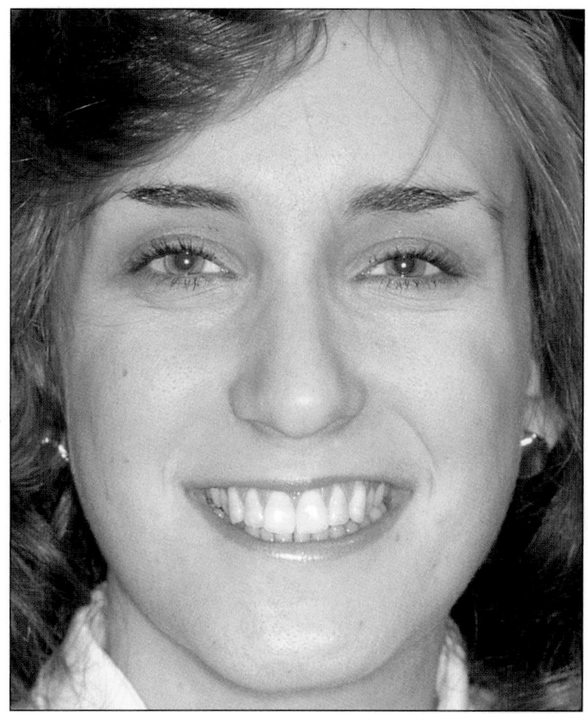

Five Treatments for Stained Teeth

Luckily, patients with stained teeth—even those that are severely discolored—can be treated successfully. Cosmetic dentistry affords these patients the opportunity to have the beautiful, natural smiles they desire with a minimum of time, discomfort and cost.

Treatment of stained teeth depends on both the cause and the degree of discoloration. Each treatment alternative has advantages and disadvantages, which are addressed more thoroughly later in this chapter. Basically, however, there are five ways to treat stained teeth. Below is a brief review of each:

• **Polishing**, the simplest method of stain removal, eliminates many food stains, the majority of which can be attributed to coffee or tea. However, excessive staining from beverages or tobacco products may require more aggressive treatment.

POLISHING IS THE SIMPLEST METHOD OF STAIN REMOVAL

• **Bleaching**, which utilizes a strong oxidizing agent to lighten the teeth, is a relatively conservative and often highly effective way to brighten the smile. Bleaching is frequently used on mild-to-moderate tetracycline and fluoride stains, as well as on those stains that result from damage to the tooth. Your dentist may recommend either in-office or home bleaching or a combination of both, depending on the nature and the severity of the discoloration.

• **Bonding** involves the application of a plastic material to the existing tooth. The composite resin bonding technique is used frequently to cover stains in a conservative and esthetically pleasing manner. This process can be particularly effective in masking tetracycline stains, white or brown spots, stains due to excessive wear and in lightening teeth that have become discolored by amalgam, the blend of metals found in silver fillings.

• **Laminating** is an extension of the bonding technique. It consists of applying a thin veneer of pre-formed porcelain, composite resin or plastic to the teeth in much the same way as an artificial fingernail is affixed to a natural nail. In the case of porcelain, both the enamel and the inside of the porcelain veneer are etched to increase adhesion. Composite resin and plastic laminates are chemically sealed to the teeth.

• **Crowning** is a longer-lasting, although less conservative, treatment alternative that requires reducing the tooth and covering the remainder with a custom-made restoration. Although it is always preferable to preserve the structure of the natural tooth, it isn't always feasible. For example, in cases where tetracycline stains are extremely dark or where amalgam stains have caused severe discoloration, crowning may be the only acceptable treatment alternative. Despite the drawbacks, crowns can be finely sculptured works of art that serve both to improve tooth shape and function while enhancing your smile.

Bleaching

Bleaching will lighten teeth in about three out of four selected cases. Teeth that tend to be yellow are the easiest to lighten.

Lower teeth typically are not bleached because they are not as visible as upper teeth. Even when they *are* more easily seen, the natural shadow of the smile tends to mask their discoloration. However, if you want your lower teeth bleached, wait until the upper teeth are completed so that you can monitor your progress by comparing the lightened upper teeth to the stained lower teeth.

Also, if you already have one or more crowns on your upper front teeth and you want to have all the teeth lightened—including the crowns—*be sure to bleach the natural teeth surrounding the crowns first.* It's much easier for your dentist to match the shade of your crowns to your new natural teeth than it is to bleach the natural teeth to match the shade of a porcelain crown. The exact shade to which natural teeth lighten is always less predictable, and thus more difficult to control.

Before

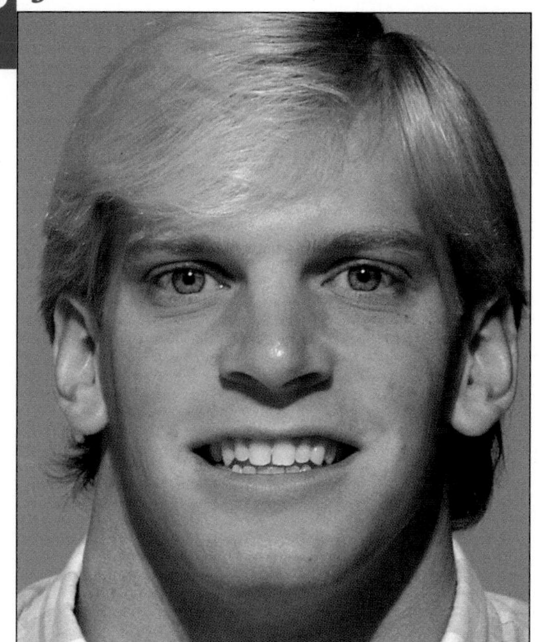

TEETH NOT WHITE ENOUGH

Although this actor had a great smile, he wanted lighter teeth.

After

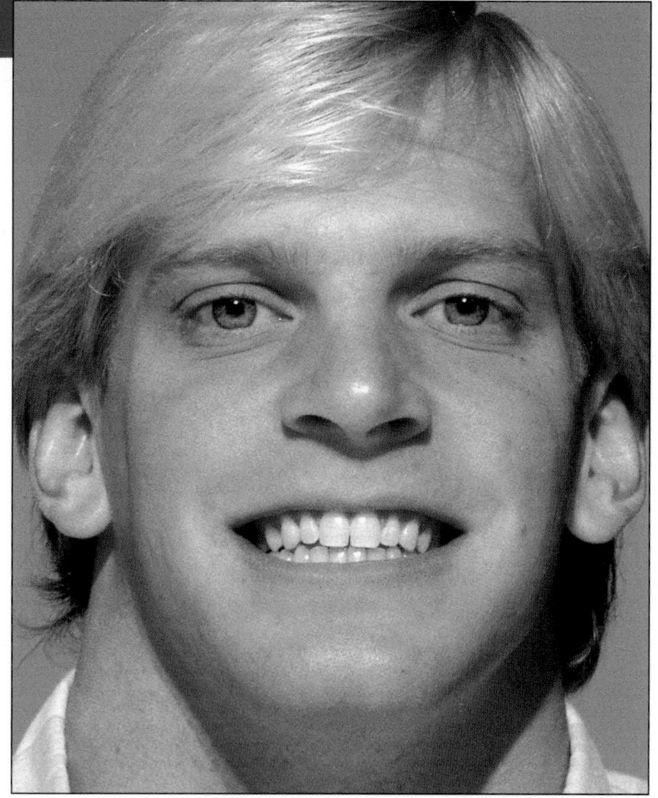

IN-OFFICE BLEACHING

Five in-office bleaching treatments were performed to help lighten this patient's teeth. Because the original shade was not dark, a successful result was achieved quickly, which helped to make a great smile even greater.

Bleaching in adults generally causes little, if any, discomfort. However, in 8- to 13-year-old children, bleaching may cause pain because the pulp chambers—the soft inner portions of the tooth where the nerves are housed—are much larger in children than they are in adults. Most discomfort, which typically occurs within the first eight hours after treatment and subsides within 24 hours, can be treated with aspirin every four to six hours. Although the number of children who experience discomfort is relatively small, it is often advisable to postpone bleaching until they are older.

Before

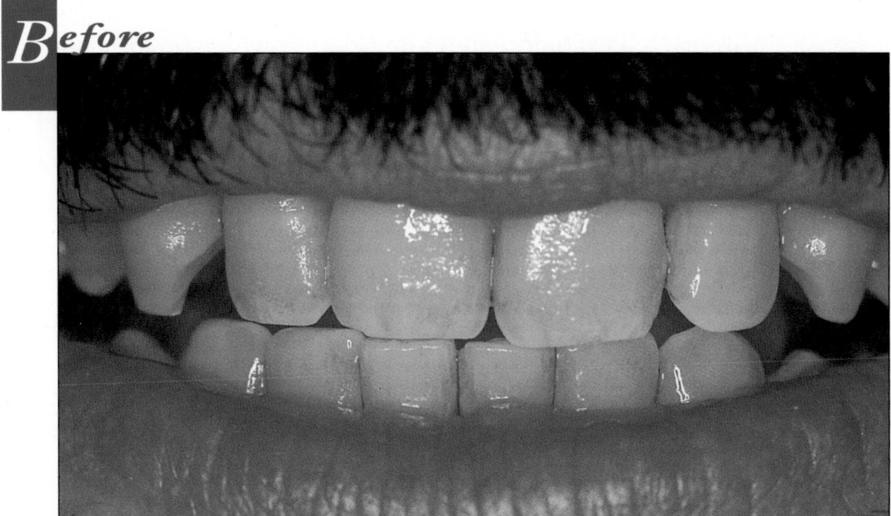

YELLOW TEETH

This 40-year-old business owner was unhappy with his dark, yellow teeth.

After

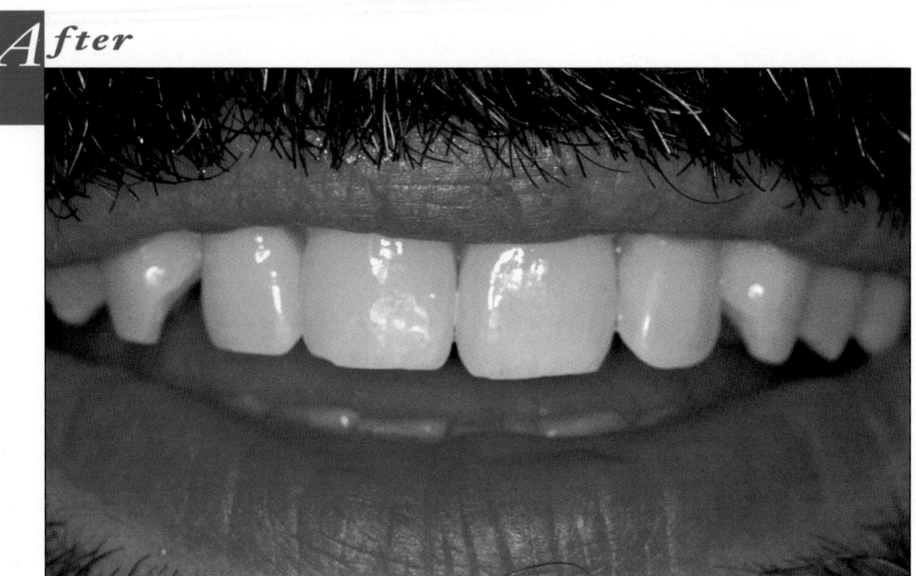

IN-OFFICE BLEACHING

Because the patient had otherwise healthy, vital teeth, bleaching was attempted to remove the yellow stain. It took six in-office treatments to achieve the color shown.

Bleaching living teeth

Bleaching "live" or vital teeth involves coating the outside of the teeth with a chemical solution—the oxidizing agent—and exposing them to heat and light for 20 to 30 minutes. First, however, the dentist usually isolates the teeth being treated with a thin rubber "dam," which protects the gums from discomfort and irritation.

If the gum tissue *does* come in contact with the bleaching solution, you may experience a light burning or tingling sensation. Inform your bleaching therapist or dentist immediately if this occurs. The affected area may also turn white temporarily. However, healing usually occurs within a few days to a week, and there are typically no short- or long-term adverse effects.

Before

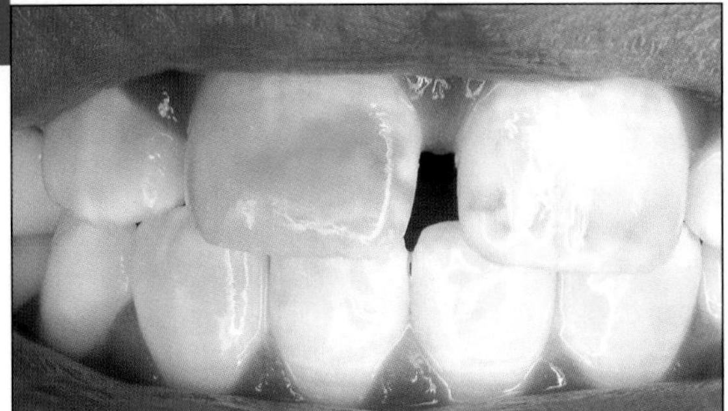

DARK STAIN ON CENTRAL INCISORS

This 11-year-old boy hated to smile because he was teased by his friends about his dark front teeth. It was believed that the child was given too much of a particular prescription drug, which was the cause of the stain.

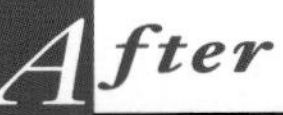

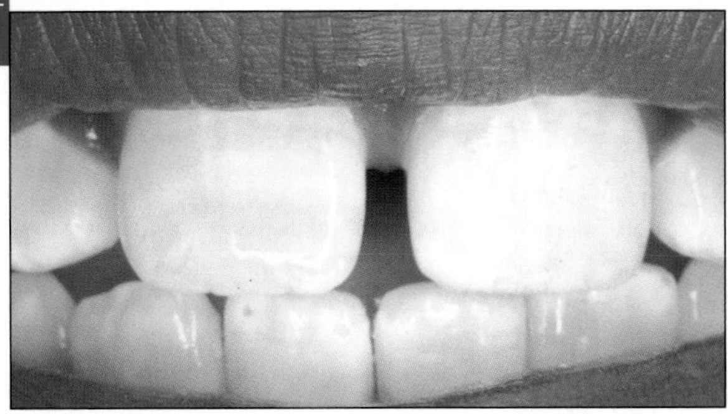

INDIVIDUAL TOOTH BLEACHING

After one bleaching treatment of the two front teeth, the stains almost disappeared. Stains of this type, however, may require several treatments to achieve optimal lightening.

Before

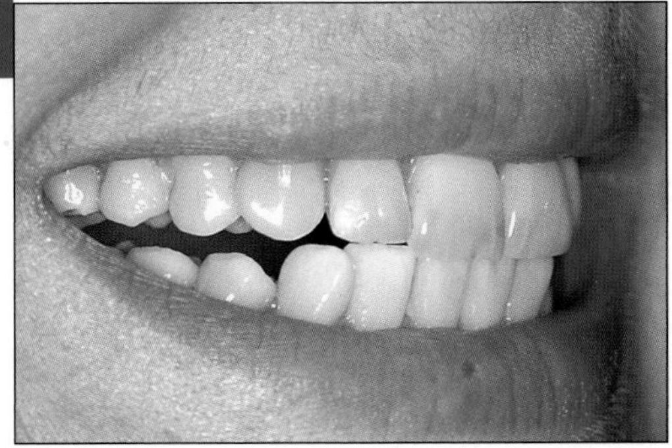

DISCOLORED TEETH

This 35-year-old woman wanted lighter teeth. Note the staining on the lower portions of her two front teeth. In addition, she was dissatisfied with the dull color that showed from the side.

After

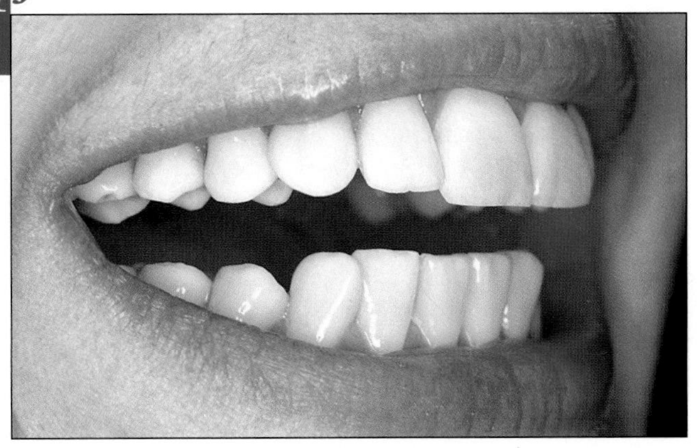

VITAL TOOTH BLEACHING

Four treatments were necessary to remove the dark stains from this patient's two central incisors. She is pleased with her new smile, which now radiates from every view.

Bleaching nonliving teeth

Teeth can be bleached even if their nerves have been removed as is the case with root canal therapy. In fact, such teeth—referred to by dentists as nonliving, nonvital, or pulpless teeth—are actually easier to bleach than vital teeth. One method of bleaching these teeth involves reopening the canal, which previously housed the nerve, placing a bleaching solution inside, and resealing the canal with a temporary filling. The bleaching process continues until the agent is removed and can be repeated until satisfactory lightening takes place. The process sometimes can be accelerated by the use of heat and/or light at the dental office.

Care should be taken to monitor the tooth closely to make sure it doesn't become *too* light. However, consider going one shade lighter than you think is appropriate, because these teeth tend to darken slightly over time. Call your dentist when you believe you have obtained the color you want. Also be sure to contact your dentist if the temporary filling loosens or falls out.

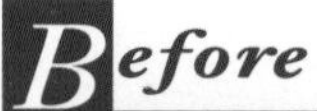

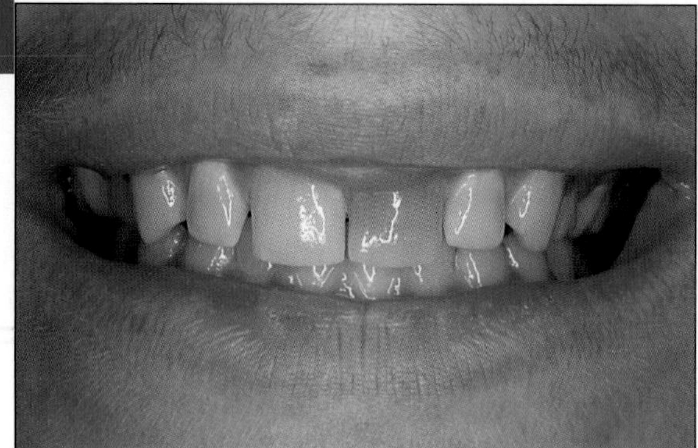

DARK FRONT TOOTH

This 16-year-old student had injured his front tooth. Although he was not concerned about his dark front tooth, his parents were aware of the difference it could make in his smile and wanted the tooth bleached.

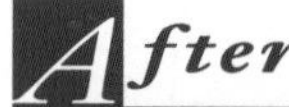

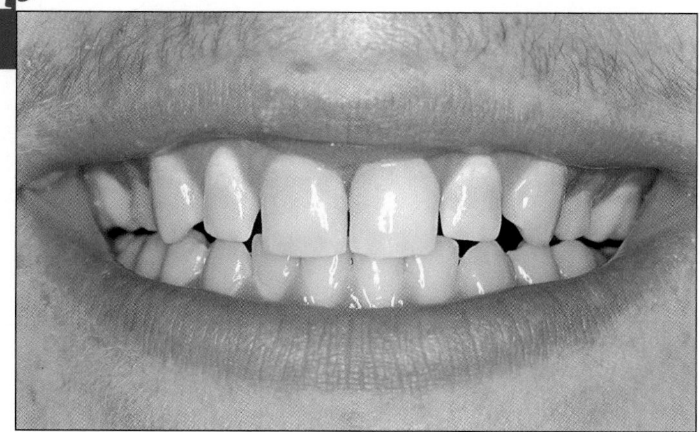

IN-OFFICE NONVITAL BLEACHING

Because the tooth had been previously treated with root canal therapy, one bleaching treatment was performed to the outside of the tooth in the dental office. Then a bleaching solution was placed into the empty pulp chamber to bleach the tooth from within, a process referred to as "walking bleach." The bleaching solution continues to work as long as the solution is sealed within the tooth. In this patient, the solution was removed after one week and a tooth-colored composite resin filling was used to seal the opening. The natural color was restored to the tooth, which helped improve his smile.

Home bleaching

Home bleaching, also called matrix bleaching or nightguard vital bleaching, is a relatively new way to whiten your teeth conveniently and cost effectively. It involves filling a plastic tray with a bleaching solution or gel and wearing it for a few hours each day or overnight. Although average treatment takes about six weeks, you may notice results after just a few days.

Lightly to moderately yellowed teeth usually respond well to home bleaching. In addition, patients who are not good candidates for in-office bleaching because of hypersensitivity, time restrictions or financial considerations can often be helped with home bleaching.

For some patients, home bleaching alone whitens the teeth to a desirable level. For others, a combination of home and in-office bleaching yields the best results. Your dentist can recommend the appropriate course of treatment for you depending on the nature and severity of the discoloration. You will also probably need a few "touch-up" bleaching sessions every six to 12 months.

As with any treatment, home bleaching isn't right for everyone. Do not use any home bleaching product if you are a heavy smoker or if you are pregnant or nursing a baby. Also keep in mind that home bleaching can have adverse side effects including tooth sensitivity, a burning sensation in the gums, soft-tissue sores or ulcers or a sore throat from swallowing the bleach. If you experience these or any other side effects, discontinue the bleaching and contact your dentist immediately. Although you may not be able to continue home bleaching, you may still be a good candidate for in-office bleaching.

If you think you'd like to try home bleaching, see your dentist first. Although there are many home bleaching kits sold over the counter, dentist-supervised products are applied in a controlled environment and use a custom-fitted mouthguard to ensure minimal contact between the gums and the bleaching agent. Follow your dentist's recommendations and instructions closely and visit the office for regular examinations.

Before

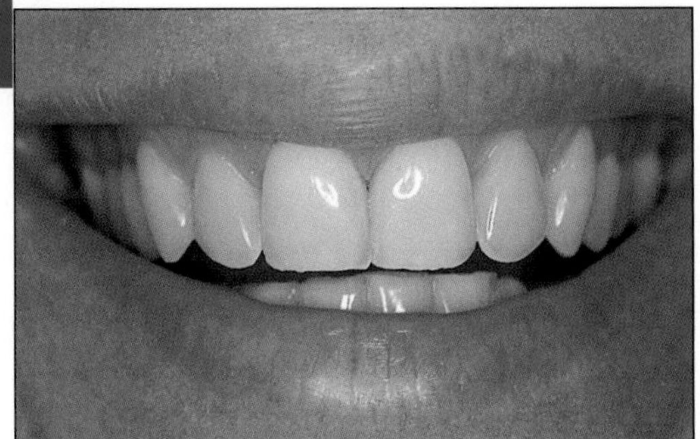

YELLOW TEETH

This patient, dissatisfied with her yellow front teeth, wanted them bleached.

After

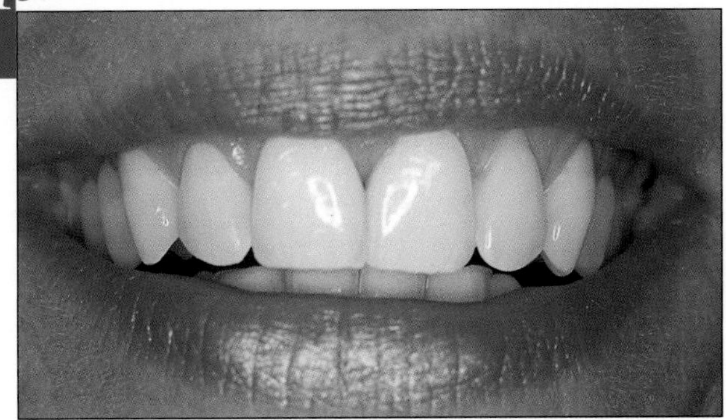

COMBINATION BLEACHING

Two in-office bleaching treatments, combined with matrix bleaching at home, produced these results within six weeks.

Before

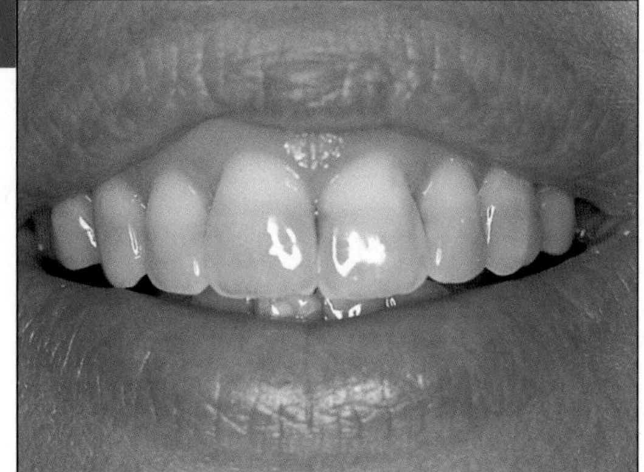

TETRACYCLINE STAINING

The teeth of this patient reveal a "ribbon effect" due to the patient having taken tetracycline during a short period in her early years.

After

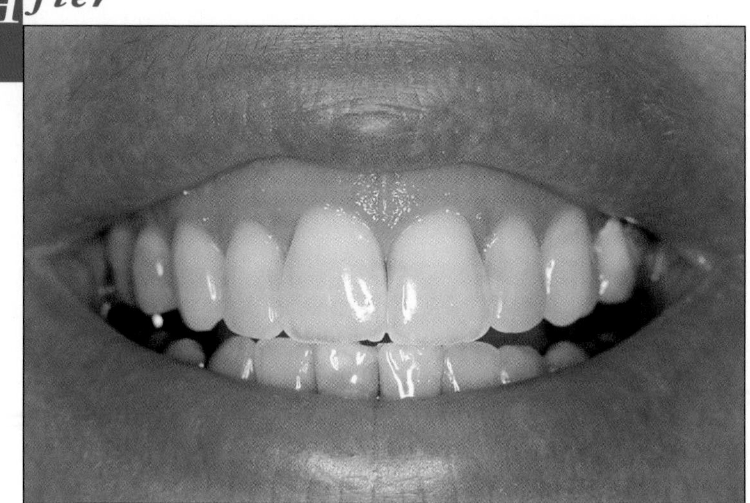

COMBINATION BLEACHING

Two in-office visits, plus an extended home matrix technique, produced these results. While the ribbon effect is still perceptible, it is much less noticeable.

Making the most of bleaching

If you and your dentist choose bleaching as a way to brighten your smile, the following tips will help you obtain the best results.

If possible, sit or lie in the sunlight with your mouth open after bleaching. The tooth structure will actually absorb some of the sun's rays, which allows the bleach to continue working. Be careful, however, not to burn your skin.

When performing home bleaching, avoid consuming citrus fruits and juices, soft drinks, and antacids. These products contain substances that when combined with the bleaching agent can slow down the tooth whitening process and cause mild mouth irritation.

Decrease your intake of refined sugars while bleaching takes place to reduce the chance of decay. Because tooth surfaces may be etched before treatment to allow greater penetration of the bleaching agent, they become more susceptible to bacteria. After treatment is completed, the tooth surfaces are polished to a natural and shiny luster. Later, nonstaining fluoride treatments can be applied to make the teeth even more resistant to decay.

Stains

Bleaching isn't always the answer

Some teeth are harder to bleach than others. Tetracycline stains, for example, are extremely resistant to bleaching because the stain is so deeply ingrained in the tooth's structure. For this reason, your dentist may suggest other treatment alternatives, particularly if no change is evident after three or four bleaching appointments.

White spots, frequently caused by a diminished calcification of the enamel, also can be difficult to treat with bleaching. These spots are often so chalky that a compatible shade cannot be achieved without creating an artificial look. Your dentist may suggest a conservative treatment called microabrasion either by itself or in combination with bleaching. The technique consists of applying a polishing agent combined with hydrochloric acid and "rubbing" it into the tooth surface. A rubber dam will probably be used to protect your gum tissue from the acid. Multiple (two to five) treatments may be necessary to make a significant difference. Both brown and white stains can be helped with this technique.

Before

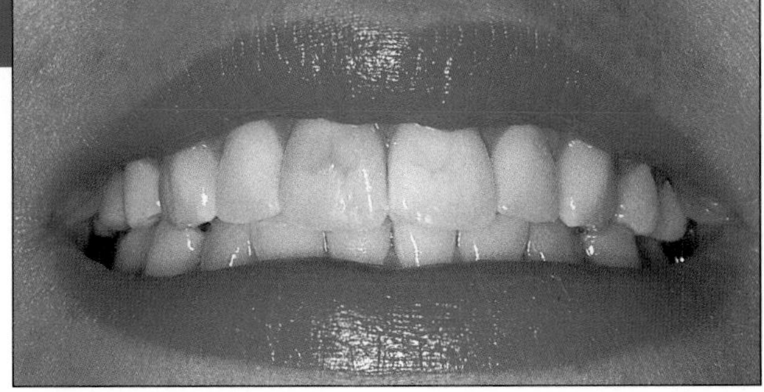

BROWN STAINS

These dark-brown stains on the central incisors marred an otherwise attractive smile.

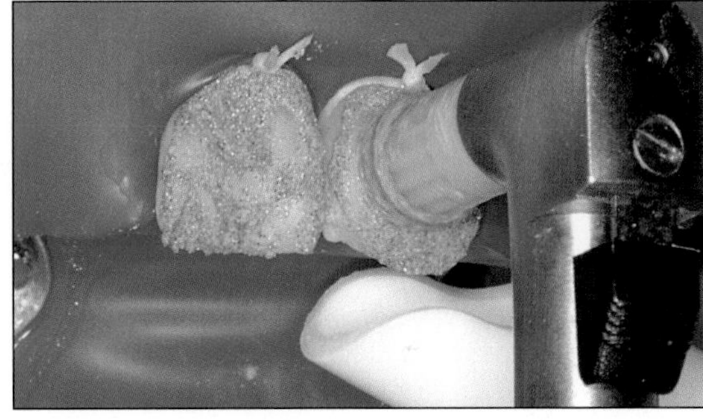

MICROABRASION

Treatment for this patient consisted of isolating the teeth with a rubber dam, applying an acid polishing paste, and tooth bleaching over three treatments.

After

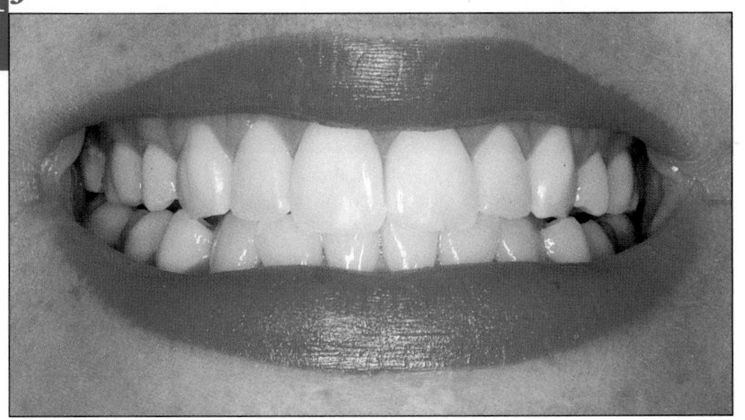

MICROABRASION PLUS BLEACHING

This prettier smile was achieved in approximately four weeks by a combination of microabrasion plus bleaching.

TREATMENT SUMMARY

BLEACHING

Treatment Time Usually three to ten treatments, lasting about thirty minutes to an hour and a half each. It is suggested that three or more professional cleanings per year be given after treatments are completed to help keep your teeth stain-free.

Patient Maintenance Thorough brushing after meals is necessary to avoid plaque accumulation. Smoking, as well as stain-causing foods such as coffee and tea, should be avoided.

Results of Treatment Deep yellow and brown stains can be considerably reduced, though teeth may not be returned to natural color.

Average Range of Treatment Life Expectancy Indefinite. Annual touch-ups may be required, but treatment may last indefinitely.*

Cost Approximately $120 to $500 per treatment.†

ADVANTAGES

1. Safe procedure
2. Painless to adults
3. No tooth reduction required
4. No anesthetic necessary
5. Least expensive of treatment alternatives

DISADVANTAGES

1. Normal tooth color may not be restored
2. Bleaching can cause discomfort in children because of their large pulps
3. Only 75 percent effective in selected cases
4. Extended treatment time may be necessary

***Treatment life expectancy** An average range of treatment life expectancy estimate is included in each treatment section summary. This estimate is based on my own clinical experience combined with three university research studies and insurance company estimates. Your own experience could be different. I have seen poor-fitting crowns and and fillings last over forty years in the mouth of a patient who cleans often and well. I have also seen well-fitting restorations last less than two years in the mouth of a patient whose diet and oral hygiene were poor. Medical factors, such as certain diseases, can also play a major role in the life of your restorations. Your experience will depend on many factors, only some of which you and your dentist can control.

†**Cost** Fees will vary from dentist to dentist based on the difficulty of the procedure, patient problems, patient history, expectations, and dentist qualifications, including technical and artistic expertise.

Finally, it may be difficult to obtain satisfactory bleaching results in teeth that display a "ribbon" effect. Although the entire tooth may become lighter, the difference will usually remain between the darker and lighter areas.

In each of these cases, bleaching may not be the best treatment alternative. Bonding or laminating, or a combined approach consisting of bleaching and bonding or laminating, often produces better results.

Bonding

Bonding, which offers a quick and easy way to mask many stains and discolorations, is often an excellent treatment alternative for patients who are not good candidates for bleaching.

Direct bonding is a relatively simple process in which a plastic fluid is molded onto the teeth. The surfaces of the teeth are etched first with a mild acid to create stronger adhesion. If teeth are darkly stained, an opaque whitish layer is also applied and a more durable coat of resin is added to mask the stain completely. The restoration is then allowed to self-cure, or it is cured with a high-intensity light.

Before

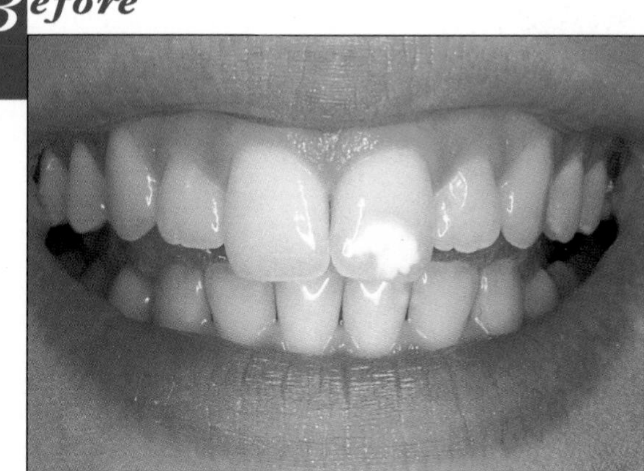

WHITE SPOT ON TOO-LENGTHY TOOTH

This 15-year-old girl had what many people call a "headlight" or white spot. Actually, it is a condition of diminished calcification of the enamel called *hypocalcification*. Note also the extra length of the two front teeth, which creates a "bunny" look to this otherwise perfect smile.

After

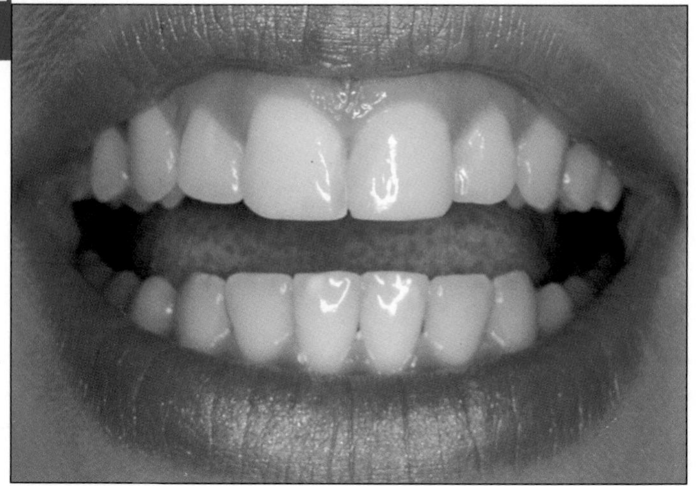

COSMETIC CONTOURING AND BONDING

The white spot was removed with cosmetic contouring, or reshaping of the natural enamel, followed by composite resin bonding in one appointment with no anesthetic. The front teeth were also shortened and reshaped to help produce a more alluring smile.

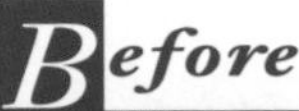

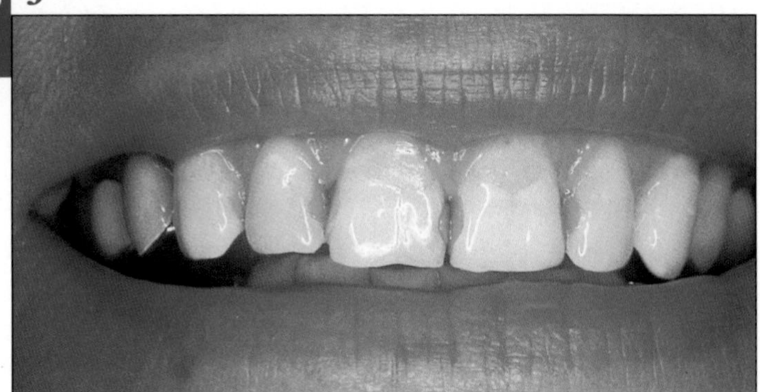

DISCOLORED FILLINGS

This 41-year-old woman was dissatisfied with her fillings, which discolored too rapidly. When front teeth have as many large fillings as these, the larger surface area is suseptible to stain each time they are replaced. Although crowning may be the final solution, an alternative to the full crown is bonding with composite resin.

After

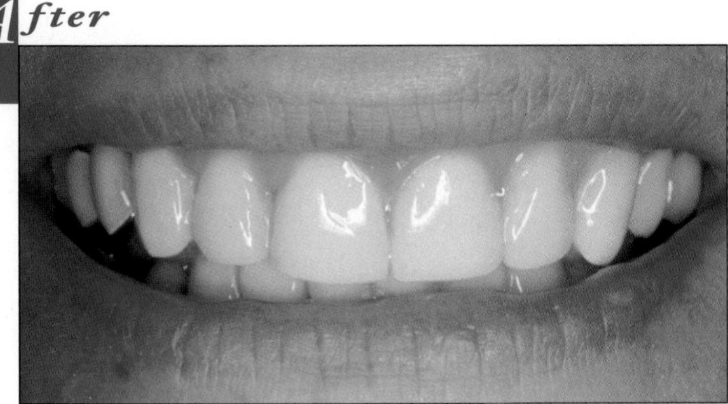

REPLACED FILLINGS

All twelve upper and lower teeth were bonded. Bonding teeth that have such large fillings may involve covering the entire front tooth surface. If the teeth were merely refilled, it would only take a short time before the junction of the filling and tooth became a site for new discoloration. In addition to the bonding, the teeth were cosmetically contoured for a more attractive smile.

How long do bonded restorations last?

Although a lifelike masking of stains can be achieved, bonded teeth—like their natural counterparts—are subject to gradual staining and discoloration, primarily around the junction between tooth and composite resin bond. Generally, however, bonded restorations generally last from five to eight years, during which time they can be repaired, if necessary, at less cost than the initial expense.

Two factors greatly influence the life expectancy of a bonded restoration. The first is the dentist's technique in preparing the bond. The second is the effort you make in home care and maintenance.

Your success in avoiding certain foods and in following proper oral hygiene is directly proportional to the esthetic life of your bonded restorations. In fact, because teeth bonded with composite resin materials are more susceptible to stains, heavy coffee or tea drinkers and heavy smokers should opt for other treatment alternatives such as porcelain laminate veneers, which do not stain. You may also want to purchase a rotary cleaning device to help remove some of the stains on your bonded restorations between professional cleaning appointments.

Before

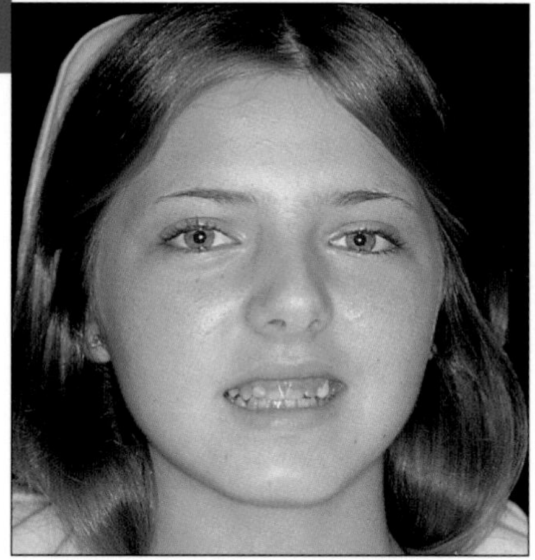

TETRACYCLINE STAIN

Children with tetracycline stain suffer from other children's cruel remarks. This 13-year-old girl said that boys called her names, referring to her tetracycline-stained teeth. Unless attention is paid to esthetic problems of young people, personality problems may develop.

After

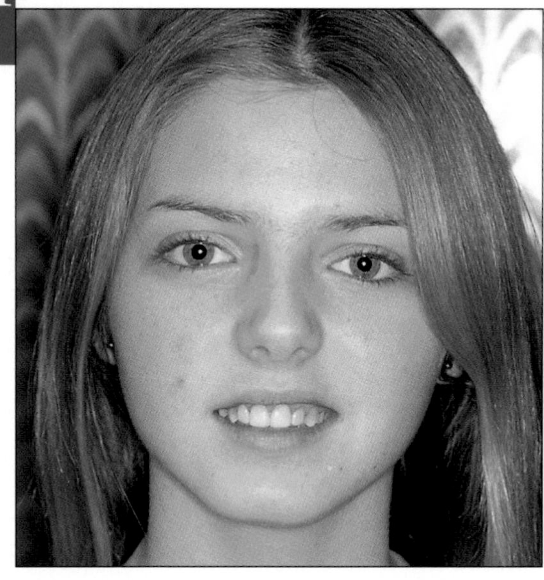

COMPOSITE RESIN BONDING

Although bleaching was attempted, it was difficult to accomplish because the pulps in a young person's teeth can be so large that the teeth may become too sensitive during the process. Therefore, the upper four front teeth were bonded with composite resin to mask the tetracycline stains. It is easy to see how one's self-confidence can be enhanced following a cosmetic improvement.

Before

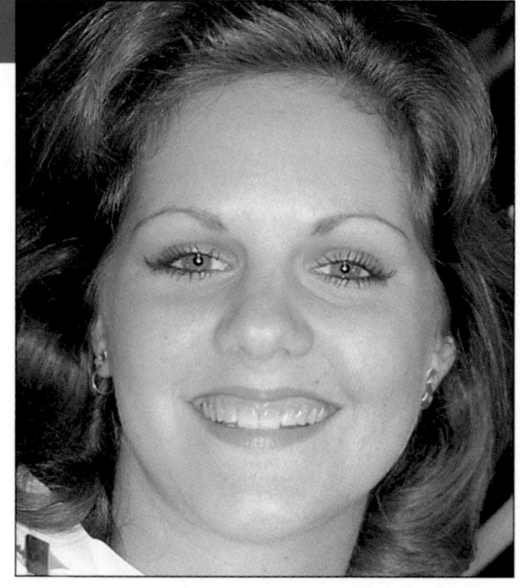

TETRACYCLINE STAIN

This young woman had discolored teeth because of the antibiotic tetracycline.

After

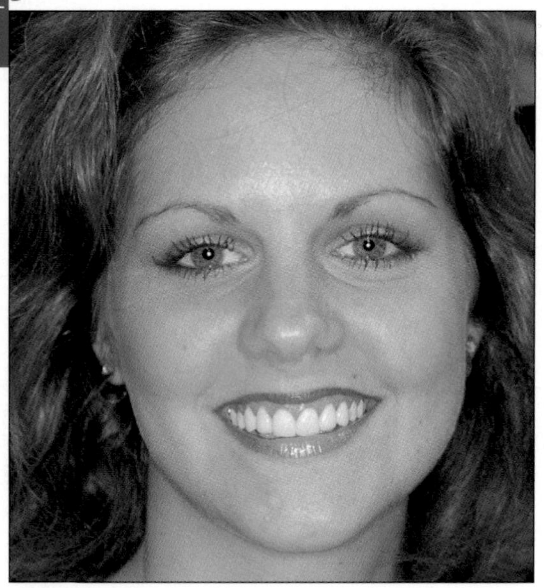

COMPOSITE RESIN BONDING

With composite resin bonding, a one-day appointment was all it took to create a more radiant smile.

Treatment Summary

Composite resin bonding

Treatment Time Usually one or two office visits. The first visit will average about one hour per tooth. If a second visit is required, it will usually take no more than one hour for touch-up and final polishing.

Patient Maintenance To keep the bonded restorations looking their best, you should have a professional cleaning three or four times a year. The reason for such frequent cleanings is to remove food stains that accumulate in microscopic spaces on the bonded surfaces of the teeth. Warn your hygienist not to use an ultrasonic scaler, which can loosen the bond, or an air abrasive spray, which can dull the polish. These bonded surfaces are not as strong as your enamel, so try to protect them by eating wisely. For instance, avoid biting down with front teeth, especially on such foods as ribs, apples, hard bagels and corn-on-the-cob. (More tips on patient maintenance can be found on p. 55.) Expect to have repolishing or repair performed as necessary.

Results of Treatment On-the-spot masking of stain.

Average Range of Treatment Life Expectancy Average life expectancy is three to eight years. May need repair or replacement more frequently. (See footnote on p. 50.)

Cost Approximately $185 to $950 per tooth. (See footnote on p. 50.)

Advantages

1. Painless
2. Immediate (one-appointment) results
3. Little or no tooth reduction
4. Generally no anesthetic required
5. Less expensive than porcelain laminates, crowning or "capping"
6. Avoids potential pulp or gum irritation that may occur when reducing tooth for full crown

Disadvantages

1. Can chip or stain
2. If orthodontic treatment is required, it should be completed before bonding
3. If orthodontic retainers are worn, holding wires should be Teflon-coated (stainless steel can cause discolorations with some types of bonding materials)
4. Extreme care must be taken to avoid metals (such as hair pins) from coming into contact with bonding
5. Bonding has a limited esthetic life expectancy
6. Certain types of stains (especially dark ones) cannot be covered well with bonding
7. May involve minor tooth reduction to remove some of the stains
8. Unless margins are finished perfectly, gum irritation can occur

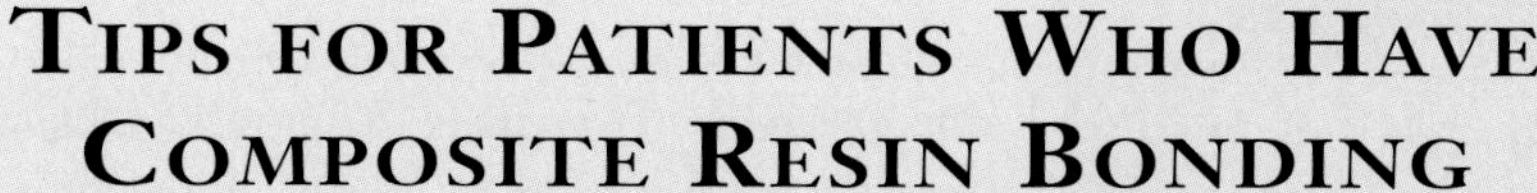

Tips for Patients Who Have Composite Resin Bonding

1. Do not chew ice.
2. Brush normally. Plaque must be removed daily! Ask your dentist about antiplaque mouthwashes and toothpastes.
3. Floss teeth at least once daily, but pull floss out horizontally, not vertically.
4. Take multi-vitamins two times daily for one month before and after treatment if gum tissue is inflamed.
5. Have your teeth cleaned at least three or four times yearly. **Be certain that the hygienist is aware of your bonded tooth or teeth and avoids using ultrasonic scaling or air abrasive on the bonded tooth surfaces.**
6. Make sure you are not grinding your teeth at night. If you are, have your dentist construct a bite guard to avoid fracturing the bonding and to minimize damage to your bonded teeth as well as your temporomandibular joint (TMJ).
7. Don't bite your fingernails! The force can crack the bonding.
8. Don't pick at a newly bonded tooth with your fingernail. You could pull open a small over-extension and shorten the life of the material. If you feel a rough edge with your tongue, return to the dentist to have the edge properly refinished.
9. Don't try your new teeth out too soon. Sometimes biting on the other side isn't wise either. Go on a soft diet for the first twenty-four hours. If your bite is not perfect, return to your dentist to have it adjusted. Never try getting used to a new bite! The bite you are used to is usually correct.
10. To prevent staining, try to avoid, or keep to a minimum, coffee, tea, soy sauce, colas, grape juice, blueberries and fresh cherries. And do not smoke!
11. To prevent fracture, avoid directly biting, with front bonded teeth, into the following foods: ribs, bones (fried chicken, lamb chops, etc.), hard candy, apples, carrots, nuts, hard rolls, hard bread, bagels or artichokes. Also try to avoid candy, mints or sugar, because acids produced by sugar can attack the junction between tooth and restoration and cause stains and premature loss of the bonded restoration.

Before

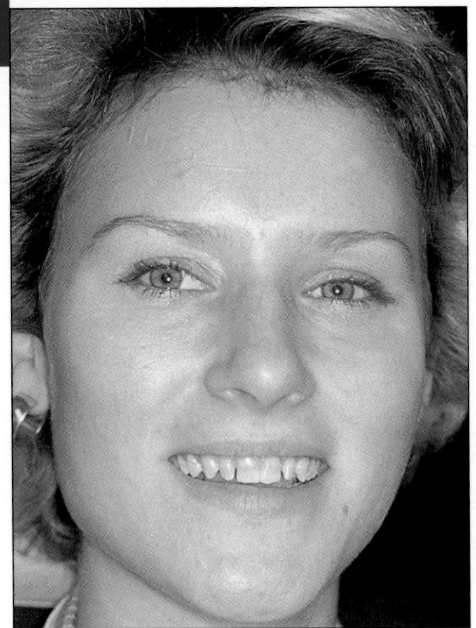

TETRACYCLINE STAIN

This 22-year-old dietician had discolored teeth due to tetracycline staining. Note the spaces that also called attention to the darkness of her smile. A series of bleaching appointments was set up to remove as much stain as possible.

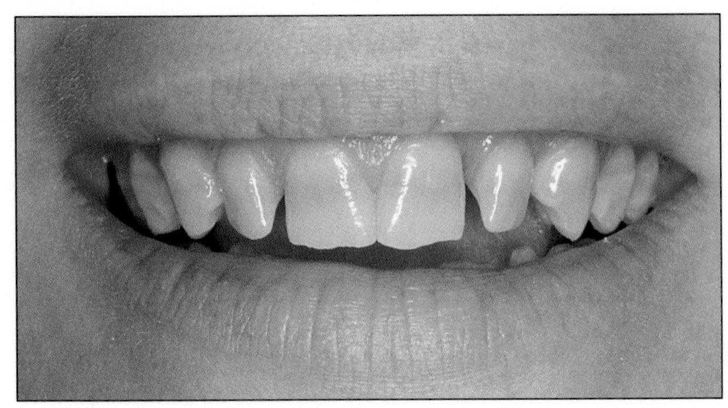

After

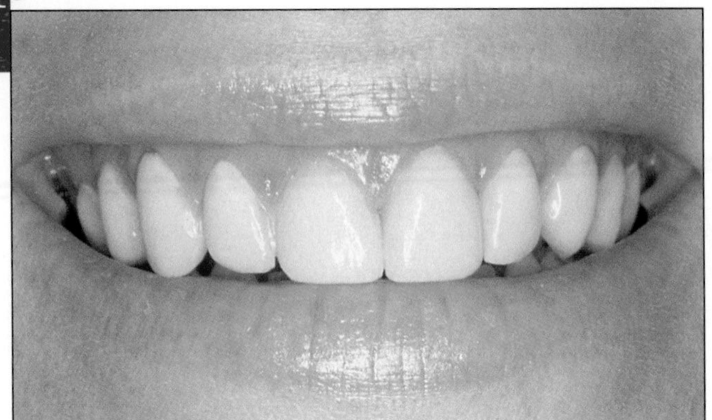

BLEACHING AND BONDING

A brilliant smile results after bleaching and composite resin bonding of ten upper teeth. The bonding permits the spaces to be closed in addition to lightening the teeth by masking the tetracycline stain. Sometimes a combination approach is best to achieve a natural look. The bleaching tends to remove the dark yellows from the teeth and permits less opaque layers of resin to be used. Therefore, the overall result is a thinner, more natural-appearing bonded tooth and a more attractive smile.

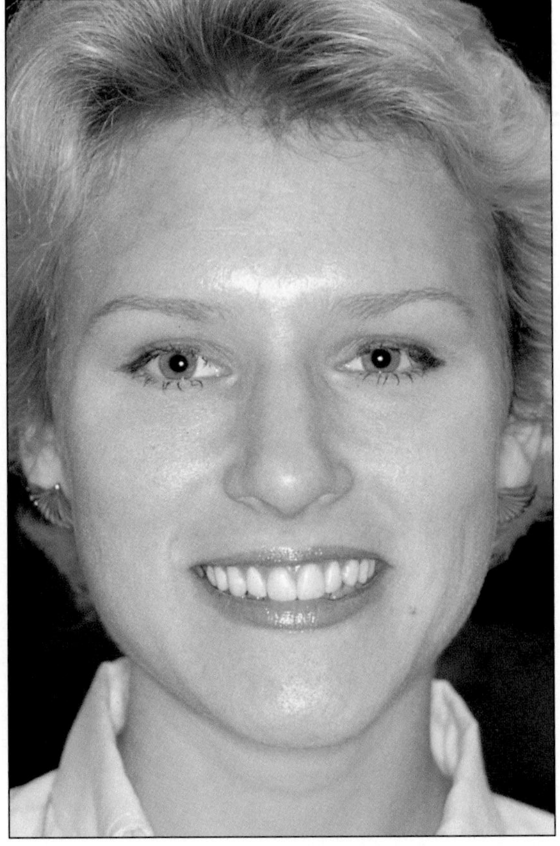

Laminating

Laminating, like bonding, consists of applying a thin veneer of pre-formed porcelain, composite resin or plastic to the teeth. Composite resin and plastic laminates are chemically sealed to the teeth. In the case of porcelain veneers, the inside of the laminates are etched to enhance their attachment to the etched enamel surfaces of the teeth. Composite resin cement is then used to bond the porcelain to the enamel.

LAMINATING CONSISTS OF APPLYING A THIN VENEER OF PORCELAIN, COMPOSITE RESIN OR PLASTIC TO THE TEETH

Although laminate veneers require less shaping and offer better polishing than direct bonded restorations, a primary disadvantage is that the laminate may chip or peel in time. As the bond loosens, discoloration may be noticed around or in the veneer, requiring that it be patched or replaced, depending on the nature of the stain. One of the newest methods of removing decay from a tooth, air abrasive technology (see p. 310), also offers an excellent method for repairing laminate veneers, eliminating much of the disadvantage.

Laboratory-constructed composite resin laminates

Your dentist may suggest masking discolored teeth with laboratory-constructed composite resin laminates. These custom-made restorations, which are mechanically bonded to the teeth, provide excellent esthetics because the lab can actually incorporate into the laminates characteristics such as greater opacity and special stains or colors that allow an almost perfect match to your own tooth structure. In addition, these laminates are easy to repair if chipping or staining occurs.

Laboratory-constructed laminates aren't without disadvantages, however. First, it takes two appointments to complete the process. The additional time, coupled with laboratory fees, means costs are typically higher for this type of laminate than for bonding. In addition, the procedure is irreversible if too much enamel is removed.

For many patients, however, the benefits of laboratory-constructed composite resin laminates outweigh the drawbacks. Discuss your expectations and treatment options thoroughly with your dentist before deciding whether or not these restorations are right for you.

Porcelain laminates

One of the most exciting techniques in cosmetic dentistry today involves bonding a thin laminated veneer made of porcelain to the etched enamel tooth surface. The primary advantages are the beauty and durability of the material. Because porcelain doesn't stain like composite resin, it remains attractive for a much longer period of time. In addition, gum tissues tolerate porcelain well, thus reducing the likelihood that gum problems will develop.

The drawbacks of porcelain laminates are similar to those of laboratory-constructed laminates. The procedure requires two office visits and costs more than conventional bonding. In addition, the restoration is more difficult to repair should the laminate crack or chip. Again, however, the many benefits of porcelain laminates often make them the treatment of choice for patients seeking long-term solutions to the problem of stained or discolored teeth.

Before

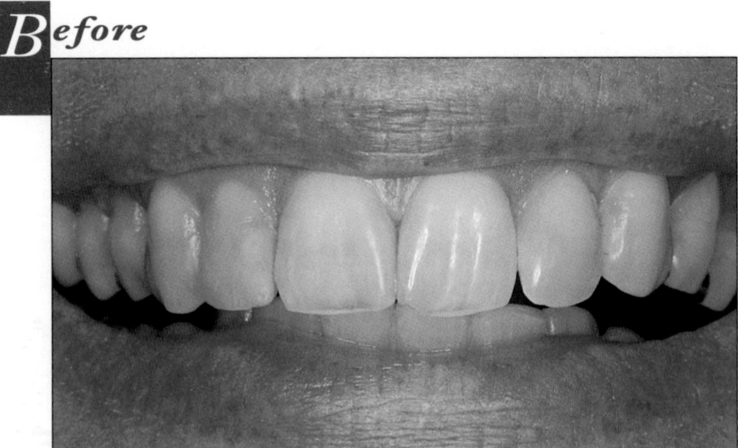

An aging smile

This woman felt her stained teeth were aging her smile.

After

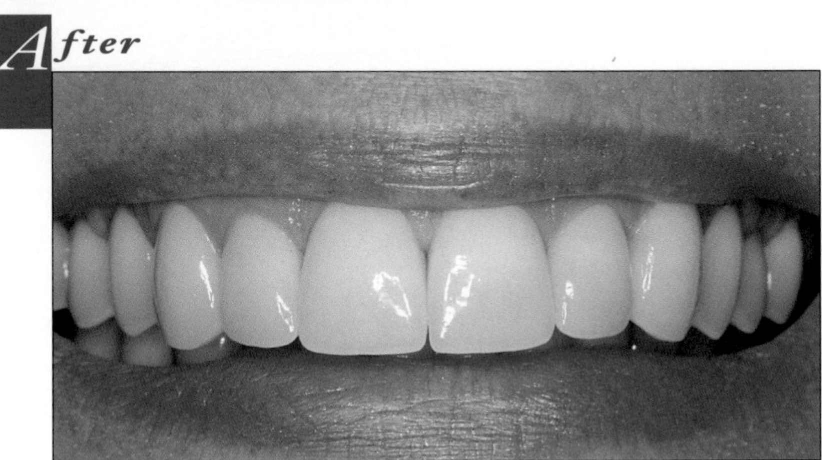

Porcelain laminates

A much lighter color was achieved by laminating the fronts of the teeth with bonded porcelain. This conservative approach saves enamel, thereby helping to preserve the health of the teeth as well.

Before

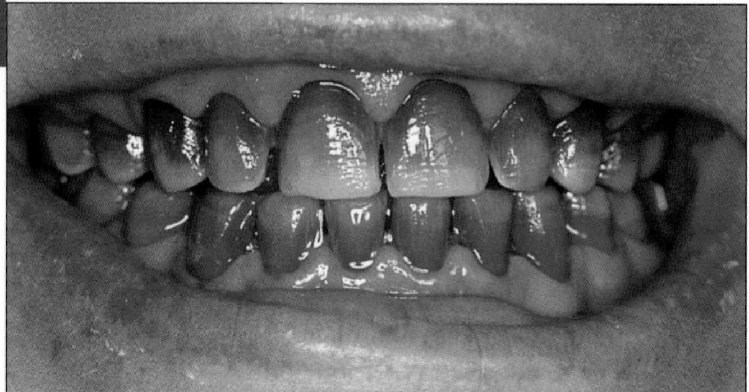

SEVERE TETRACYCLINE STAIN

The dark teeth of this professional dancer are the result of severe tetracycline staining.

Stains

After

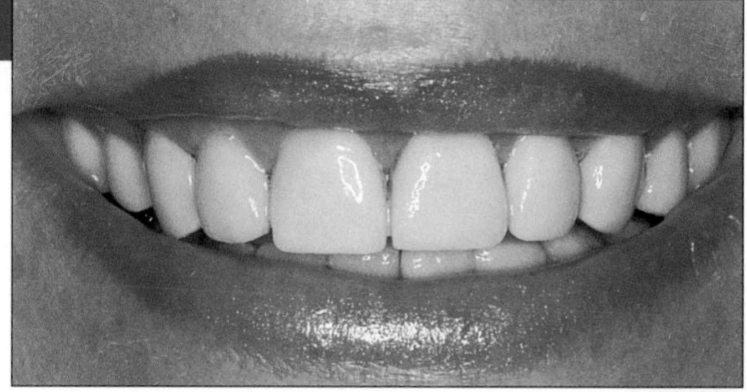

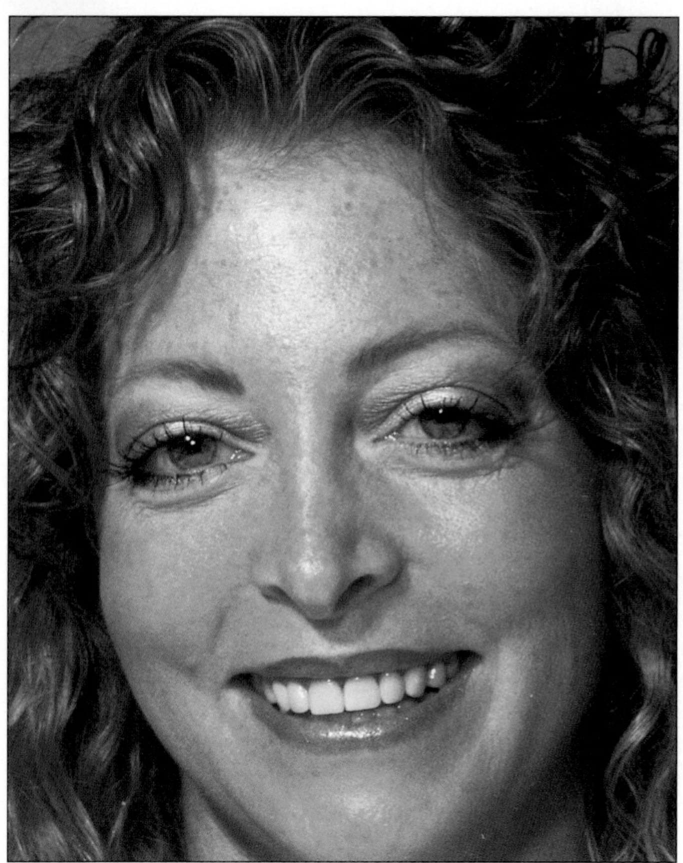

PORCELAIN LAMINATE VENEERS

It required twenty porcelain laminates to successfully mask this woman's severely stained upper and lower teeth. To create a natural look, it is important to restore all teeth that show during the widest smile.

Enamel reduction: to remove or not to remove?

Regardless of which bonding or laminating system you choose, you and your dentist must first decide whether or not to remove enamel from the front surfaces of the teeth, and if so, how much.

The purpose of reducing enamel is to make room for the bonding material or laminate. The replacement should blend in naturally rather than appear as bulky and "overbuilt."

When enamel is reduced, approximately half of its thickness is left intact. This enhances the laminate bond to the tooth. Because there are no nerves in enamel, this amount of tooth structure can usually be reduced without anesthesia.

Although most dentists have a personal preference regarding enamel reduction, you should play an integral role in the decision-making process. The following is a list of the advantages and limitations of enamel reduction.

Enamel Reduction

Advantages

1. Less chance the tooth will look too bulky
2. Better tooth form usually means greater gingival health
3. Greater chance for successful esthetic result

Disadvantages

1. The procedure is generally not reversible
2. If the underlying dentin surface is stained because of tetracycline use, the tooth may appear darker as more enamel is reduced

How a Laminate Veneer Is Attached

Patient's left central incisor is too dark to respond well to bleaching, so a porcelain laminate will be constructed for this tooth.

Shown is the inner view of the constructed porcelain laminate with the etched surface that will help hold the laminate to the tooth. The laminate is then turned to line it up with the tooth *(arrows)*, and a resin cement is applied to the etched surfaces of the tooth inside the laminate. The laminate is then placed on the tooth.

Approximately one half of the front surface enamel is reduced to help make room for the new laminate without overbuilding the tooth.

Approximately one half of the enamel surface is left intact to help bond the laminate to the tooth. Now an impression of the prepared tooth can be made so that the porcelain laminate can be constructed in the dental laboratory.

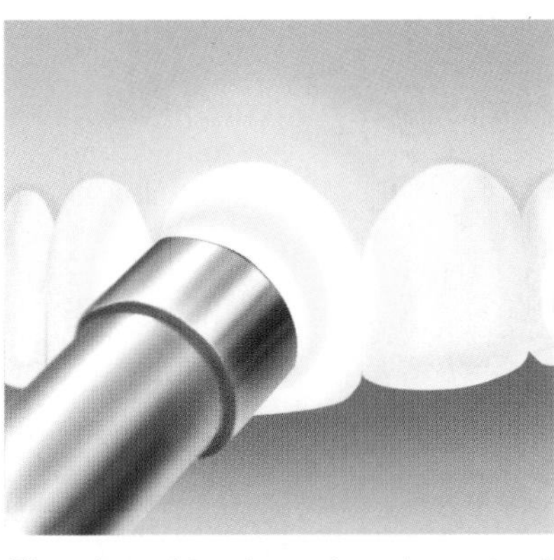

The placed laminate is polymerized (cured) by high-intensity light, which accomplishes final hardening in sixty seconds.

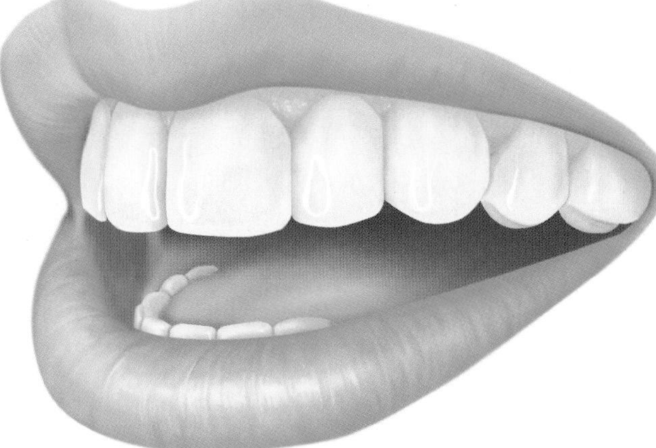

The final laminate is polished. It appears just like a natural tooth, with tissue looking healthy around the laminate.

Before

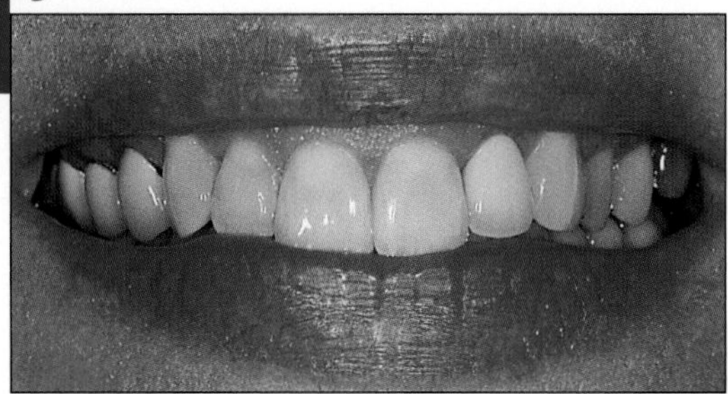

STAINED TEETH, HIGH LIPLINE

This woman desired a more appealing smile. Showing a disproportionate amount of gum tissue around the necks of the front teeth kept her smile from looking its best.

After

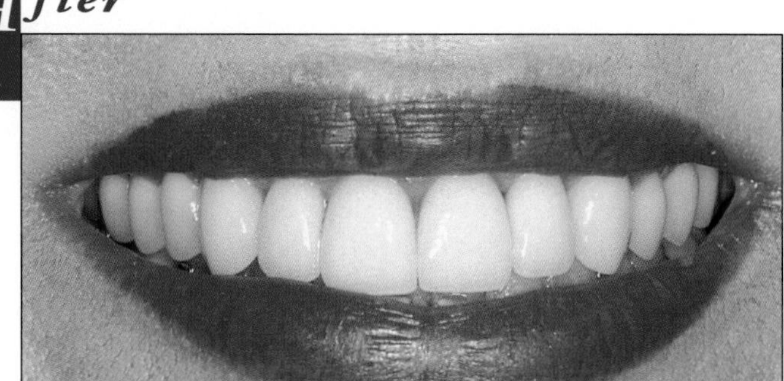

COMBINED THERAPY

Orthodontic treatment was followed by the placement of full crowns, porcelain inlays and onlays and an implant-supported crown. The final result, which took approximately twenty-four months to achieve, was well appreciated by the patient.

TREATMENT SUMMARY

LABORATORY-CONSTRUCTED COMPOSITE LAMINATES

Treatment Time Two visits. Impressions made after tooth preparation. On second visit, dentist will fit and place laminates.

Patient Maintenance Same as bonded tooth. (See p. 54.)

Results of Treatment Attractive result that masks stain.

Average Range of Treatment Life Expectancy Three to ten years. (See footnote p. 50.)

Cost $350 to $1500. (See footnote p. 50.)

ADVANTAGES

1. Can mask dark stains more esthetically than direct bonding
2. No anesthetic usually required
3. Can easily be repaired in the mouth if and when staining or chipping occurs
4. More conservative—less tooth reduction than crowning
5. Usually less expensive than crowning
6. Color change possible

DISADVANTAGES

1. Requires two visits
2. Greater expense than bonded composites
3. Can chip or fracture
4. Can be an irreversible procedure if much enamel is removed
5. Not as strong as porcelain laminates
6. Greater wear than porcelain laminates

TREATMENT SUMMARY

Stains

PORCELAIN LAMINATES

Treatment Time Two office visits. The teeth will be prepared and an impression made during the first visit, which can take from one to four hours. The laminates will be fitted and inserted at the second visit, which may also take the same amount of time. Expect to spend more time for more extensive treatment.

Patient Maintenance The teeth should be professionally cleaned three to four times yearly. Warn your hygienist not to use ultrasonic scaling or air abrasive. Some precautions on eating habits: as with bonding and crowning, take special care when biting into or chewing hard foods with your laminated teeth, because they will not be as strong as enamel. Margins eventually need resealing.

Results of Treatment A polished, natural-appearing result that effectively masks stains.

Average Range of Treatment Life Expectancy Average life expectancy is five to twelve years. (See footnote p. 50.)

Cost Approximately $450 to $2500 per tooth.* (See footnote p. 50.)

ADVANTAGES

1. Less chipping than bonded restorations
2. Etched porcelain provides an extremely good bond to enamel
3. Wears less than the composite resin laminate
4. Less stain—less chance of loss of color or luster
5. More conservative—less tooth reduction than crowning
6. Lasts five to twelve years as compared to plastics (three to eight years)
7. Gum tissue tolerates porcelain well
8. No anesthetic may be required
9. Color change possible

DISADVANTAGES

1. More costly than conventional bonding
2. More difficult for dentist to produce a polished surface after contouring in the mouth
3. More difficult to repair if the laminate cracks or chips
4. Can be an irreversible procedure if much enamel is removed

*Expect to pay extra for esthetic temporaries or ceramics.

Crowning

Crowning or "capping" is the most aggressive form of treatment for staining and discoloration. The entire tooth surface must be reduced and replaced with an artificial material.

There are several types of esthetic crowns. Some are made entirely of high-strength porcelain or cast glass; others combine metal and porcelain. The type of crown you and your dentist choose will depend on a number of factors, including the location of the tooth or teeth being crowned, the type and severity of the discoloration, and overall health of the surrounding gums. Generally speaking, however, the ceramic-metal crown is the best choice because the metal provides added strength.

Regardless of the type of crown you choose, your dentist will first reduce the teeth approximately one-third in size. Impressions are then made of the teeth and life-size models built from hard stone. A dental technician who specializes in working with porcelain and metals then constructs the actual crowns from these models. When you go to the office for your "try-in" appointment, each crown is fitted and colored to the desired shade.

WHEN DONE CORRECTLY, CROWNING CAN PRODUCE NEAR-PERFECT ESTHETIC RESULTS

When done correctly, crowning can produce near-perfect esthetic results. However, because many teeth may be involved in cases of staining or discoloration, both the cost and the number of office visits required may make this treatment prohibitive for some patients.

How a Tooth is Crowned or "Capped"

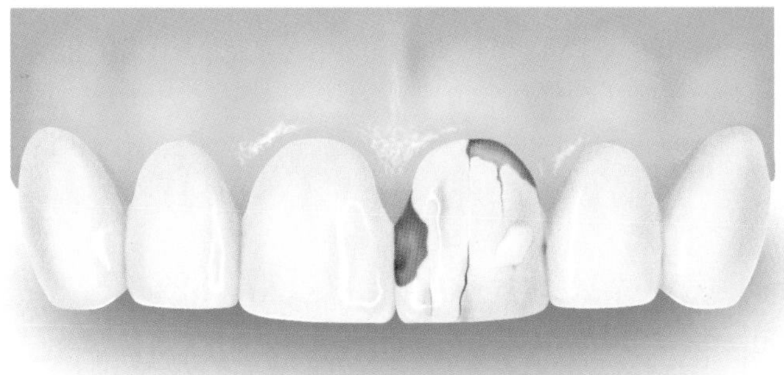

Front view of the tooth to be crowned.

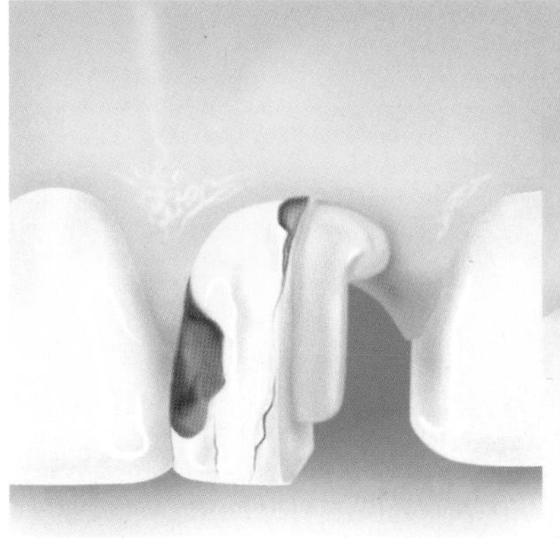

One half of the tooth has been prepared so you can see approximately how much tooth structure has been reduced.

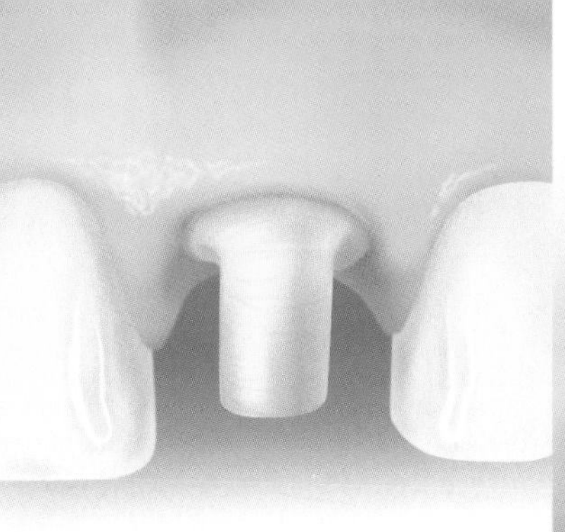

The tooth has now been fully prepared to make room for the porcelain (and most times an underlying layer of metal for support). Then two sides of the tooth are prepared with only a slight taper to help hold the crown in place.

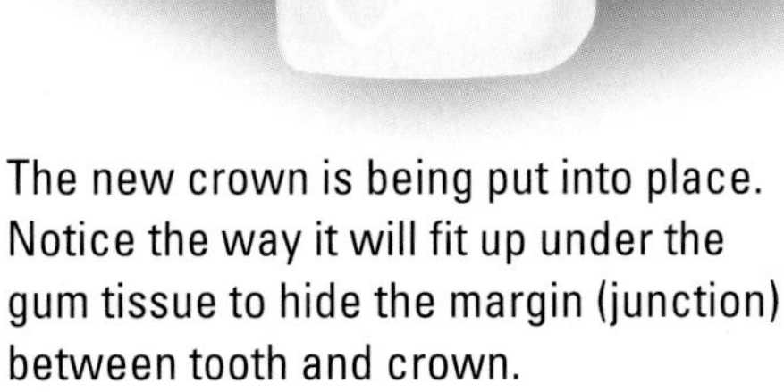

The new crown is being put into place. Notice the way it will fit up under the gum tissue to hide the margin (junction) between tooth and crown.

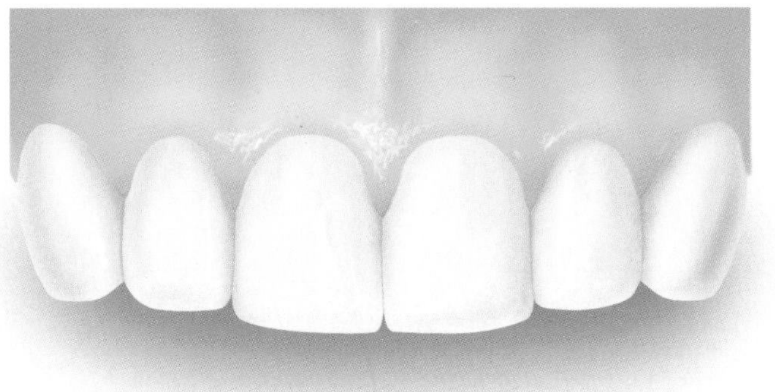

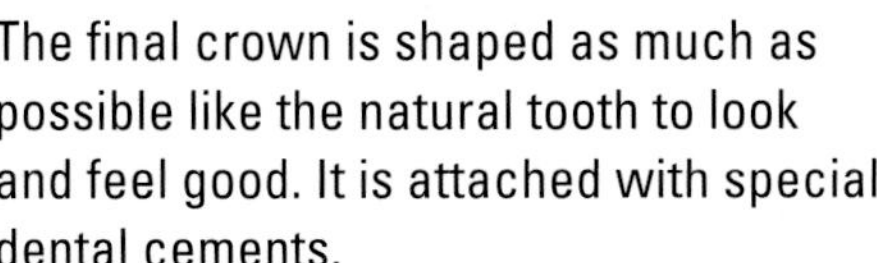

The final crown is shaped as much as possible like the natural tooth to look and feel good. It is attached with special dental cements.

Temporary crowns can help you decide

Temporary crowns made of acrylic typically are used while final restorations are being made. These "temporaries" can help you become accustomed to having a new shape in your mouth if teeth are being lengthened or if a new bite is formed. They also can help you decide—in advance—if you like what you see and if you think you can live with it. Certain types of temporary restorations can even be used to shift teeth slightly, particularly before and after gum surgery. In such cases, teeth that are loose due to bone loss may be repositioned and held in place during the healing process.

If you'll be wearing temporaries for any length of time, consider paying more for better ones. They most likely will be double- or triple-lined with plastic and possibly combined with metal for greater strength. Although the additional time required to create more esthetically pleasing restorations costs more, the results are usually worth it.

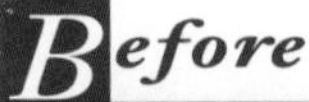

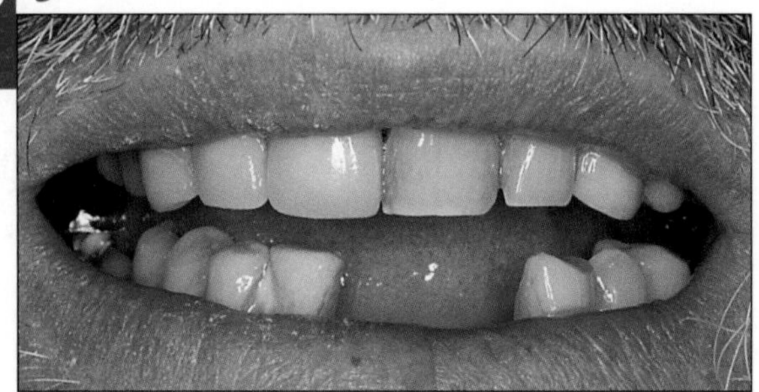

DISCOLORED AND MISSING TEETH

An aging smile motivated this fifty-seven-year-old artist to seek a bright new look.

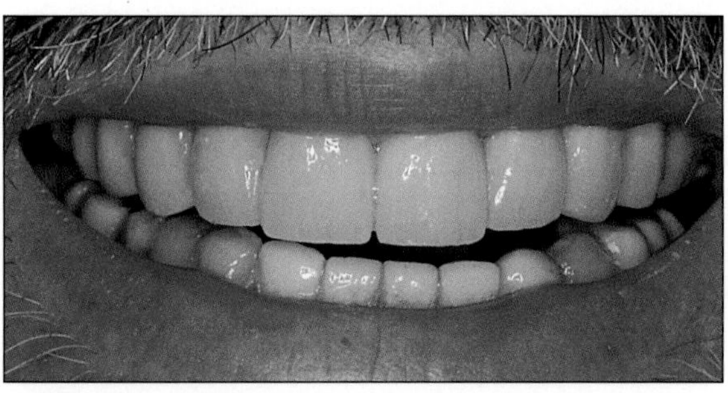

TEMPORARY ACRYLIC CROWNS AND FIXED BRIDGE

Well-fitting temporary acrylic full crowns were made to make sure the patient would like his new look.

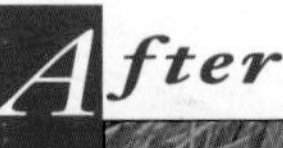

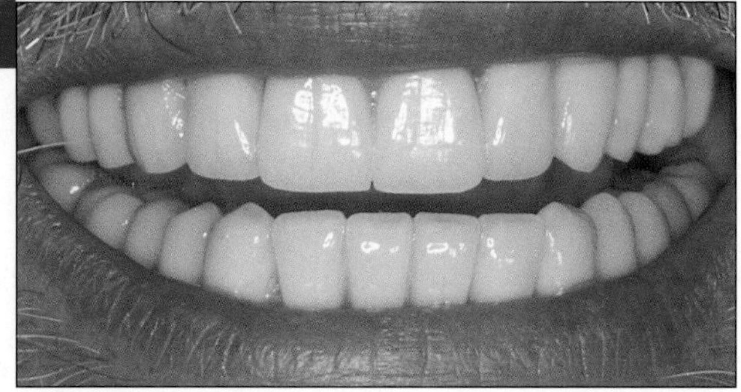

PORCELAIN CROWNS

After wearing the temporary crowns for several months, the new porcelain crowns were placed. It was important to the patient to have a much brighter smile, and his satisfaction can be seen in his winning grin.

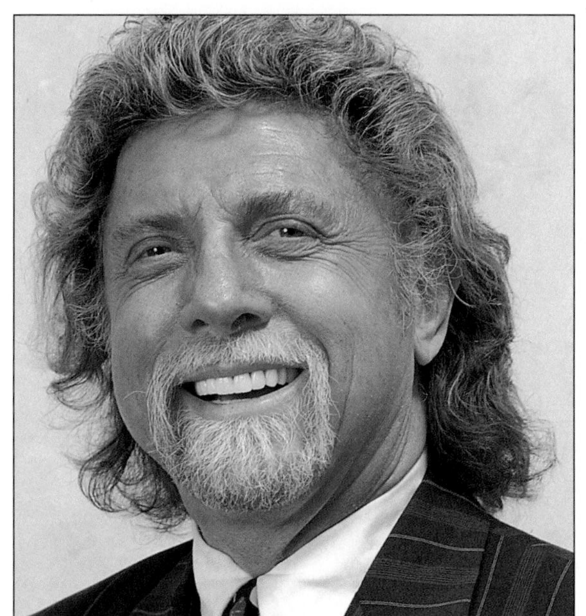

Before

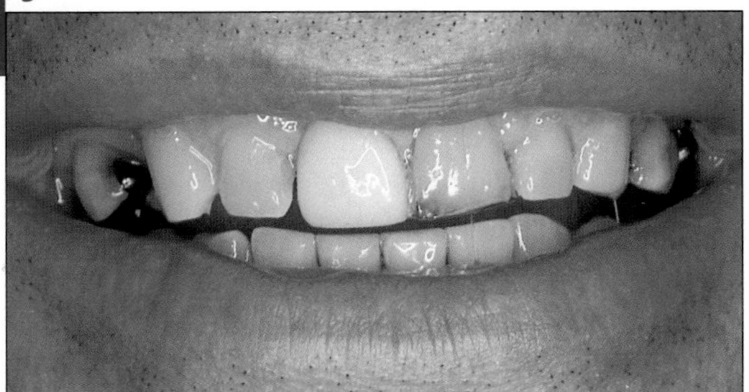

Stained and missing teeth

This man was a few years from retirement, and he thought looking good was important for a second career. A missing right front tooth (central incisor) had been replaced with a tooth that was much whiter than the adjacent teeth, and the patient wanted to lighten the other teeth to match that tooth. There were also missing teeth, as well as spaces between the other teeth and wear on the biting edges on the left side.

After

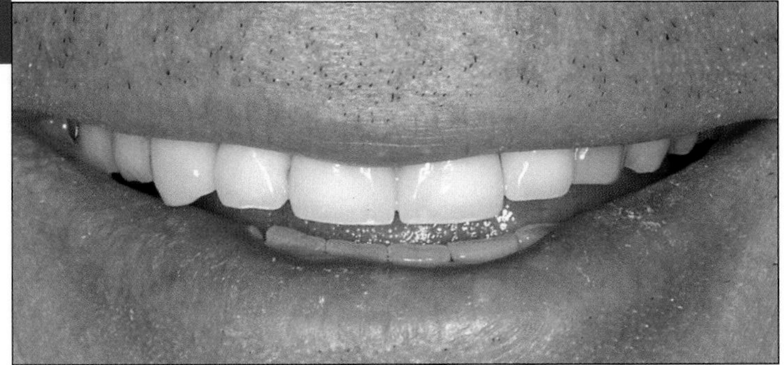

Crowns and bridges

All the upper teeth were either crowned or bridged to restore proper tooth form and a lighter color. A more youthful smileline was created by lengthening the front two teeth with crowns. Slight staining was done between the front teeth to make the crowns look more natural. Opaque whitish areas were placed on the bottom edges of the front teeth to help create "highlights" for better light reflection. Note the various colors used in the tooth to give a "third dimension" of naturalness to the smile. Remember, the average person sees you from about a three-foot distance from which the porcelain must look natural. This treatment was done in stages, so the patient could take advantage of his insurance policy, which covered only a certain amount each year.

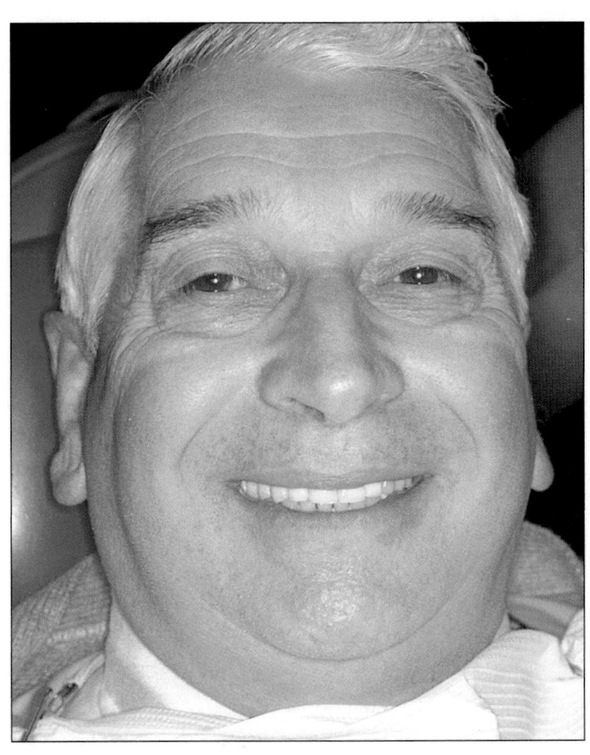

The esthetic try-in appointment

When crowns are made, a "try-in" appointment is usually scheduled to make sure that you will be happy with your new restorations. This appointment often means the difference between average and excellent cosmetic results.

At the try-in appointment, avoid anesthesia if possible so that your lipline can be seen in its natural condition. Ask for a large mirror that shows your entire face and hold it at arm's length to get an idea of how your smile is seen by others. (Few people will be scrutinizing your teeth any more closely!) Look at the restorations from various angles and in different types of light using expressions that are natural for you.

Don't make split-second decisions at the try-in appointment. Look at the restorations long enough to grow accustomed to them, and take someone with you to provide a second opinion. Also consider your dentist's opinion, as well as your own, when making value judgments at the try-in appointment. *Above all, be honest.* If you aren't happy with what you see, now is the time to make necessary changes. If you are in doubt about the length, shape or color of your new teeth, consider reimaging on the computer. Any number of proposed alterations can be easily made without destroying the artistry that has thus far gone into the making of your new restorations.

The esthetic factors that you and your dentist should consider at the try-in appointment appear in the checklist on p. 70. Feel free to use it to convey what you want to your dentist.

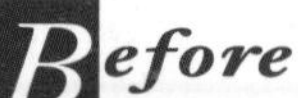

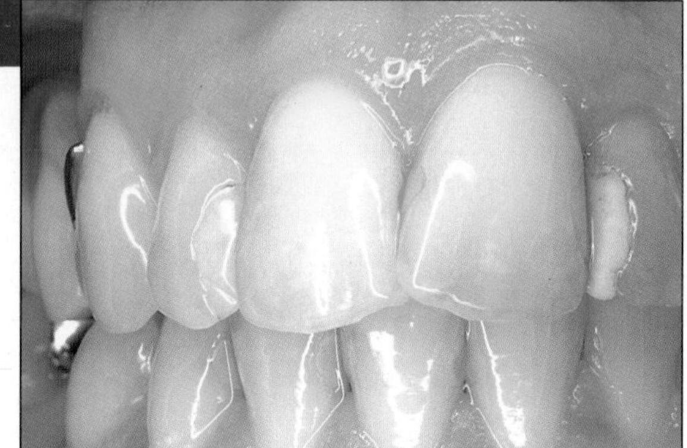

STAINED AND CROWDED TEETH

This 25-year-old hair stylist had discolored and crowded upper teeth.

After

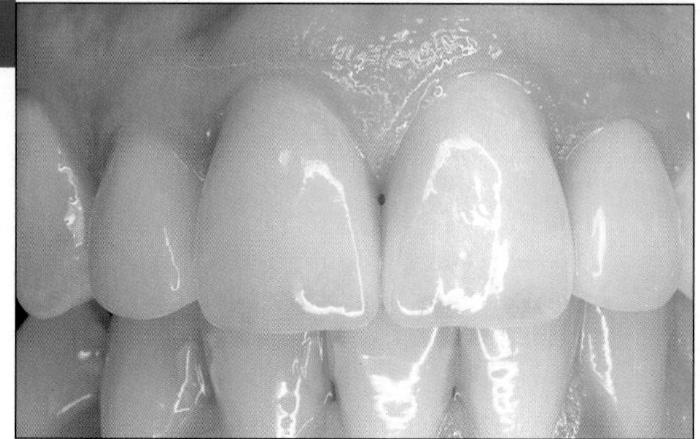

FULL CROWNS

The upper front teeth were crowned with full porcelain to provide a life-like look. Note how the crowns fit under the healthy gum tissue to hide the junction or margin between tooth and crown.

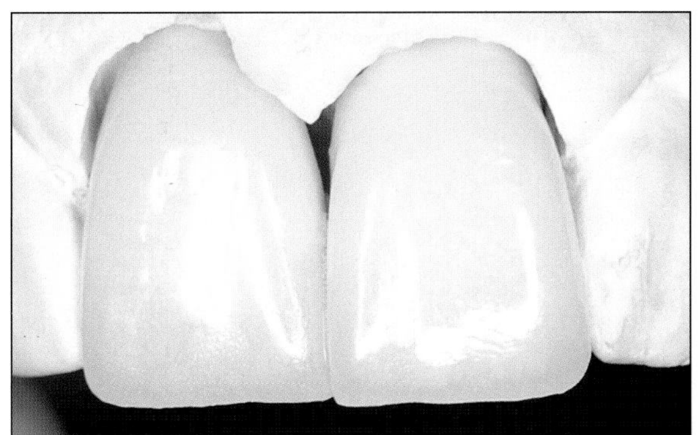

TWO CROWNS ON THE CONSTRUCTION MODEL

These two central incisor crowns were constructed on a stone model.

NATURAL-APPEARING CROWNS

These are the same two front teeth as they appear in the patient's mouth. Notice how well they blend with the natural teeth on each side.

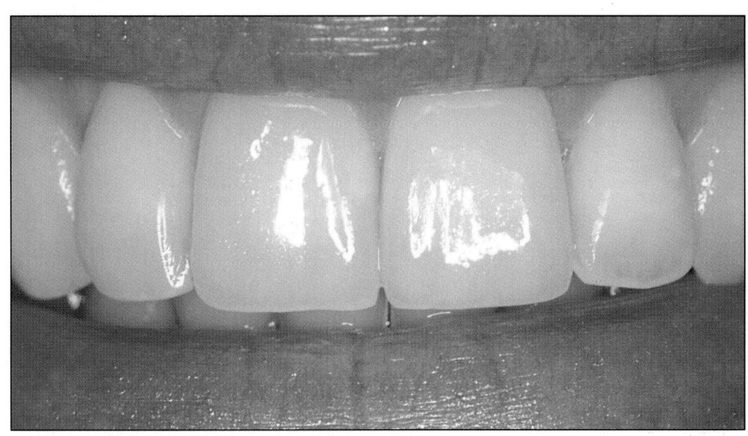

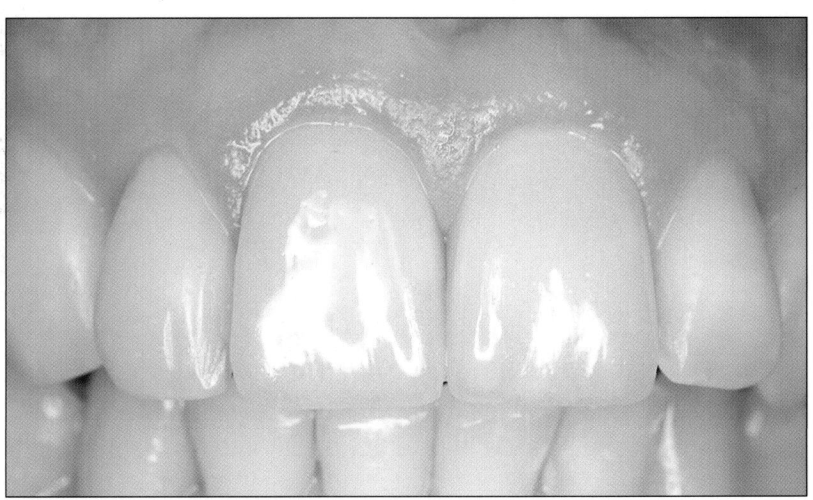

HEALTHY-LOOKING TISSUE AROUND THE NEW CROWNS

This final result shows how healthy gums look around crowns. Note the absence of dark lines or metal showing at the gum line around the two central incisors.

Esthetic Checklist for Your New Crown

- ❑ **Color**
  Will the color blend in with the rest of the teeth, or do you want the crowns to stand out by being lighter? In general, it is better for the front teeth to be the same shade since light makes the teeth stand out and dark makes them recede. The color varies, but it should match or blend in with the surrounding teeth. The objective is to make the crown look as natural as possible. Younger people usually have more translucence, and sometimes spots of blueness appear toward the biting edge of the upper front teeth. The degree of translucency or opaqueness will vary with the materials used to make the crown. Expect less translucency with porcelain-fused-to-metal crowns. The most translucency will be evident with the all-porcelain or glass crowns, but they may lack the strength that the metal provides.

- ❑ **Length**
  Are they too long or too short? Ideally, the biting edges of the upper teeth should just touch the bottom lip when you say "forty-five." Remember, if you want a younger smileline, the two front teeth or central incisors should be slightly longer than the two lateral incisors. If the front teeth can't be lengthened, consider having the laterals shortened slightly or rounded to give the illusion that the front teeth are slightly longer. Computer imaging is a good alternative to having the dentist cut away the porcelain or add length by baking new porcelain; it can give everyone a preview of the proposed change. Then if everyone agrees change is required, it becomes easier to predict that the treatment result will be favorable.

- ❑ **Gums**
  Make sure the gum tissue looks healthy. It should outline each tooth in a half-moon shape. Red, puffy or bleeding gums are unhealthy.

- ❑ **Midline**
  An imaginary vertical line drawn between the two front upper teeth should be in line with the middle of the face. If not perfectly in line, it should be parallel to the facial midline, at least.

- ❑ **Shape**
  Shape is one of the most important aspects of a crown since it must duplicate the form of the natural tooth. Bring in old photographs of yourself if you have them to help the dentist create the best form for you. Your tooth should not be too bulky, and it should not look like the gum is pushing it out of the mouth. It should slide right under and fit flush with the gumline.

- ❑ **Texture**
  If you want a natural-looking tooth, it is important to match the surface characteristics of adjacent teeth. If the adjacent tooth surface has ridges or other irregularities on the front surface, they should be included when the porcelain is glazed in order to make the light reflect the same way as it would off the natural tooth.
  Warning: When discussing the type of materials to use in your crown, take into consideration your gumline. For strength, you may choose a porcelain-fused-to-metal crown. However, if you have a high lipline, a metal margin can eventually show if the gum recedes. There is a compromise solution: metal on the inside and porcelain in the front, sometimes called a porcelain butt joint. This is a good example of trading off some function for esthetics, since the porcelain butt joint may not be quite as strong as a metal margin, but the esthetic result can be more pleasing.
- ❑ **Adjacent teeth**
  Look at the teeth on either side to see if they can be improved with cosmetic contouring or a new filling before the new crowns are placed.
- ❑ **Arrangement of teeth**
  Does the tooth placement look natural? Sometimes an addition of a little porcelain or a slight reshaping can make a tooth look a bit irregular and more natural.

Final note: Take your time and do not be too rushed to consider each of the above factors. In addition to viewing your restorations close up, be sure to hold the mirror at arm's length to see how others will see your new smile.

Communication is essential

When extensive esthetic changes are required, you may be asked to sign a written statement of approval when you are satisfied with your appearance at the try-in appointment. Treatment should not progress until you, your dentist and anyone else involved is pleased with the appearance of the restorations at this stage.

If you want a particular "look," be sure to discuss it with your dentist from the start. Once the teeth are ready for a try-in, it's too late to make radical treatment changes. If you're the type of person who values certain other people's opinions very highly, be sure to bring them to the try-in appointment. You don't want to regret having consented to a treatment because someone significant to you was not present at try-in.

Although the most successful cosmetic dental treatment is the result of a thorough analysis and accurate interpretation of your age, sex and personality, remember that there is no "right" or "wrong." There is only esthetic interpretation. You will always be more attractive to some people than you are to others. In the final analysis, you are the one who must be satisfied.

Basic Types of Esthetic Crowns

Advantages	Disadvantages
Ceramo-metal*	
Strongest type of esthetic crown	Metal may be visible if tissue shrinks
Doesn't fracture or chip as easily as alternative esthetic type crown	Metal may be visible if tissue is thin
Usually most economical esthetic crowns	Metal may affect color of porcelain
	Possible bluish tint of gum if gum tissue is thin and metal shows through
Ceramo-metal crown with porcelain butt joint*	
Esthetic	Metal usually visible from inside view only
No metal shows from front	Underlying metal may affect color of porcelain
Strong	Porcelain margin more susceptible to chipping than metal
	More costly to make
All-porcelain or cast glass†	
Most esthetic throughout crown life	Not as strong as ceramo-metal crown
No metal shows	Margin may be more susceptible to chipping
	More costly to make

*See p. 73 for illustrations.
†See p. 73 for illustrations.

Getting Used to Your Crowns

Don't expect your new restorations to feel normal overnight. Your tongue, cheeks, lips and brain need time to adjust, which typically takes a week or two, particularly if drastic changes have been made such as closing large spaces. Relax and try to get your mind off your mouth. With a little time, you can grow accustomed to almost anything new.

If your bite doesn't feel right, however, see your dentist immediately. If allowed to persist, a bad bite can cause pain, as well as damage the temporomandibular joints.

What Happens if Your Gum Shrinks?

Crown type	*Gum shrinkage*	*Repair*

A ceramo-metal crown with an all-metal margin.

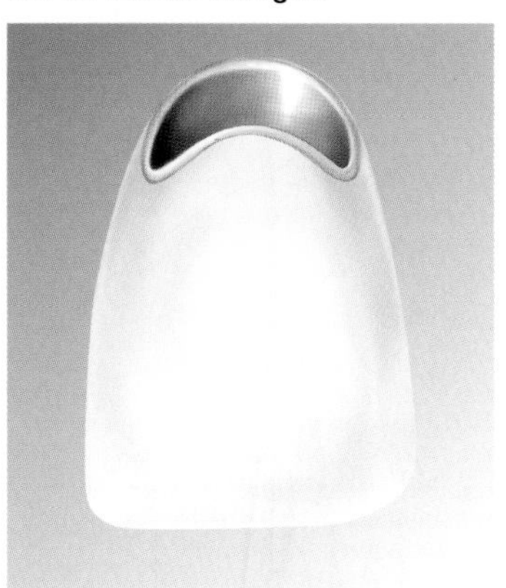

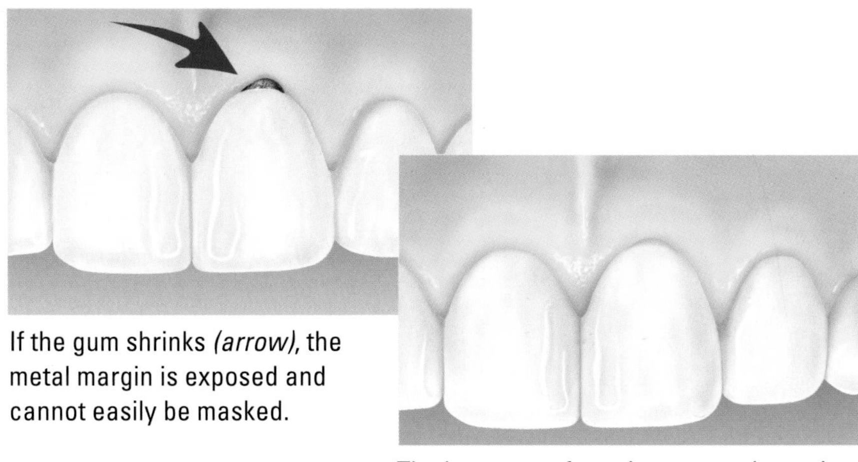

If the gum shrinks *(arrow)*, the metal margin is exposed and cannot easily be masked.

The best type of repair to a metal margin.

A porcelain butt joint.

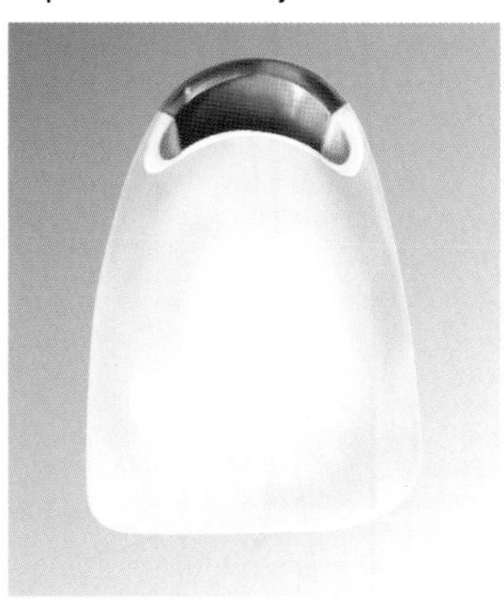

If the gum shrinks *(arrow)*, the root is exposed, but it can be esthetically masked with composite resin if necessary.

Porcelain butt joint repair.

An all-porcelain crown.

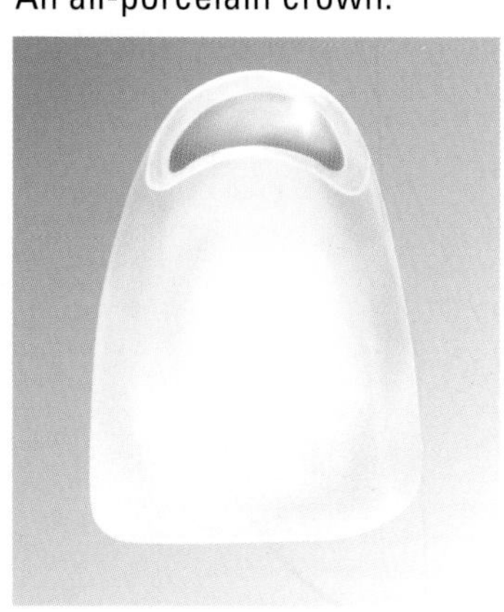

If the gum shrinks *(arrow)*, the root is exposed, but as with a porcelain butt joint, the root can be esthetically masked with composite resin if necessary.

Repair of a porcelain crown.

Before

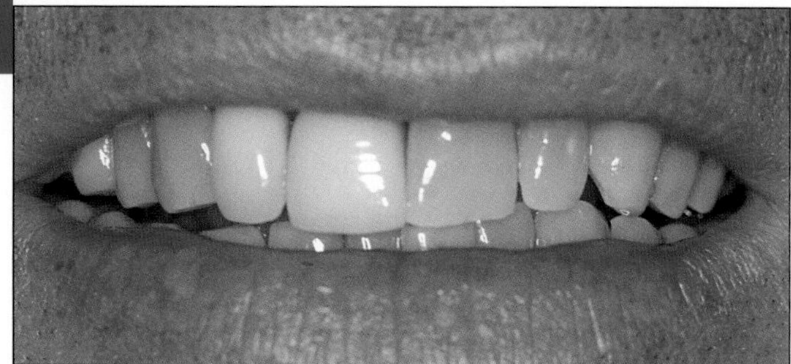

CROWNS TOO LIGHT

This 46-year-old man wanted a more uniform color in his smile. The first decision he had to make was to choose a color he could be happy with.

After

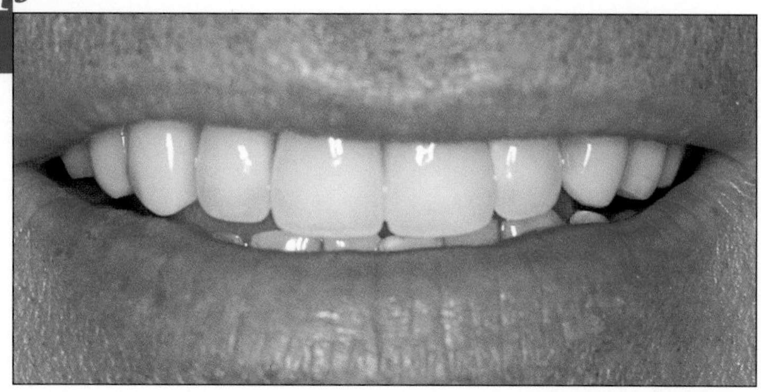

ALL-CERAMIC CROWNS PLUS COMPOSITE RESIN BONDING

The four front teeth were crowned with a high-strength all-ceramic material. Three teeth on either side of the four anterior crowns were bonded with a lighter shade of composite resin. This permitted a brighter, more even-appearing smile for this patient.

Before

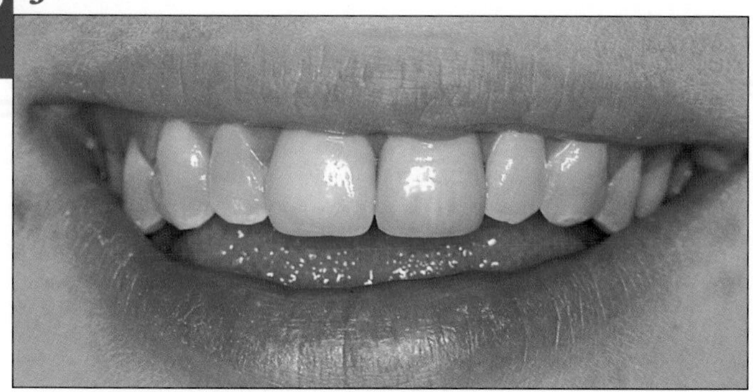

CROWNS TOO DARK

Although the natural teeth were discolored, the two front teeth on this young lady were too bulky, making them look protruded.

After

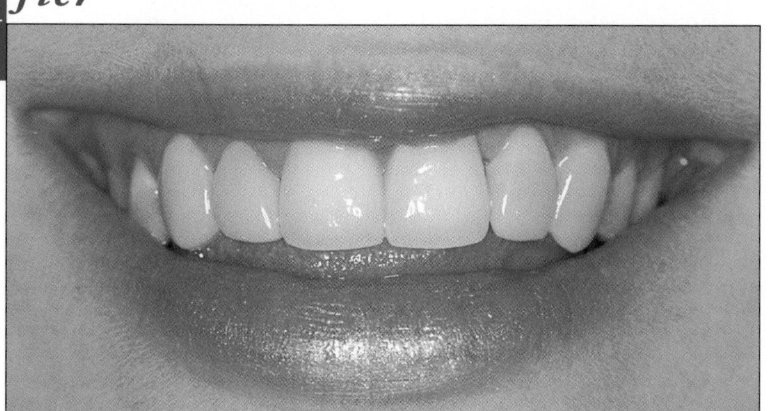

ALL-CERAMIC CROWNS PLUS COMPOSITE RESIN BONDING ON FOUR TEETH

After five appointments, the patient's smile was much brighter, and her wedding smile six months later was radiant.

TREATMENT SUMMARY

Stains

CROWNING

Treatment Time Usually two appointments of approximately one to four hours each for up to four teeth. Expect to spend more time as additional teeth or more extensive treatment are involved.

Patient Maintenance Crowns are designed to look and feel like real teeth. As with your original smile, however, care must be taken to avoid tooth fractures. Biting down on hard things like peanut brittle or ice is strictly prohibited. A caries-free or decay-free diet—a diet that reduces intake of refined sugars—is imperative to prevent the cement that helps hold the crowns in place from washing away because of decay. Have a professional cleaning at least three or four times yearly. Fluoride treatments should be given once a year. Ask your dentist to recommend a fluoride toothpaste and mouthwash for you to use at home to help prevent future decay. Usually, these products can be bought over the counter, but be sure to choose well-tested products carrying the American Dental Association Seal of Acceptance. Flossing at least once per day is essential for crowns. The most beautiful results with full crowns can be destroyed if your teeth beneath the crowns decay.

Results of Treatment Crowning can achieve the ultimate in shade control, tooth shape and size.

Average Range of Treatment Life Expectancy The average esthetic life of the full crown is about five to fifteen years. Life expectancy is directly proportional to three things: fracture, problems with tissues, and the hidden danger of decay. (See footnote on p. 50.)

Cost Approximately $550 to $3000 per tooth.* (See footnote on p. 50.)

ADVANTAGES

1. Teeth can be lightened or whitened to any desired shade
2. The dentist can improve shapes of teeth during this process
3. Some realignment or straightening of teeth is possible
4. Longest life of any restoration

DISADVANTAGES

1. Ceramic crowns can fracture
2. Crowning requires an anesthetic
3. Original tooth form is altered (possibly involving the nerve)
4. If tissue shrinkage occurs, it can expose the junction between tooth and crown, allowing for the possibility of an unsightly line
5. Crowning is not permanent; there is limited esthetic life expectancy
6. Crowning requires much greater expense than bonding

*Expect to pay extra for esthetic temporaries or ceramics.

Stained Fillings: Should You Bond, Laminate or Crown?

Although crowns were once the treatment of choice for teeth with large stained fillings, today's ideal solution is often bonding or laminating. Composite resin restorations are both cosmetically appealing and cost effective. In addition, they provide a healthy alternative to complete crowns because they allow preservation of more natural tooth structure, thus reducing the chances of gum problems and pulpal irritation.

Alternatively, a treatment combining laminates with full crowns may be preferable. This option allows you to conserve as much of the enamel as possible while still obtaining a beautiful result.

Before

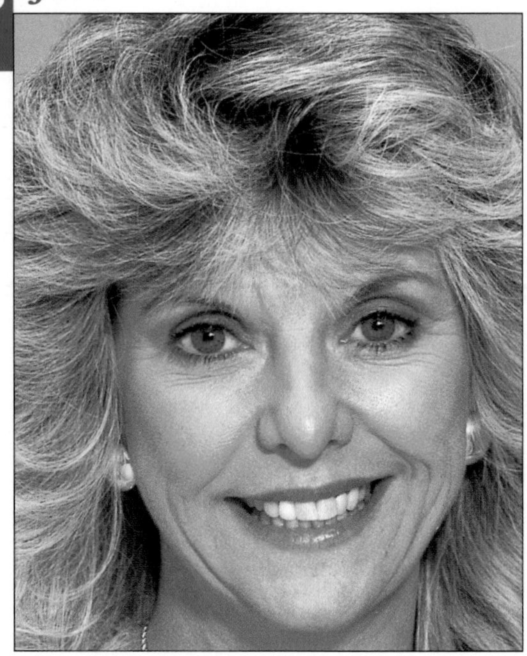

Stained Teeth and Nonmatching Crowns

This woman had a smile marred by stained front teeth and false-looking crowns that did not match.

After

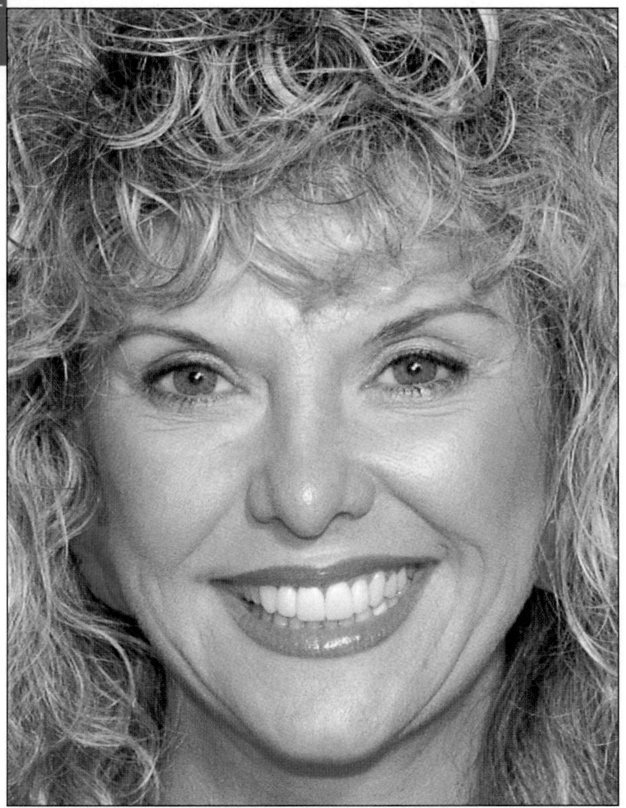

Porcelain Laminate Veneers and Crowns

A combination of new crowns and porcelain laminate veneers conserved this patient's enamel while providing a strong, beautiful result.

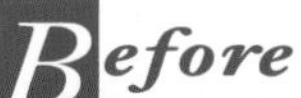

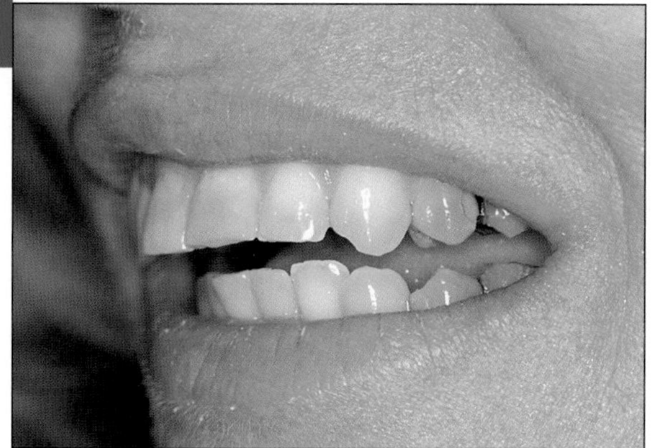

DARK BACK TOOTH

This state government worker was unhappy with her discolored side teeth. The main cause of the staining was her old silver fillings, which were leaking through the dentinal tubules and discoloring the enamel.

After

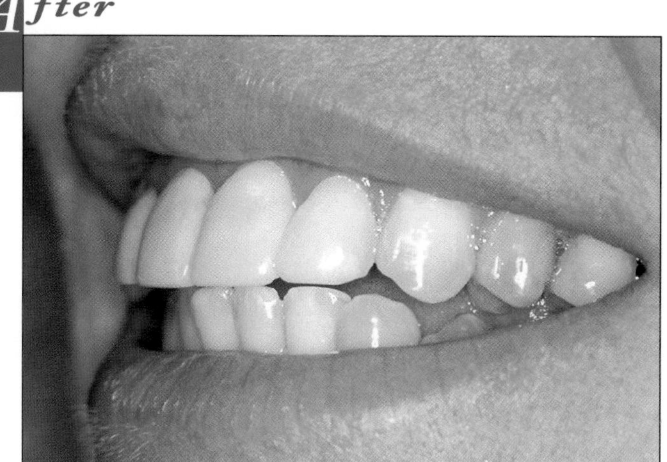

COMPOSITE RESIN BONDING

Replacing the old silver fillings with one of the newer posterior composite resins immediately restored the tooth to its natural color. The main problem with these new restorations is that their estimated life expectancy may be much less than that of silver or gold. Porcelain or composite resin inlays are a better solution but more costly. In this case, the patient opted also for treatment of the front teeth.

REPLACING OLD FILLINGS

In addition to advanced decay, old or defective silver fillings often cause the teeth to become discolored and unsightly. If you have this problem, several alternatives are available. To determine which is best, I believe all old filling material should be removed. You and your dentist then may decide to:

• ***Replace the defective filling with a new silver filling.*** Before inserting the new filling, the dentist often "seals" the tooth with a liner to prevent the problem from recurring.

• ***Replace the defective filling with a tooth-colored composite resin.*** If the area isn't too large, composite resins can provide a cosmetically appealing filling alternative, particularly in lower back teeth that show when you smile or laugh. Keep in mind, however, that these restorations probably won't last as long as silver fillings, and they are more expensive. Estimated cost is $75 to $420.

• ***Replace the defective silver filling with a gold inlay or onlay.*** Inlays and onlays are particular types of fillings made of porcelain or gold. Inlays are custom-made to fit the prepared cavity and are then cemented into place. Onlays actually cover the entire chewing surface of the teeth. One advantage to using gold over silver is that gold doesn't discolor or stain the teeth. It also has a longer life expectancy than silver and can be placed esthetically into upper back teeth where it doesn't show. The primary disadvantage of gold is its cost, which ranges from $435 to $1850 per tooth.

• ***Replace the defective silver filling with a porcelain or cast glass inlay or onlay.*** Because porcelain and cast glass inlays and onlays have etched surfaces, the cement bond to the tooth is increased. In fact, research shows that bonded porcelain inlays and onlays can equal the strength of natural teeth, making them particularly attractive choices when both esthetics and strength are required. However, extra stress can fracture both porcelain and cast glass just as it can natural teeth. If the inlay or onlay is made by a computer (CAD/CAM, see p. 307), the entire procedure can be accomplished in one appointment. The cost of these restorations is equivalent to that of a gold inlay or onlay, approximately $435 to $1850 per tooth.

Before

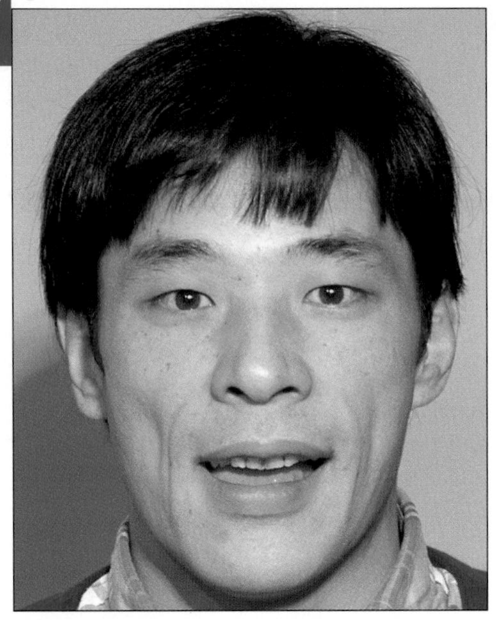

DISCOLORED AND DECAYED TEETH

This 34-year-old engineer hesitated to smile fully because of his discolored, decayed and chipped front teeth.

After

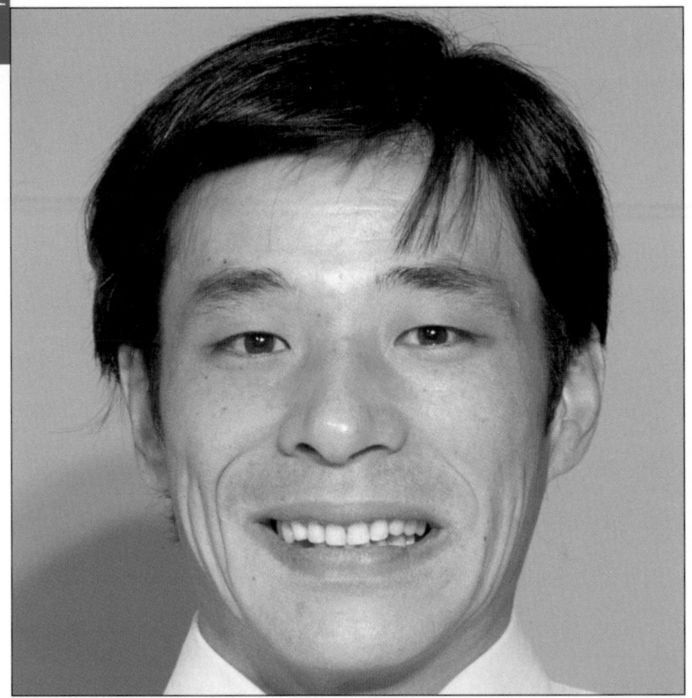

COMPOSITE RESIN BONDING AND COSMETIC CONTOURING

The teeth were professionally cleaned before they were restored with composite resin. Finally, reshaping (cosmetic contouring) of the teeth to obtain a straighter look helped to produce a more handsome smile.

Before

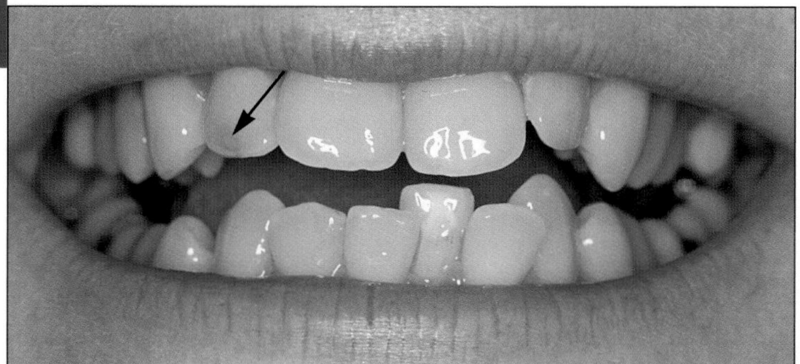

Discolored (Gray) Lateral Incisor

This woman was concerned about her lateral incisor (arrow), which was discolored because of a silver filling.

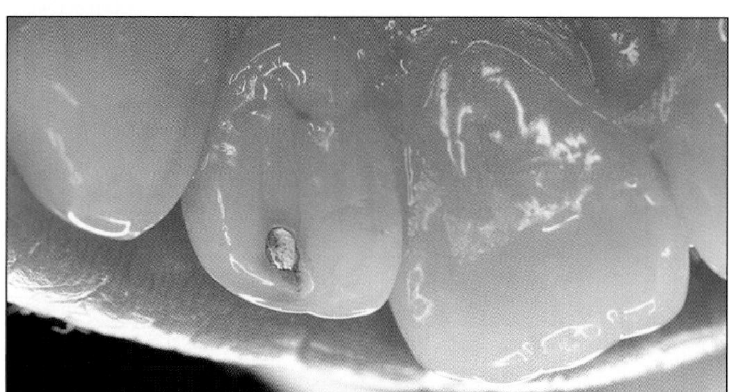

All of these treatments involve removal of the offending silver filling and replacing with one that will restore the original color to the tooth. In the event that the tooth color does not return to its natural shade, three other options remain: masking the stain through composite resin bonding, laminating with porcelain or composite resin, or crowning.

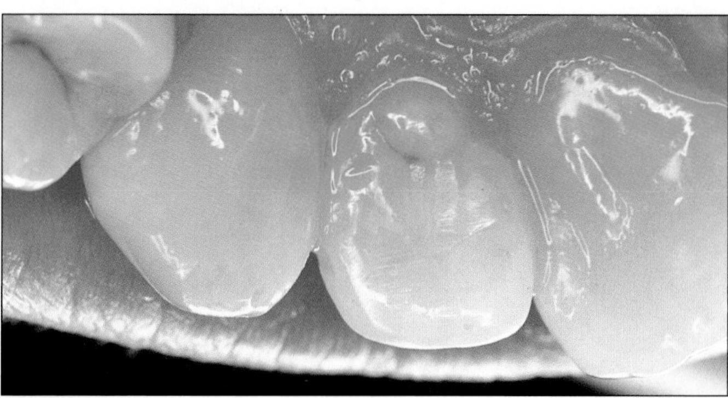

After

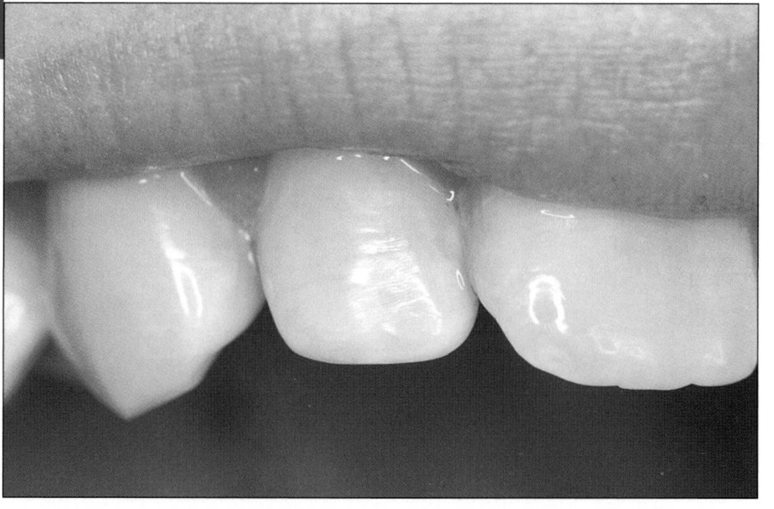

Tooth-Colored Filling

Replacement of the defective amalgam filling with composite resin helped to restore proper color to the tooth. In the front of the mouth, it is generally advisable to use tooth-colored filling materials when possible.

Four Popular Ways Back Teeth Are Rebuilt

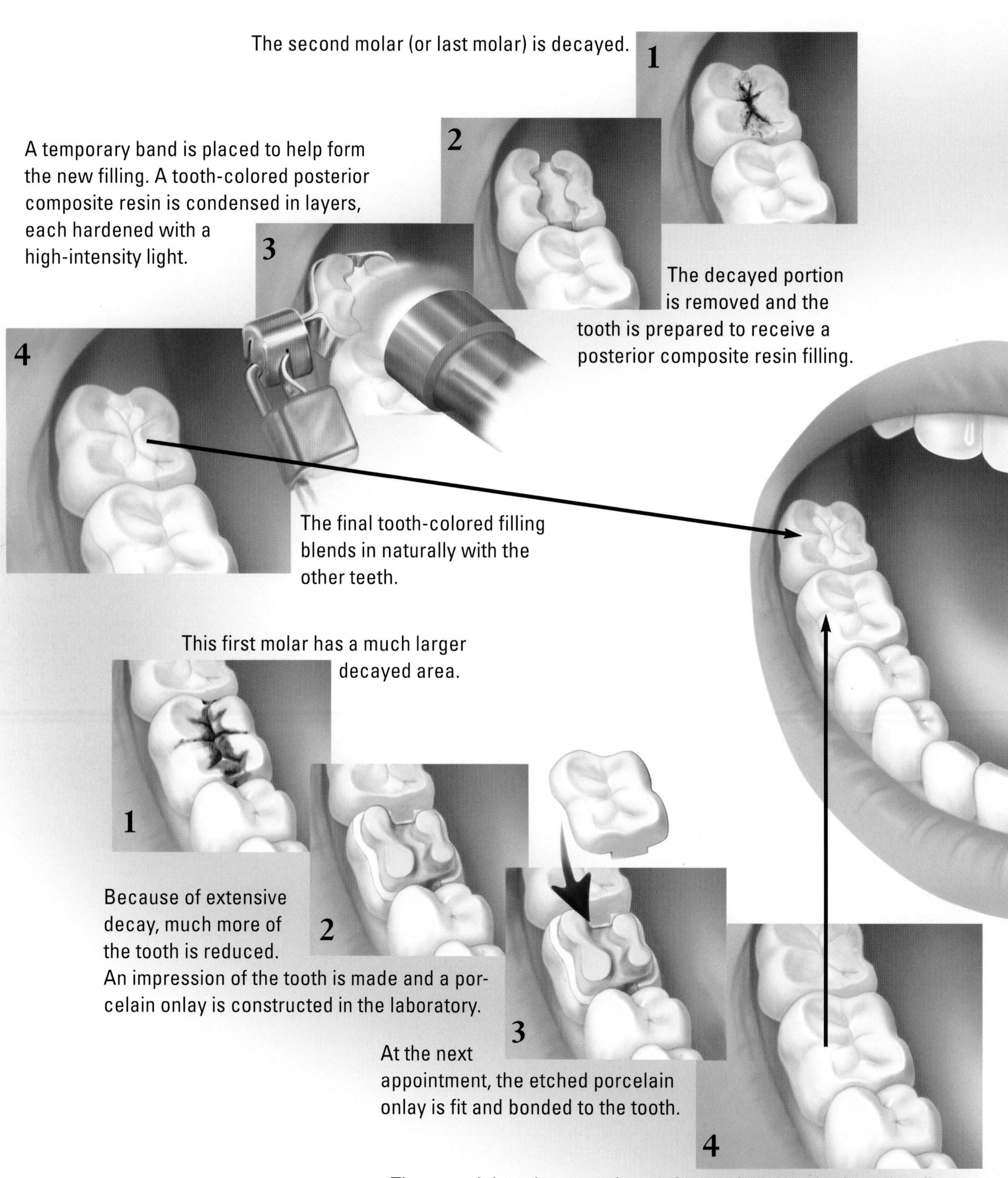

The porcelain onlay was chosen for maximum esthetics as well as tooth support. Note how beautifully it blends in with the natural tooth. (This onlay could have been made of gold for longer life expectancy.)

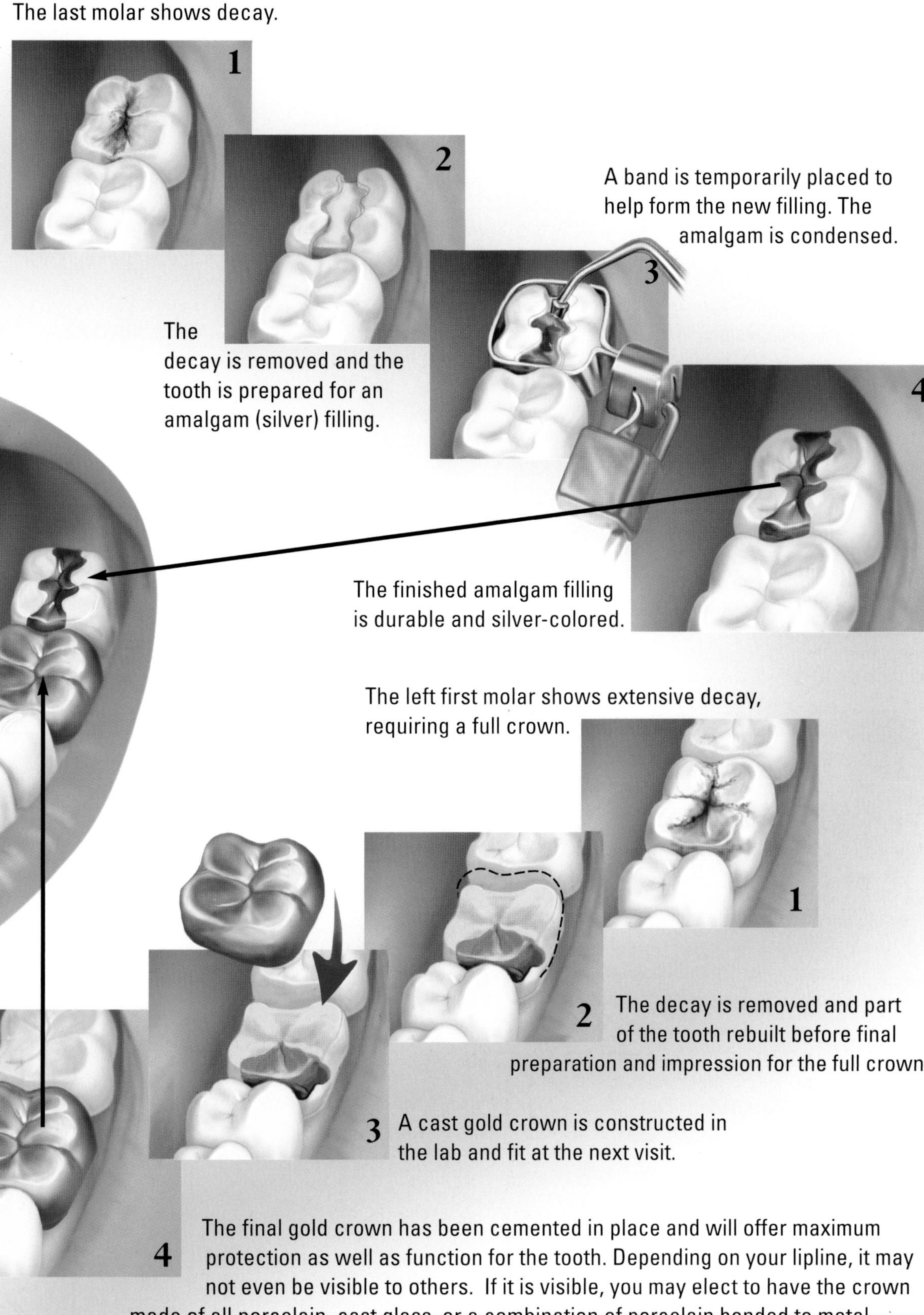

The last molar shows decay.

The decay is removed and the tooth is prepared for an amalgam (silver) filling.

A band is temporarily placed to help form the new filling. The amalgam is condensed.

The finished amalgam filling is durable and silver-colored.

The left first molar shows extensive decay, requiring a full crown.

2 The decay is removed and part of the tooth rebuilt before final preparation and impression for the full crown.

3 A cast gold crown is constructed in the lab and fit at the next visit.

4 The final gold crown has been cemented in place and will offer maximum protection as well as function for the tooth. Depending on your lipline, it may not even be visible to others. If it is visible, you may elect to have the crown made of all porcelain, cast glass, or a combination of porcelain bonded to metal (ceramo-metal).

TREATMENT SUMMARY

POSTERIOR PORCELAIN INLAY/ONLAY

Treatment Time Two appointments of approximately one to two hours each per tooth.

Patient Maintenance Avoid biting hard objects in order not to fracture the porcelain. Professional examination and cleaning two to four times per year. Daily flossing and brushing same as natural teeth.

Results of Treatment Porcelain inlays/onlays can successfully achieve both esthetic and functional results in restoring discolored posterior teeth.

Average Range of Treatment Life Expectancy Five to fifteen years. Life expectancy is directly proportional to problems with tissues, fracture and danger of decay. (See footnote on p. 50.)

Cost Approximately $385 to $1850 per tooth, depending on size and difficulty. (See footnote on p. 50.)

ADVANTAGES

1. Highly esthetic
2. No metal shows
3. Strong once bonded to tooth
4. Long lasting

DISADVANTAGES

1. Can chip
2. Greater cost over amalgam or composite resin
3. Can wear opposing tooth if you grind your teeth
4. Takes two appointments

This 43-year-old man was unhappy that his old silver and gold restorations showed when he smiled widely. The old restorations were removed and four porcelain inlays/onlays were constructed for his lower right side. Shown are the new porcelain restorations on his right side compared to the older silver and gold restorations on his left side.

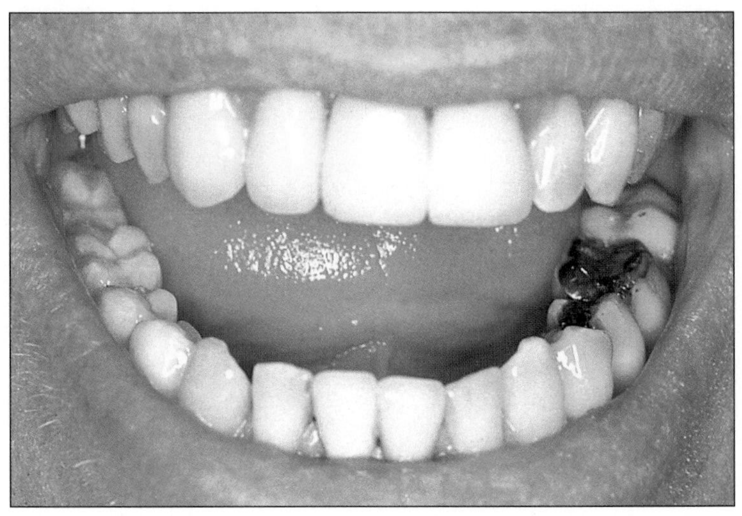

Stains

TREATMENT SUMMARY

POSTERIOR COMPOSITES

Treatment Time One appointment of approximately one hour per filling.

Patient Maintenance To keep resin-bonded restorations looking their best, you should have a professional cleaning three or four times a year. Frequent cleanings remove food stains that accumulate in microscopic spaces on the bonded surfaces of the teeth. These bonded surfaces are not as strong as your enamel, so try to protect them by eating wisely. For instance, avoid most foods that stain. (More tips on patient maintenance can be found on p. 55.) Expect to have some repolishing or repair as necessary.

Results of Treatment Posterior resin bonded composites can restore as well as esthetically match the natural tooth.

Average Range of Treatment Life Expectancy Average life expectancy is three to eight years. May need repair or replacement more frequently. (See footnote on p. 50.)

Cost Approximately $60 to $550 per tooth, depending on size and difficulty of restoration. (See footnote on p. 50.)

ADVANTAGES

1. Tooth colored
2. More economical than crowning or porcelain inlay/onlay
3. Produces an effective immediate seal from restoration and enamel surface that can bond weak or cracked teeth together
4. Permits less tooth structure reduction

DISADVANTAGES

1. Wears faster than silver, gold or porcelain restorations
2. Can fracture
3. Shorter life expectancy compared to gold, silver, or porcelain
4. Less suited for large cavities
5. Can stain

TREATMENT SUMMARY

GOLD INLAY/ONLAY

Treatment Time Usually two appointments, one to two hours per tooth.

Patient Maintenance Normal brushing/flossing every day. Watch diet to avoid large amounts of refined carbohydrates and chewy foods such as caramels and other candies that can eventually eat away at the cement line and possibly cause decay under the gold restoration. Use fluoride mouth rinse and toothpaste.

Results of Treatment Best functional and longest lasting method of restoring teeth, but does tend to show metal of large restoration. However, can be "antiqued" or sanded to dull gold reflectance.

Average Range of Treatment Life Expectancy Five to twenty years. (See footnote on p. 50.)

Cost $435 to $1850. (See footnote on p. 50.)

Treatment Summary

Amalgam

Treatment Time One appointment, approximately one half hour to one hour per tooth.

Patient Maintenance Normal brushing and flossing every day. Limit refined sugars, such as candy, which can attack margins, causing decay around and under fillings. Use fluoride mouth rinse and toothpaste.

Results of Treatment Still the most common of posterior filling replacements. Not as technique-sensitive as other materials. Silver color may be visible depending on where and how large the restoration is.

Average Range of Treatment Life Expectancy Five to twelve years. (See footnote on p. 50.)

Cost $65 to $420. (See footnote on p. 50).

Treatment Summary

Posterior crowns

Treatment Time Two to three appointments, approximately one to two hours per tooth.

Patient Maintenance Normal brushing and flossing. Fluoride mouth rinse and toothpaste as prescribed by your dentist. Same dietary restrictions as above for longest restorative life.

Results of Treatment Crowning can achieve the ultimate in shade control, tooth shape and size.

Average Range of Treatment Life Expectancy Five to fifteen years. (See footnote on p. 50.)

Cost Approximately $460 to $2500 per tooth. (See footnote on p. 50).

The Four Most Popular Posterior Restorative Materials

	Advantages	Disadvantages
Gold inlays/onlays	Longest lasting Wears more like tooth structure Will not fracture Well suited for large cavities	Metal can show Takes two appointments More costly than amalgam or composite resin Noninsulative (conducts heat and cold)
Silver amalgam	One appointment Least costly Predictability Long life	Metal can show Tooth may discolor Can corrode Contains mercury Not sealed to tooth Noninsulative Less suited for large cavities (ie, covering a cusp)
Posterior Composites	Esthetic (tooth colored) Insulative One appointment Well-sealed to tooth (bonds to tooth structure) More economical than crowning or porcelain inlays	More costly than amalgam Wear faster Can stain Can chip or fracture Shorter life expectancy compared to silver, gold or porcelain Less suited for large cavities
Porcelain inlays/onlays	Esthetic (tooth-colored) Stronger than posterior composite resins Well-sealed to tooth Will not stain Insulative Well suited for large cavities	More costly than amalgam or composite Can fracture Porcelain takes two appointments (except CAD-CAM, which can be done in one appointment) Possible wear of opposing natural tooth

Combined Treatment Therapy for Posterior Teeth

Treatment	Treatment time	Patient maintenance
Gold inlay/onlay crowns	Usually two appointments, one to two hours each per tooth.	Normal brushing/flossing every day. Watch diet to avoid large amounts of refined carbohydrates and chewy foods such as caramels and other candies that can eventually "eat away" at the cement line and possibly cause decay under the gold restoration. Use fluoride mouth rinse and toothpaste.
Amalgam	One appointment approximately one half to one hour per tooth.	Normal brushing and flossing every day. Limit refined sugars such as candy, which can attack margins causing decay around or under fillings. Use fluoride mouth rinse and toothpaste.
Posterior composites	One appointment approximately one hour per tooth.	Normal brushing and flossing. Use fluoride mouth rinse and toothpaste as prescribed by your dentist. Avoid biting on extremely hard foods such as bones and ice.
Porcelain or glass onlay/inlay	Usually two appointments, approximately one to two hours per tooth.	Normal brushing and flossing. Use fluoride mouth rinse and toothpaste as prescribed by your dentist. Same dietary restriction as above for longest restorative life.
Porcelain, cast glass or ceramo-metal crowns	Two to three appointments, approximately one to two hours each per tooth.	Normal brushing and flossing. Use fluoride mouth rinse and toothpaste as prescribed by your dentist. Same dietary restriction as above for longest restorative life.

RESULTS OF TREATMENT	LONGEVITY	COST
Best functional and longest lasting method of restoring tooth, but does tend to show metal of large restoration. However, can be "antiqued" or sanded to dull gold reflectance.	Five to twenty years	$435 to $1850
Still the most common of posterior filling replacements. Not as technique sensitive as other materials. Silver color may be visible depending on where and how large the restoration is.	Five to twelve years	$35 to $125
Esthetic replacement of old amalgam (silver) fillings or new decay areas, which can be kept quite small. Tooth-colored filling materials, usually not perfect color blend, but much improved over metal surfaces. More conservative than full crown.	Five to eight years	$65 to $350
Can be highly esthetic replacement for discolored or metal posterior filling materials, although may not be a perfect color match. More conservative than full crown.	Five to fifteen years	$450 to $1850
Crowning can achieve the ultimate in shade control, tooth shape and size.	Five to fifteen years	Approximately $450 to $2500 per tooth

Extending the Life of Your Restorations

Nothing lasts forever, including dental restorations. Not only are dental materials subject to chipping and fracturing, they are also subject to everyday wear and tear. Some people grind their teeth; others brush too vigorously. Even normal chewing eventually causes breakdown. The materials used to bond the restorations to the teeth can also deteriorate when exposed to oral fluids over long periods of time.

If you have dental restorations, avoid foods that may cause damage to the bond of the restoration to the tooth, such as mints, chewing gum, candies, and other sticky refined carbohydrates. Also make sure you don't clench or grind your teeth. Nothing causes more harm to new fillings or crowns. Although we tend to do this in our sleep, it also can occur subconsciously during the day when we are concentrating or tense. (See p. 178.)

Buyer Beware!

No commercial product can compare to professional dental treatment for correcting stained or discolored teeth. In fact, some products can even harm the teeth with excessive amounts of cleaning abrasive. The ingredients may remove the surface stains on your teeth—but they may remove some enamel too!

Don't be misled by slick magazine ads and television infomercials either. Lots of products promise whiter teeth. But do they really have the chemical bleaching capabilities to do more than remove simple food stains?

The best rule of thumb: Never use a product for the treatment of stained teeth unless your dentist recommends it. The American Dental Association's seal of acceptance is also a good sign that a product will perform as advertised.

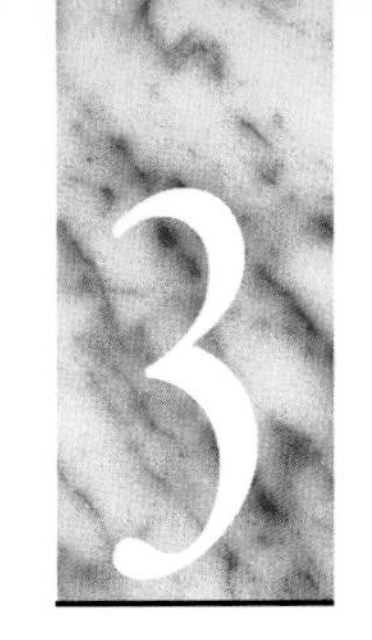

Repairing Fractured Teeth

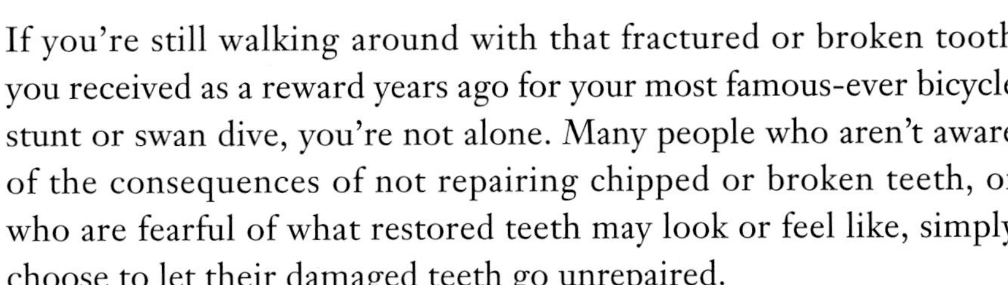

If you're still walking around with that fractured or broken tooth you received as a reward years ago for your most famous-ever bicycle stunt or swan dive, you're not alone. Many people who aren't aware of the consequences of not repairing chipped or broken teeth, or who are fearful of what restored teeth may look or feel like, simply choose to let their damaged teeth go unrepaired.

The purpose of this chapter is to set the record straight. A damaged tooth can be saved and repaired to look and feel like the real thing—perhaps even better! There are several treatment options available. The more informed you are, the more likely you are to be pleased with the results.

When Teeth Break

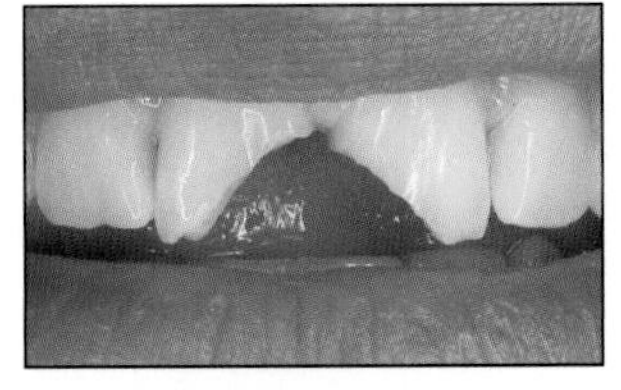

Some people assume that dentists won't be needed once science eliminates tooth decay and gum disease. Not so! Accidents account for a large share of every general dentist's practice. Countless tooth fractures result from traffic accidents, bicycle falls, sports mishaps, blows to the face and chewing hard objects such as ice. And while a fractured tooth may look cute in the mouth of a tousled-haired youngster, it can evolve into a source of embarrassment for the appearance-conscious adolescent or adult.

When a tooth gets chipped or fractured, the first consideration must be whether the pulp—the vital, living portion of the tooth—has been damaged. If a fracture is sensitive, painful or uncomfortable, it may be because the pulp is exposed. Ultimately, the condition of the pulp and the amount of remaining tooth structure will determine the choice of treatment.

MINOR FRACTURES ARE USUALLY SIMPLE TO REPAIR

MINOR FRACTURES, such as small chips off the biting edges of the teeth, are usually simple to repair. If the chipped tooth is of sufficient length so that shaping it with a sandpaper disc won't harm the smile line, it may be cosmetically contoured. Often, the neighboring teeth are also contoured so that no one tooth stands out from the rest. Or, an acid-etch bonding technique may be used to "fill out" the defect. Avoid crowning in cases of minor fracture whenever possible. Remember that it is always best—at least initially—to try simple therapies that preserve the color, shape and health of the tooth.

SERIOUS FRACTURES, which are often caused by accidents, usually are best treated with the least amount of additional stress possible. Your dentist may choose to bond some teeth and crown others, especially when he needs time to determine whether the nerves in the teeth can be saved. If you experience a serious fracture, see your dentist immediately, even if you aren't experiencing any pain. Often, the only sign of pulpal damage is tooth discoloration. In such cases, the first step is to replace the damaged nerve structure with a root canal filling. Then, because much of the natural tooth structure is gone, full crowns typically are placed.

In cases of VERTICAL ROOT FRACTURE, there may be no practical way to save the tooth, making extraction the only answer. However, *all possibilities should be considered before any tooth is extracted.* The function of dentistry is to maintain the integrity of the dental arch and to preserve the natural tooth as much as possible.

PORCELAIN CROWNS AND BRIDGES can also fracture. Keep an eye on your metal-bonded crowns to see if dark outlines appear at the gumline. If a dark outline gradually appears, you may have a fracture of the crown or shrinkage of the gum tissue. If a fracture has occurred, the loss of porcelain at the gumline may weaken the remaining restoration, making it susceptible to additional damage. Eventually, the entire crown may have to be replaced. When detected early, however, some of these minor fractures can be repaired simply by smoothing the chipped porcelain or bonding composite resin to the area.

COSMETIC CONTOURING: IDEAL FOR MINOR DAMAGE

Cosmetic contouring is an ideal treatment for small fractures and chips because anesthesia is not required and the amount of tooth reduction involved is minimal—just enough to "smooth out" the rough edges. Once treatment is complete, no replacements or touch-ups are necessary. The cost and time involved are minimal, as well.

In some situations, however, cosmetic contouring may not be the best treatment alternative. For example, contouring can damage the smileline if a chipped tooth is shortened and its neighbors are brought down to match. Because the natural aging process flattens the smile line, the result may be an older look.

In such cases, bonding is a preferable alternative. Why add years to your smile unnecessarily?

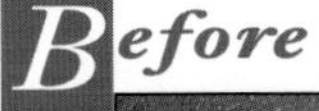

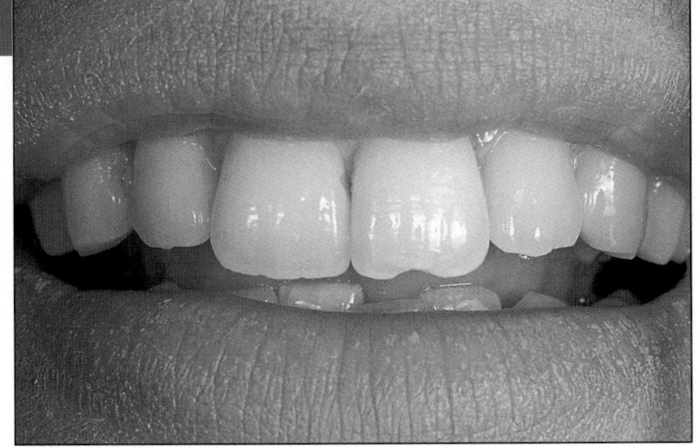

CHIPPED FRONT TOOTH

This 23-year-old woman chipped her front tooth on a metal object. She did not like the thought of losing more enamel or the potential for the constant maintenance that can be required with a bonded restoration.

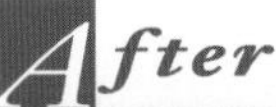

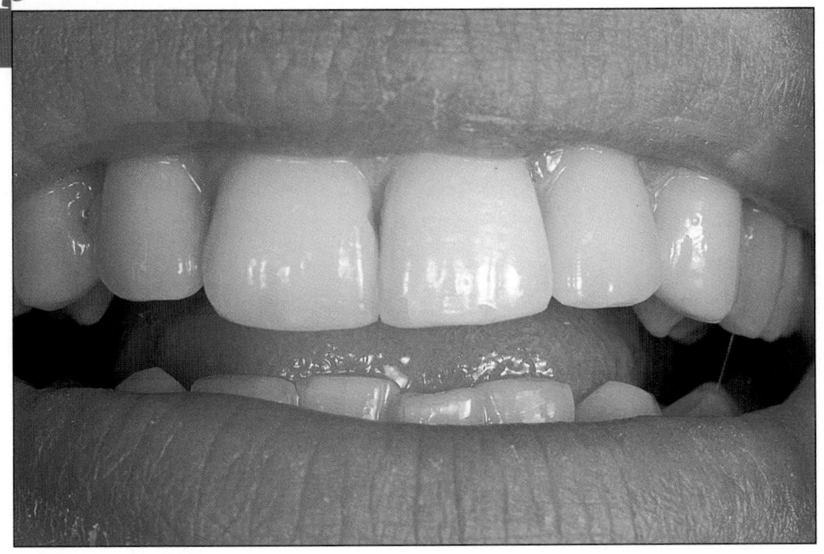

COSMETIC CONTOURING

Since the two front teeth were more than adequate in length, it was determined that cosmetic contouring, or reshaping, of both central incisors would be the ideal long-range treatment.

TREATMENT SUMMARY

COSMETIC CONTOURING

Treatment Time 15 to 60 minutes.

Patient Maintenance Normal cleaning.

Results of Treatment Teeth can appear straighter immediately after treatment.

Average Range of Treatment Life Expectancy Indefinite. (See footnote on p. 50.)

Cost $100 to $950 per arch. (See footnote on p. 50.)

ADVANTAGES

1. No anesthesia is required
2. Permanent solution
3. No maintenance
4. Most conservative
5. Quickest solution

DISADVANTAGES

1. Too much reduction can alter the appearance of the smileline and may be unattractive
2. Bite may limit how much of the tooth can be removed
3. In rare instances sensitivity may be a problem

BONDING: NEW HOPE FOR BROKEN TEETH

In years past, chipping a tooth meant replacing it with a crown, unless the chip was small enough to be cosmetically contoured. With bonding, however, the process of repairing broken teeth has been revolutionized. Now, a new tooth can be formed simply by applying moldable plastic to its remaining structure. This rebuilds the tooth to its original shape, and often makes it look even better! The procedure also can be performed inexpensively and quickly—typically in no more than an hour per tooth.

Bonding also can be used as a stop-gap measure in cases of complex fracture. By immediately sealing off exposed nerve endings with a sedative dressing and bonding material, your dentist may be able to preserve the nerve system in the tooth. This technique should be used in lieu of crowning whenever possible, particularly on front teeth.

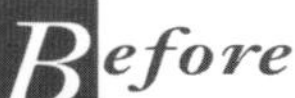

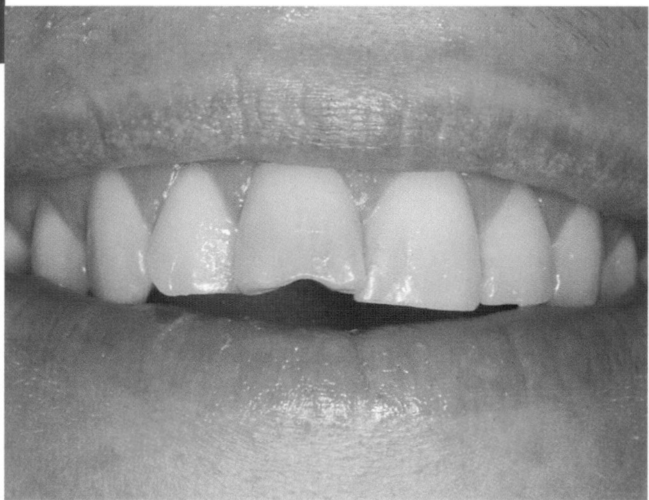

Fractured and protruding front tooth

As a young boy, this television and movie actor was chosen for roles partially based on his appearance. As he grew older, the fractured tooth began to detract from his smile and he decided to have it corrected.

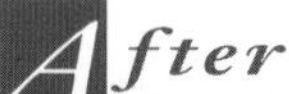

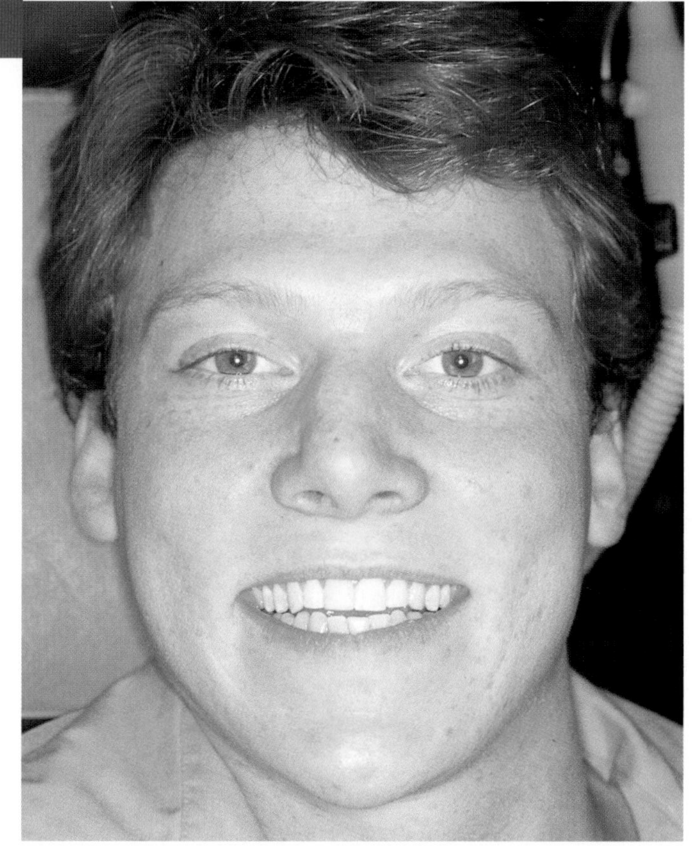

Cosmetic contouring and composite resin bonding

Since the right central incisor was not only fractured, but slightly protruded, the tooth was first reshaped through cosmetic contouring to make it look straighter. Next, the missing part of the tooth was repaired by bonding with composite resin. This one-appointment procedure restored this actor's smile and made it possible for him to compete for a wider range of roles.

Before

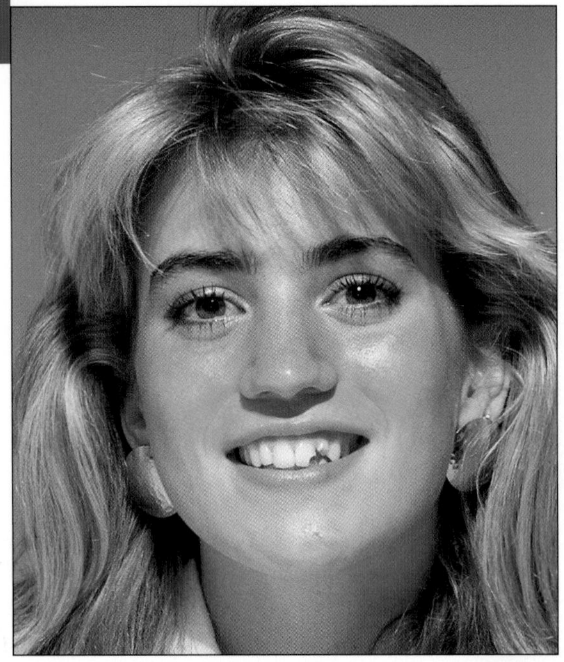

EMERGENCY FRACTURE

This young model fractured her upper left central and lateral incisors.

After

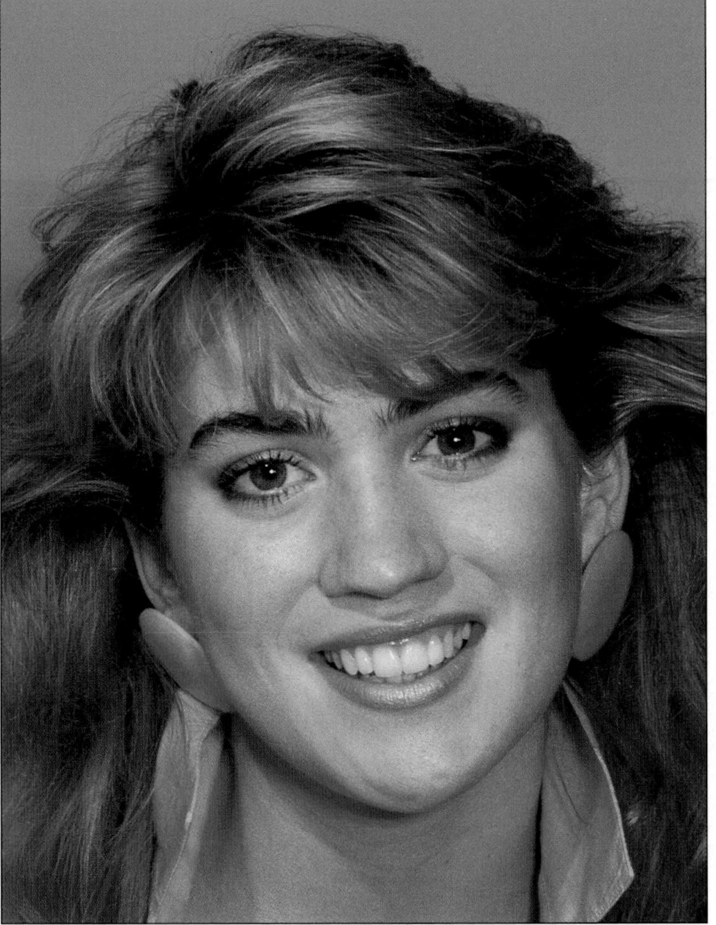

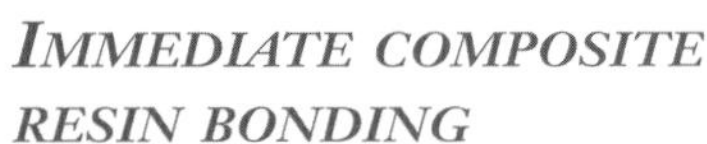

IMMEDIATE COMPOSITE RESIN BONDING

Composite resin bonding was an excellent stop-gap measure to help preserve the nerve in the tooth until it could be determined if root canal treatment would be necessary.

Before

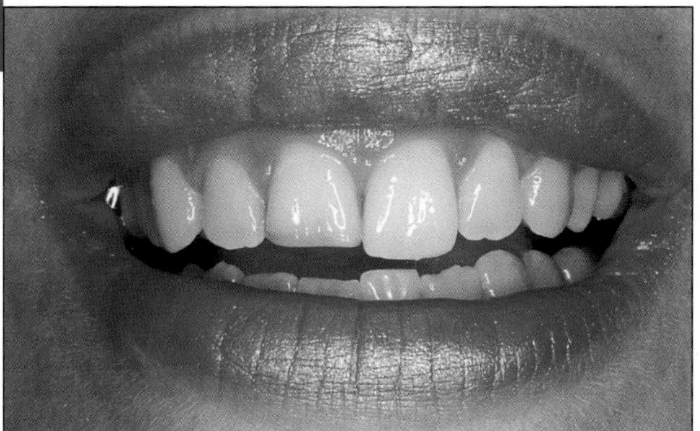

HORIZONTAL FRACTURE

This 18-year-old model suffered a horizontal fracture of her left right central incisor. In such cases, there are two choices: shorten the adjacent tooth through cosmetic contouring, or bond the fractured tooth.

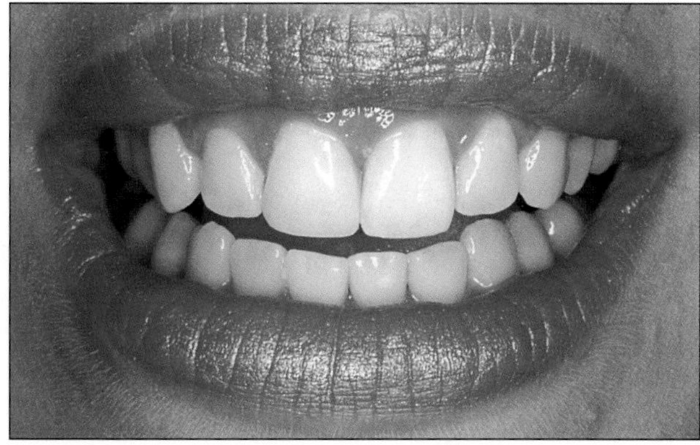

COMPOSITE RESIN BONDING

Shortening the longer tooth would have meant changing the smileline and giving this model a less youthful look, so composite resin bonding was chosen to repair and lengthen the right front tooth.

After

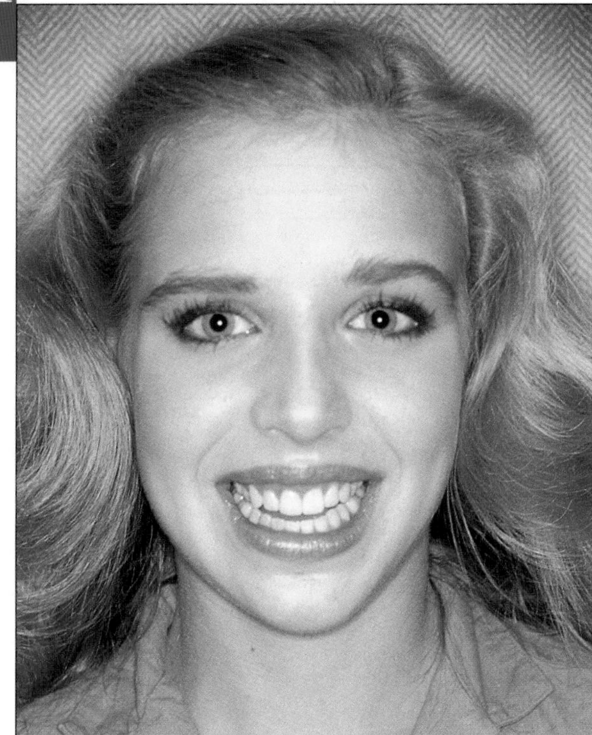

*B*efore

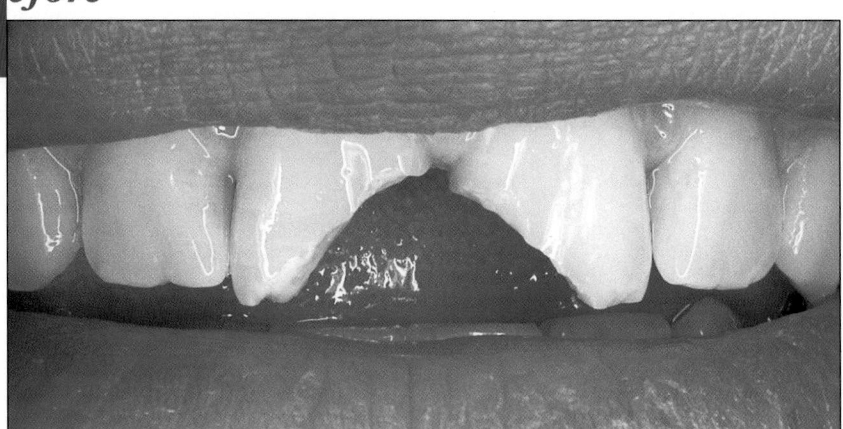

Two fractured incisors

This 17-year-old student and model fractured her two front teeth on the edge of a concrete swimming pool. Although the teeth were sensitive, the nerves remained intact.

*A*fter

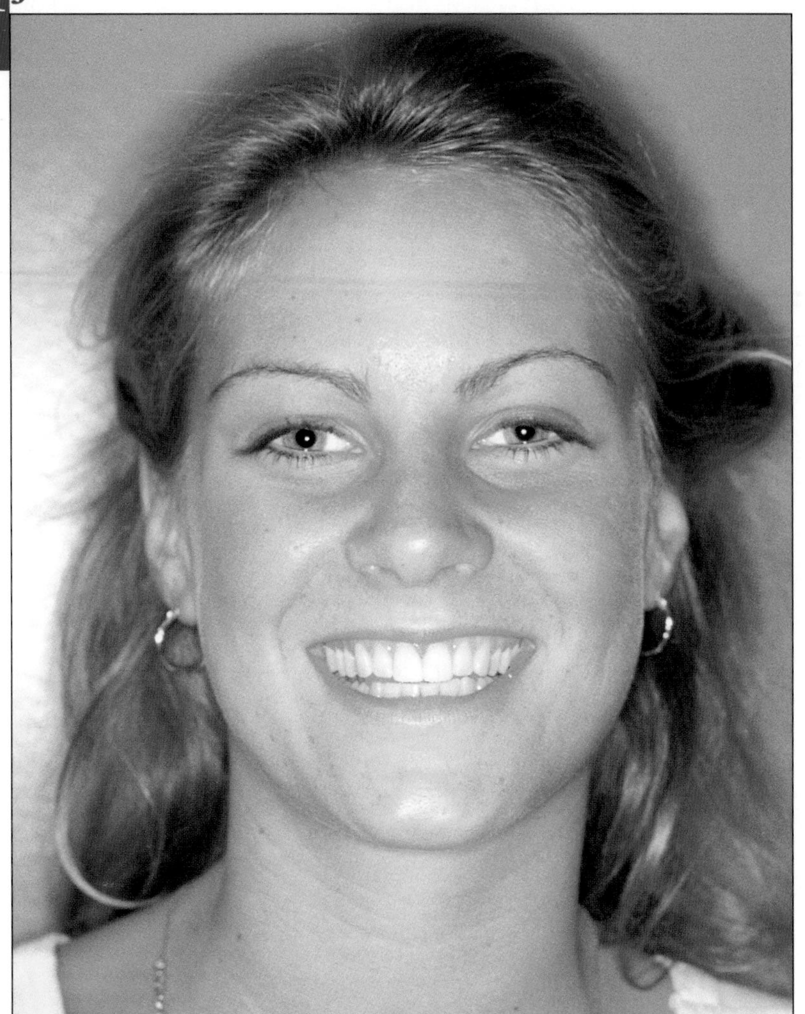

Composite resin bonding

No anesthetic was required to slightly reshape and replace the missing parts of the teeth with composite resin bonding material.

A bonded fractured tooth has a life expectancy of five to eight years, but it may need some maintenance during that time. Since bonding is the least traumatic procedure in repairing a fractured tooth, it is preferred as an emergency procedure before deciding if a tooth will need further nerve (root canal) treatment. Five years later, no additional treatment had been required for these teeth other than to replace the bonding once.

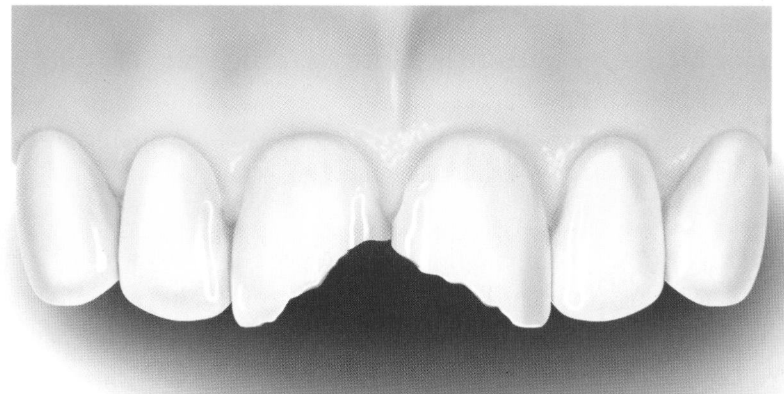

The process of composite resin bonding involves the physical attachment of the resin to the tooth, which requires a mild etching of the outer layer of enamel.

This figure shows the enamel etched in preparation for the attachment of the composite resin.

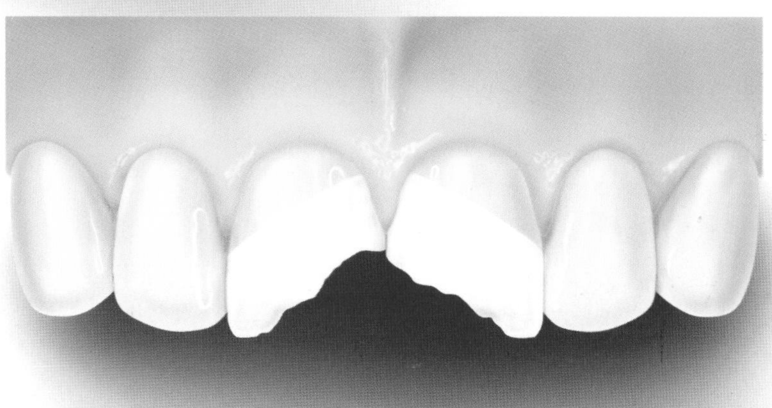

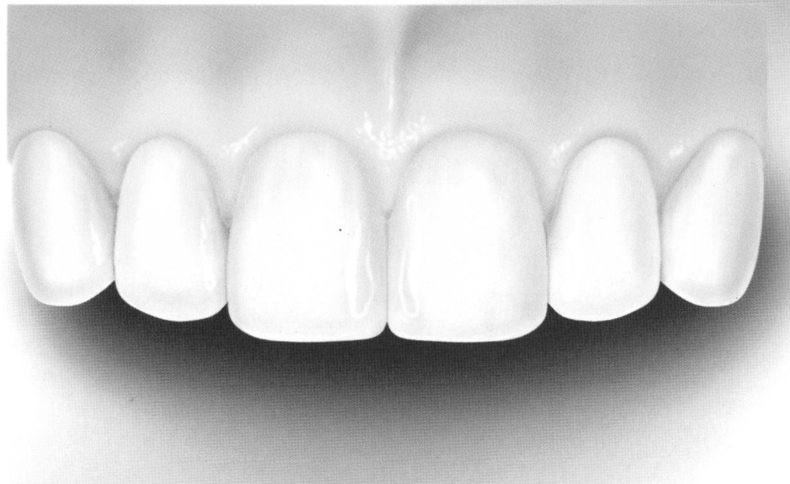

Composite resin bonding, which is painless, can usually be accomplished in one appointment.

There are times, of course, when bonding *isn't* the best solution, even on front teeth, for example, when a fracture is located in a high bite-pressure position. Although a metal post could be placed for added strength prior to bonding, the odds are great that the metal would show through the shallow material. When a tooth is this weak or when it has little enamel left, crowning may be a preferable treatment alternative.

Bonding also can be used to repair fractures in porcelain crowns, although this usually provides only a temporary solution. Gold acrylic veneers that show at the gumline also can be "touched up" with bonding so that cracking is avoided and the look for the tooth is improved. However, most fractured porcelain or acrylic veneer crowns look better if they are remade.

Bonding is by far the most desirable treatment when the tooth can be rebuilt without harming the smile line. Its primary drawback is that it must be repeated every 5 to 8 years because of stain and wear. However, improved bonding materials are constantly being developed and introduced in the dental market. If your tooth structure is still intact, these materials may provide you with stronger, longer-lasting and more stain-resistant restorations in years to come. Once your tooth is reduced for a crown, on the other hand, you no longer have this alternative.

TREATMENT SUMMARY

BONDING

Treatment Time 1 to 2 hours per tooth.

Patient Maintenance Professional cleaning three or four times a year. Eat wisely as these teeth can chip easily. Floss in and pull it through rather than popping it out. Because staining or chipping can occur, expect to have some repolishing or repair as necessary.

Results of Treatment Most fractures and chips can be easily repaired with bonding.

Average Range of Treatment Life Expectancy Five to eight years, with professional finishing once every few years. (See footnote on p. 50.)

Cost $350 to $900 per tooth. (See footnote on p. 50.)

ADVANTAGES

1. No anesthesia required
2. Little tooth reduction required
3. Immediate results
4. Teeth can also be lightened
5. Less expensive than crowning

DISADVANTAGES

1. Can chip or stain
2. Bonding has a limited esthetic life
3. May not work for severe fractures

What About Porcelain Laminates?

Although bonding is a quicker and more cost-effective treatment alternative than porcelain laminates for chipped and broken teeth, if your adjacent teeth have been rebuilt in porcelain, your fractured tooth should be restored in porcelain. Esthetically, the fractured tooth will match the adjacent teeth much more closely because the same material has been used. (See p. 63 for a treatment summary and a listing of porcelain laminates' advantages and disadvantages.)

Before

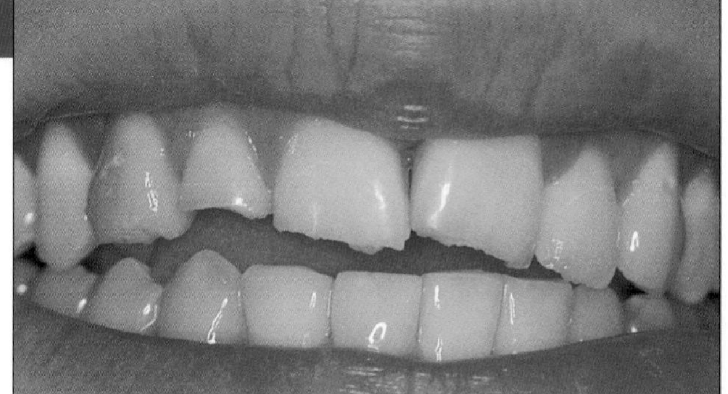

Multiple fractured teeth

This 21-year-old student sustained multiple tooth fractures in an automobile accident.

After

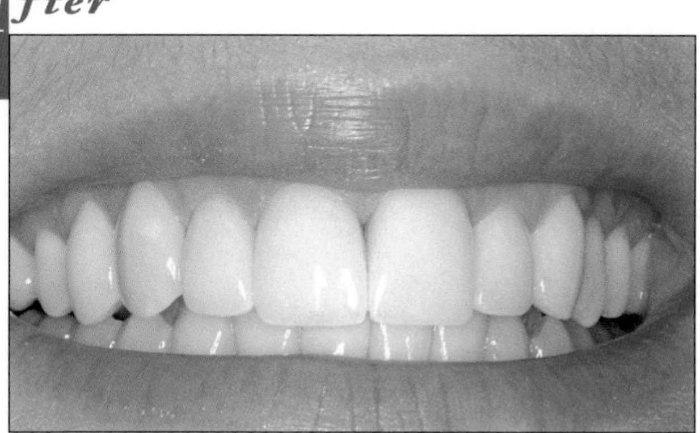

Emergency bonding

Emergency bonding with composite resin was maintained for a year to first determine which, if any, teeth would need root canal therapy. Later, ten porcelain laminate veneers were constructed for this patient.

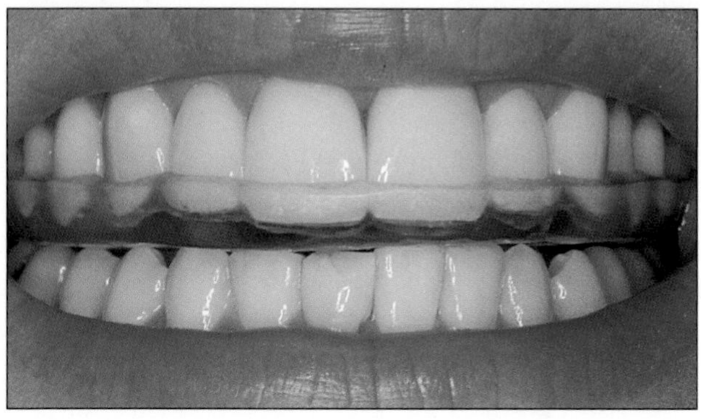

Protective night appliance

A "soft-touch" bite guard is worn at night to help protect the porcelain laminates from the effects of possible clenching or grinding during sleep.

Crowning: Often the Only Answer

If you fracture a front tooth so badly that there is little tooth structure left, crowning is probably the treatment of choice. The procedure should be performed immediately, however, because the pulp is exposed and living nerves are unprotected.

If a back tooth fractures, it also may be best to restore it with a crown. Just remember that, while porcelain-fused-to-metal crowns can look just like natural teeth, the porcelain can chip and fracture. Therefore, if you have porcelain or all-glass crowns, avoid hard foods such as hard apples, and give up bad habits such as chewing ice.

The science of dentistry awaits a porcelain that will not fracture or break its metal bond. In the meantime, however, there will be fractures to repair and crowns to replace. If you fracture a crown that has a metal substructure, it is often more practical and less expensive to build a new crown around the old one—just as you would with a real tooth—instead of repairing it. By making the porcelain-fused-to-metal segment the appropriate size, facings sometimes can be replaced. Just keep in mind that such repairs may not last as long as the original.

Before

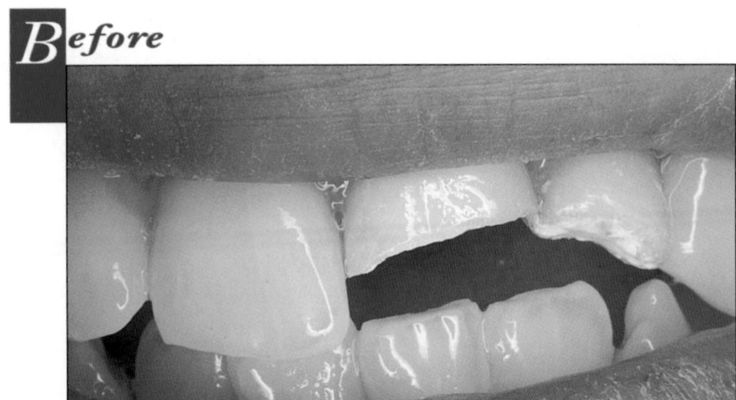

Two fractured incisors

This 19-year-old student fractured her two upper left teeth to such an extent that the nerves in both teeth had to be removed to save the teeth.

After

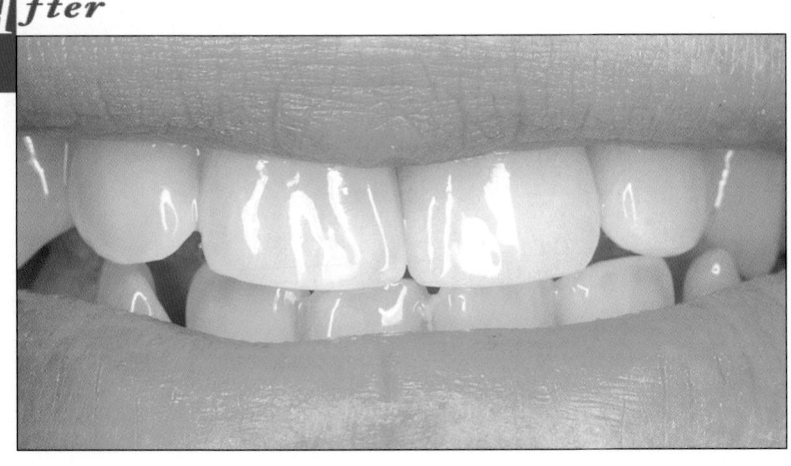

Porcelain crowns

Cast metal posts were constructed to strengthen and help prevent future fracture of these teeth. After insertion of these two gold posts, two full porcelain crowns were made for the two fractured teeth. Note how form, texture and highlights are used to match the corresponding teeth in the arch to create a natural appearance.

Before

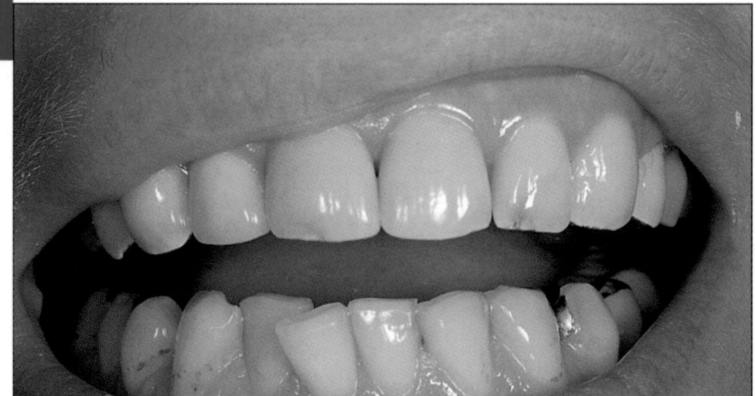

CHIPPED PORCELAIN CROWNS AND CROWDED LOWER TEETH

This 31-year-old leading vocalist was concerned because her crowned teeth were beginning to chip and fracture. She also wanted lighter-colored teeth since her profession required her to be under stage lights much of the time. She was also unhappy with the appearance of her crowded lower teeth.

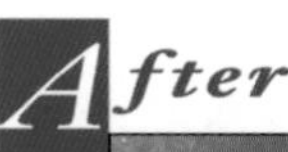

After

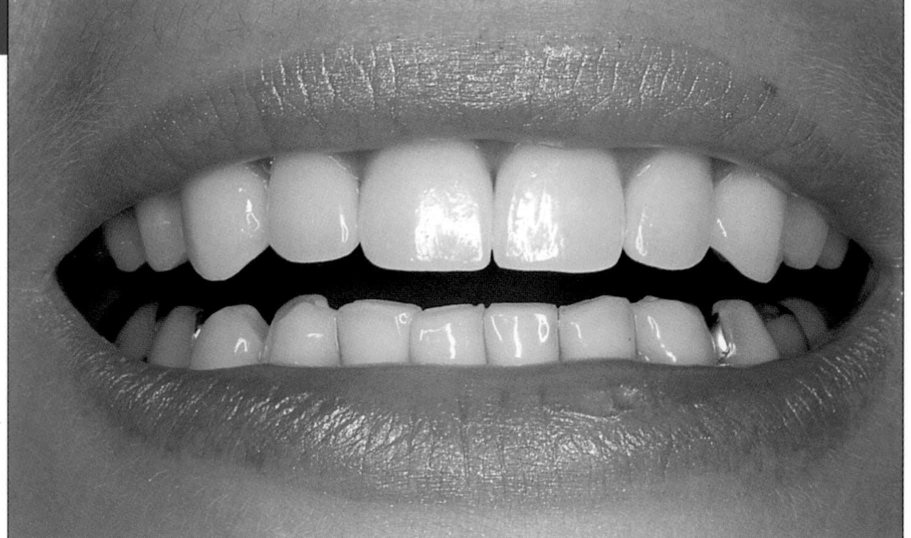

FULL PORCELAIN CROWNS AND REMOVABLE ORTHODONTIC APPLIANCE

The six new crowns were constructed entirely of porcelain rather than a combination of metal and porcelain. They were carefully textured to give maximum reflection of light. Although the metal-reinforced porcelain crown is stronger than an all-porcelain crown, the latter type usually provides greater translucency. The lower front teeth were straightened with a removable appliance.

Spare Set Is the Best Bet

Because crowns invariably seem to break on weekends or during vacations—never when it's convenient to see a dentist—it's a good idea to have a backup.

If you have an accident and it is determined that porcelain crowns are needed, a spare set can be fabricated at the same time for about half the cost. **If budget constraints prohibit you from purchasing an extra set, consider keeping temporaries on hand which any dentist can place as an interim "fix."**

The advantages to keeping a spare set of porcelain crowns are numerous. It often costs less to replace chipped crowns in this way because the expense of fabricating and fitting new temporary restorations is avoided. And although the color of the two sets will never be exactly the same, they will blend so that no one will notice that the spare is different from the original. It also can be a comfort to know you won't be caught running around with only a "stump" of a tooth if your crown should break unexpectedly. This is particularly true if you travel frequently. At the very least, ask your dentist either to save the mold from which your crown was made or give it to you to keep. Many times this mold can be reused. And although this alternative is more costly than having a spare crown fabricated, time and money may be saved because an impression for a new mold may not have to be made.

TREATMENT SUMMARY

SPARE CROWNS

ADVANTAGES

1. Less expensive than starting over
2. You get instant replacement in case of fracture
3. You can save the cost of a temporary or an extra office visit
4. You could beat inflation; your crowns could cost more later

DISADVANTAGES

1. Your initial cost is more
2. You may never need the extra set
3. Your tooth underneath may change drastically with time and then the spare crowns would not fit properly
4. If your gum line changes around the neck of the tooth over the years, the spare crowns may be useless

Treatment Summary

Crowning

Treatment Time Usually two appointments of approximately one to four hours on up to four teeth. Expect to spend more time as additional teeth or more extensive treatment is involved.

Patient Maintenance Crowns are esthetically designed to look and feel like "real teeth." As with your original smile, however, care must be taken to avoid tooth fractures. Yearly fluoride treatments may be advised. Flossing every day is as essential with crowns as with natural teeth.

Results of Treatment Badly fractured teeth may be repaired and reshaped as desired.

Average Range of Treatment Life Expectancy Five to fifteen years. Life expectancy is directly proportional to problems with tissues, fracture and danger of decay. (See footnote on p. 50.)

Cost Approximately $550 to $3000 per tooth. (See footnote on p. 50.)

Advantages

1. The dentist can repair the chipped or fractured tooth
2. Teeth can be lightened to any shade
3. Some realignment or straightening of the teeth is possible

Disadvantages

1. Crowns can fracture
2. Procedure requires anesthesia
3. Original tooth form is altered
4. It is not permanent
5. It is more costly than bonding

Tips for handling a broken crown

If your crown breaks, see your dentist as soon as possible, particularly if your tooth is sensitive. The inside portion of the tooth may be exposed or the tooth may be damaged, necessitating immediate treatment.

If you have a spare crown or temporary, use it to replace the broken one. Just don't neglect to get another spare to replace the one you're now wearing! If you don't have a spare crown or temporary, save the fractured piece of porcelain. Although your dentist doesn't always have a lab technician available, he or she generally has cement on hand! Hopefully, the fractured piece of porcelain can be bonded into place until a new crown is made.

Support of Restored Fractures: Pins vs Posts

Fractures often leave teeth weak and in need of underpinnings for support. In such cases, pins and posts can be placed in the tooth to provide added strength and create a core around which to build a restoration.

Pins are sometimes used in back teeth to add retention for filling materials. They typically are *not* used with composite resins, however. Pins may be cemented, tapped or screwed into place to add support when nerve removal is unnecessary. They generally cost between $45 and $125 per pin.

Posts are often placed inside a tooth when the nerve has been removed. Using them depends on how much chewing force will be exerted on the bite and how much tooth structure is left.

An additional fee is charged for placement of a post, typically $160 to $550 per tooth.

Before

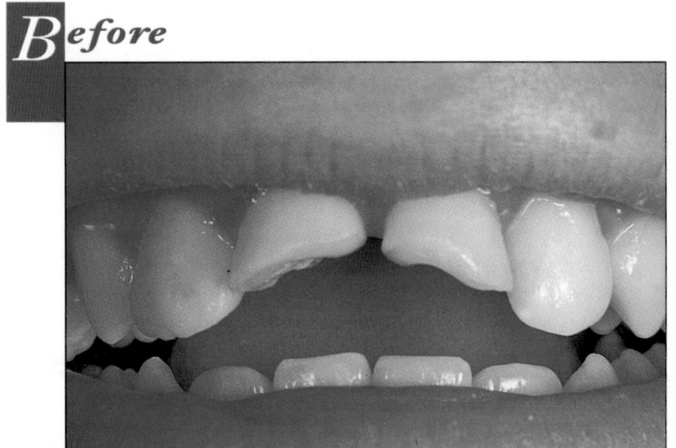

Fractured Teeth in a Young Child

This 12-year-old girl fractured her two front teeth in an accident and was referred to an oral surgeon to have the teeth removed. Fortunately for her, the oral surgeon felt the teeth could and should be saved. He then referred the patient to a specialist, who removed the nerves from the teeth and performed periodontal (gum and bone) surgery.

After

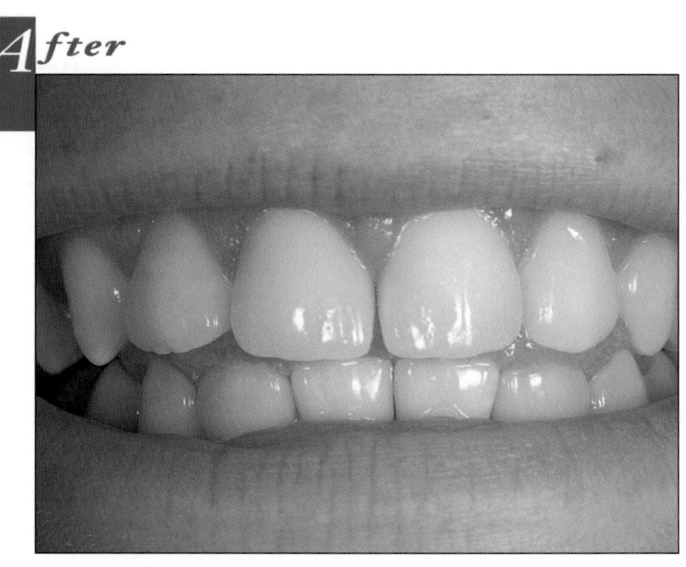

Gum Surgery, Root Canal Treatment and Full Crowns

Following surgery, two metal posts were constructed to reinforce the teeth. Finally the front teeth were crowned with porcelain to produce the beautiful new smile shown. Never assume that severely fractured teeth have to be extracted—it may be possible to save them. The function of dentistry is to maintain the integrity of the dental arch and to preserve the living structure. For this patient, this goal was achieved. One reason for saving the individual tooth is that it is much easier to clean an individual tooth than to clean underneath a bridge.

WHO SHOULD HANDLE REPAIRS?

If you fracture a bridge or temporary restoration, save the pieces. Although it's a long-shot, your dentist may be able to repair it.

Do not attempt to repair restorations yourself unless you have had dental training. Some of the glues on the market can dissolve in your mouth. Moreover, if you use a cyanoacrylate-based glue, your dentist may not be able to separate the glue from the tooth in order to reposition it more precisely.

Because most fractures seem to happen at the most inopportune times and places, you may not be able to see a dentist immediately. In such cases, continue to brush your teeth as usual, avoiding any sensitive areas. Otherwise, bacteria can build up and aggravate your problem. Then, see a dentist as soon as possible. Postponing treatment can result in additional damage.

Before

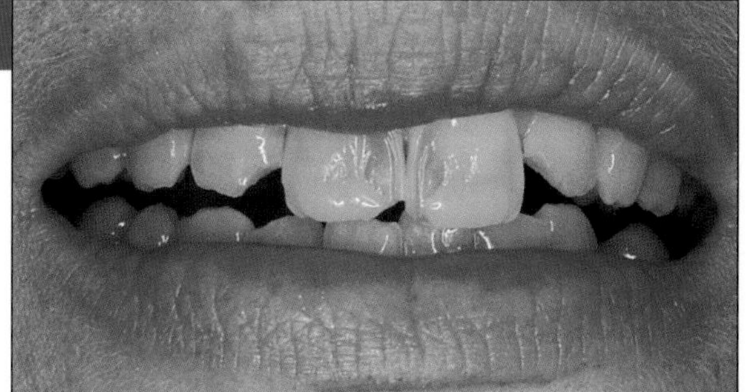

FRACTURES OF MULTIPLE TEETH

This 36-year-old woman had a serious bicycle accident in which 22 teeth were injured.

After

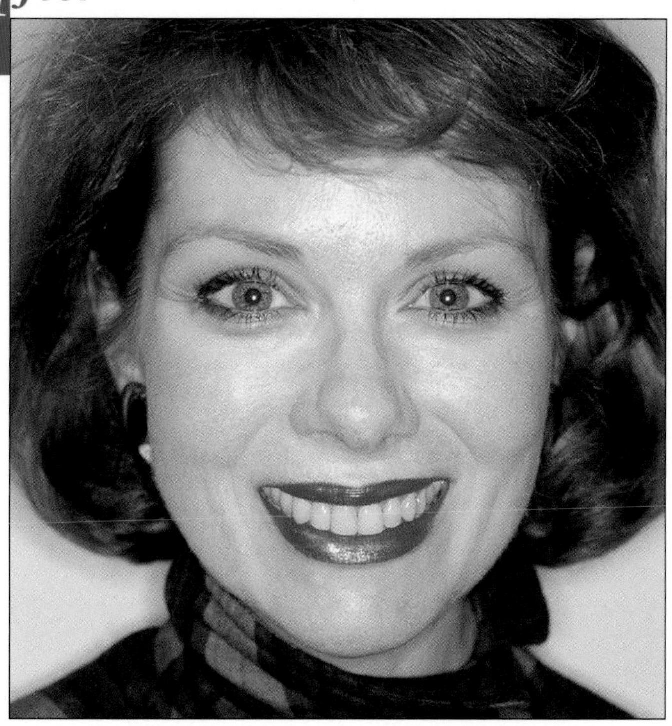

COMPOSITE RESIN BONDING AND FULL CROWNS

Although 13 of the back teeth had to be crowned, the six front upper teeth were bonded with composite resin. Note the improvement in color of the newly bonded teeth. Composite resin bonding is particularly helpful to reinforce the fractured tooth if sufficient enamel is present for the resin to bond to. If necessary, root canal treatment can easily be done through the bonded surfaces later.

If a Tooth is Knocked Out

Don't assume that a knocked-out tooth can't be reimplanted. The handy reference below, provided by the American Association of Endodontists, outlines the steps to be taken when a tooth is lost. Parents, teachers and sports officials, in particular, should keep this information handy.

1. Remain calm while you try to locate the tooth.
2. Pick up the tooth gently, being careful to handle it by its crown and not by its roots.
3. Gently remove any debris from the tooth. Do not scrub or use any cleaning agents on the tooth.
4. Look for fractures in the roots. If there are no fractures, carefully replace the tooth in its socket or keep it moist in a glass of water or milk. If no water or milk is available, place the tooth in the mouth next to the cheek.
5. See a dentist immediately, preferably within 30 minutes.

An Ounce of Prevention . . .

There's no way to anticipate most of the events that cause tooth fractures. Sports, however, are the exception. If you or someone you care about is involved in any type of contact sport, ask your dentist about a bite guard. When designed and worn properly, bite guards substantially reduce the risk of tooth fractures.

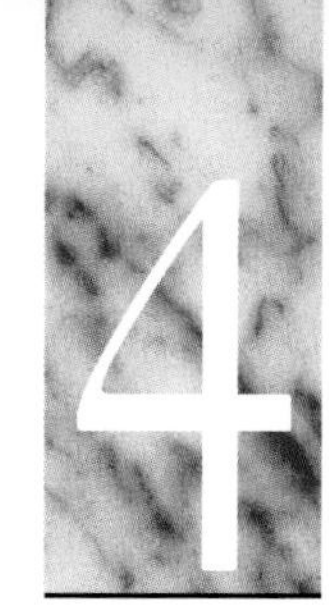

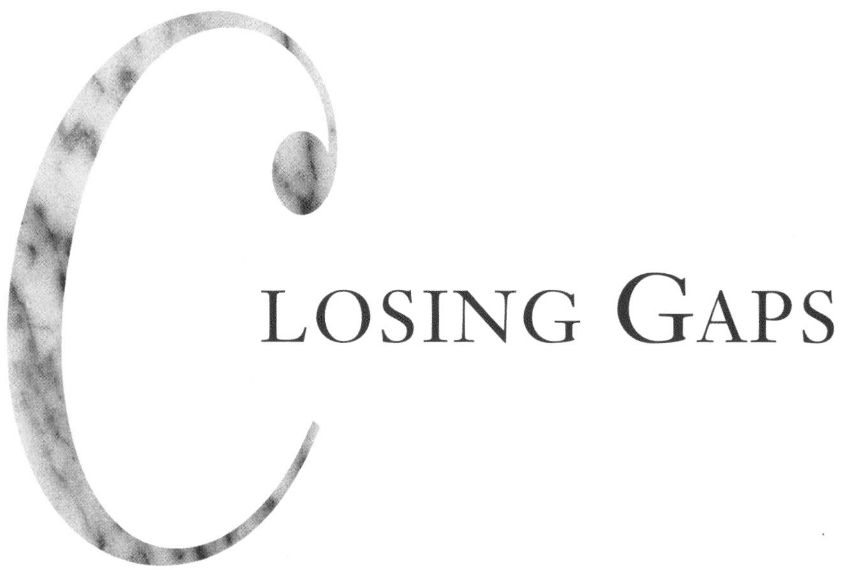

Closing Gaps

The first time I realized how a space between the front teeth can affect the face was when I closed one on a man in his 40s. Although the corrective procedure—crowning the upper front teeth—was routine, the affect on this man's life was extraordinary.

A week after I crowned his teeth, the patient was back in the office for a checkup. When I asked him what kind of comments he had received, he said, "You wouldn't believe it. Some of my friends thought I had a new hairstyle. Others actually thought I'd had a facelift! They don't realize that the only thing different is that the space between my front teeth is gone."

Since that time I've seen the same phenomenon over and over again. Why? Because for the first time, people are actually looking at the patient's face instead of being distracted by that space between his or her teeth. If you have a space between your teeth that you don't like, but you haven't had it closed because you were told it would take years of orthodontic treatment, this chapter is for you.

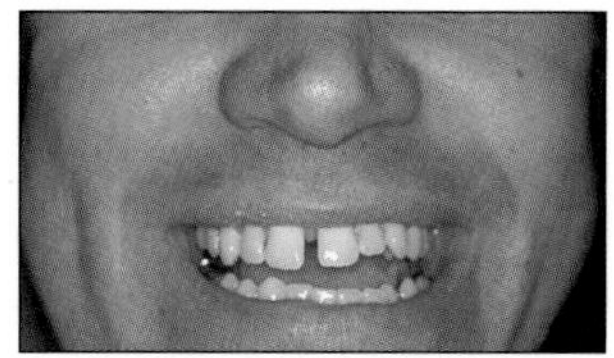

Spaces between teeth can be corrected with bonding, porcelain laminates, crowns, bridges and implants. Treatment will not only improve your self-image, but it will allow people to look at your face without being distracted by the irregularity in your smile. But don't be surprised if people don't recognize exactly what's different about you. Just get ready for comments like, "You look terrific!"

What Causes Gaps?

Spaces between the teeth are most often caused by heredity. However, they also may be caused by personal habits such as tongue thrusting, or by abnormal tongue or swallowing movements. Constant probing with the tongue, for example, can push teeth apart.

The loss of supporting bone under the gum tissue can also cause teeth to separate. Sometimes teeth are extracted due to infection or decay, and an unattractive space results. Loss of the back teeth often transfers chewing activity forward, forcing the teeth to spread.

The cause of the space has a lot to do with how it is treated. For a patient with gum disease, for example, the underlying problem must be controlled before the space is corrected.

Closing Gaps with the Help of the Three Rs

There are several ways to close unsightly gaps, depending on the cause of the space, its size, its location and the condition of adjacent teeth. Both cost and your personal needs will play a significant role in your choice of treatment.

Correcting space problems, however, usually involves one of the three Rs: **Repositioning** the teeth with orthodontics; **restoring** the teeth through bonding, laminating or crowning; or **removal** of the teeth, followed by replacement with a bridge or implant. Removal is the least desirable alternative and is used only as a last resort.

WHEN TEETH ARE ATTRACTIVE AND HEALTHY, REPOSITIONING IS THE IDEAL TREATMENT

When teeth are attractive and healthy, repositioning is the ideal treatment, as it involves no loss of enamel. Some alternatives, like full crowns, require sacrificing healthy tooth structure for cosmetic correction.

However, patients frequently prefer immediate results. In such cases, bonding or laminating may be the answer. In other cases, a combination of therapies offers the best results.

After you read this chapter, you will be in a much better position to talk with your dentist about which option is best for you. Just keep in mind that the goal of treatment is always to fill the spaces with as little natural tooth loss as possible.

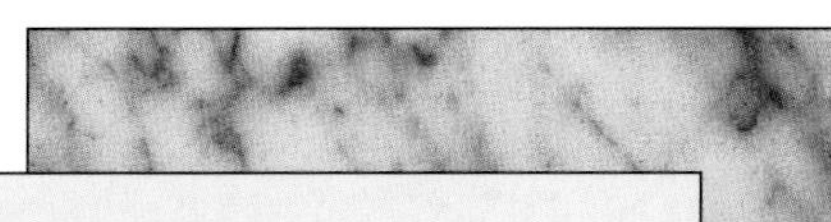

Solutions for Spacing Problems

- Orthodontics to reposition teeth
- Bonding or laminating to restore teeth
- Crowning or "capping" to restore teeth
- Removable acrylic overlay
- Bridges to replace missing teeth
- Implants to replace missing teeth

Orthodontics: Not Just for Kids

Braces aren't just for children anymore. In fact, adults now comprise approximately 30 percent of patients who seek the help of an orthodontist to straighten teeth, close gaps or just improve their smiles. In some cases, treatment consists of nothing more than removable appliances or retainers. In others, clear plastic brackets, instead of traditional metal ones, can be used.

Orthodontic treatment has the advantage of leaving the natural teeth intact

One of the most exciting developments in moving teeth is lingual braces, appliances that are mounted *behind* the teeth and which are virtually imperceptible to others. There are limited situations where lingual braces can be used, however, and treatment can also cost more and take longer than with other devices. Nevertheless many adults who otherwise would not have undergone orthodontic treatment have changed their smiles with these "hidden" appliances. *In the long run, orthodontics is the best solution for most people. Even if full crowns eventually will be needed, teeth should be aligned properly first.*

And although orthodontic treatment requires regular checkups and requires the most time of the alternatives—usually taking six months to two years to complete—it has the advantage of leaving the natural teeth intact and being closest to a permanent solution. Bonding, laminating or crowning, on the other hand, will usually require repair or periodic replacement.

You may also consider a compromise solution for your space problem . . . sometimes you can have the teeth moved to a more favorable position in just a few months, and then bond or laminate the teeth in this improved position. The advantage to this is being able to better proportion the teeth.

Of course, no treatment is problem-free, and orthodontics is no exception.

Before

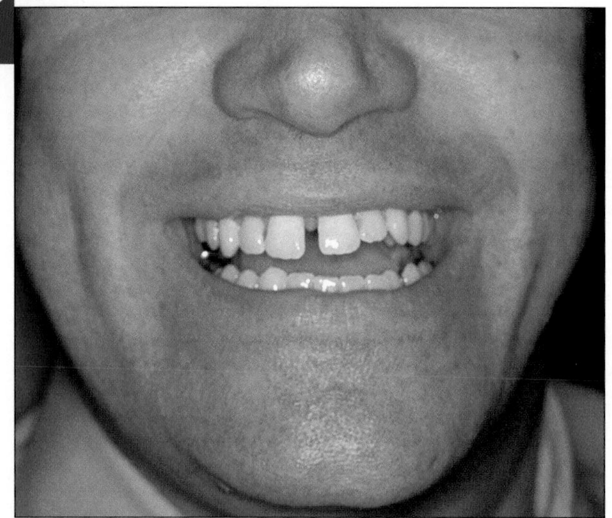

Diastema (Space) and Midline Deviation

This network television correspondent had a large gap between his front teeth. The teeth were off center and caused a midline deviation. Because television tends to magnify the size of a space, it was desirable to have the space closed. The space also called more attention to the midline deviation and facial asymmetry.

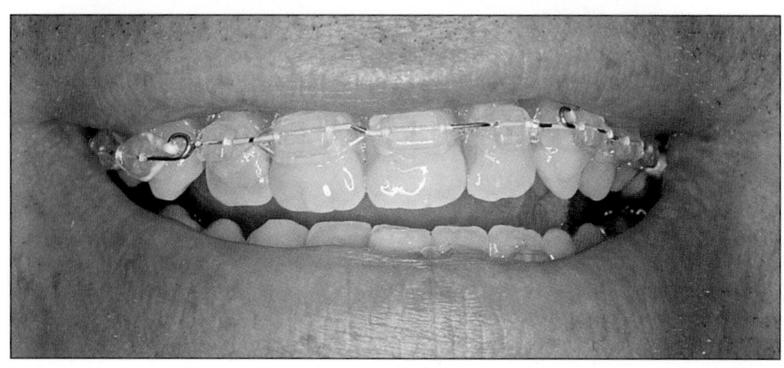

Tooth-colored wire and plastic brackets were used because of the esthetic demands of this patient's vocation. During the time he was undergoing orthodontic treatment, viewers did not even realize it due to the almost invisible appearance of these appliances from a distance.

After

Orthodontics and Bonding

About eighteen months were required to produce this more flattering smile. Notice how no attention is called to the now seemingly minor midline deviation when the teeth are together. The final procedure was to bond the front teeth together with composite resin to keep the space from recurring. Orthodontic movement improved his smile as well as his bite.

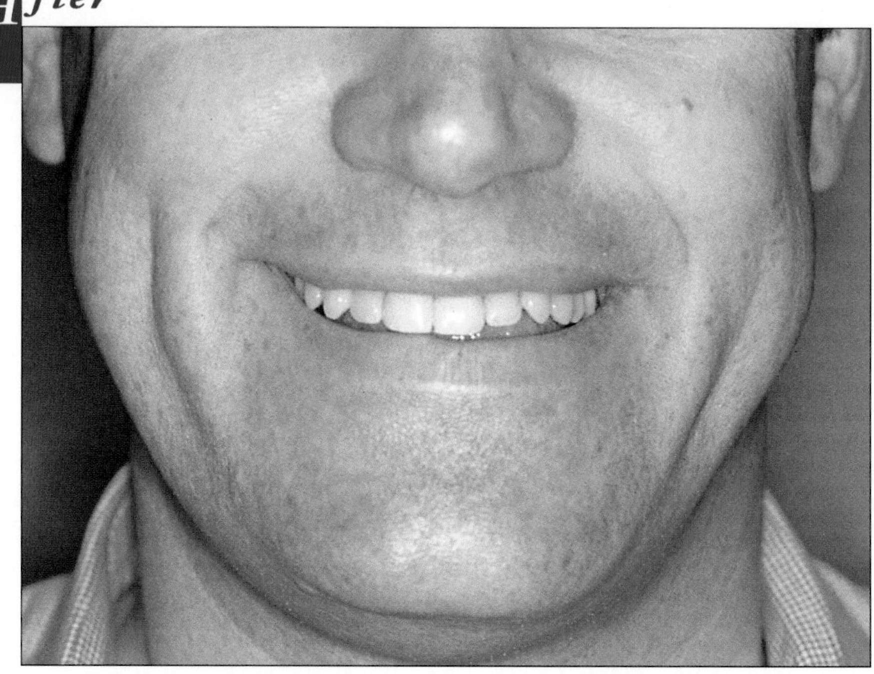

In some cases, the teeth shift back to their original positions unless retainers are worn. And occasionally, loose bands create decalcified areas where decay can begin. However, new techniques involving the bonding of brackets to the teeth minimize this problem.

If you have a discrepancy between the midline of your face and the midline of your teeth, it will be even more apparent if there is also a gap in the front of your mouth. If possible, close the space through orthodontics, and the midline deviation will not be nearly as evident.

Before

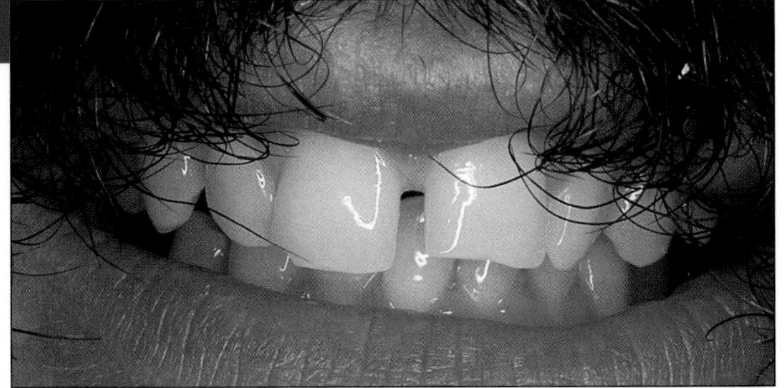

Space with Deep Overbite

Orthodontics is generally the best way to close a space in the front of the mouth. This 26-year-old clothing executive had not only spaced but crowded front teeth complicated by a deep overbite. He strongly resisted orthodontic treatment for esthetic reasons.

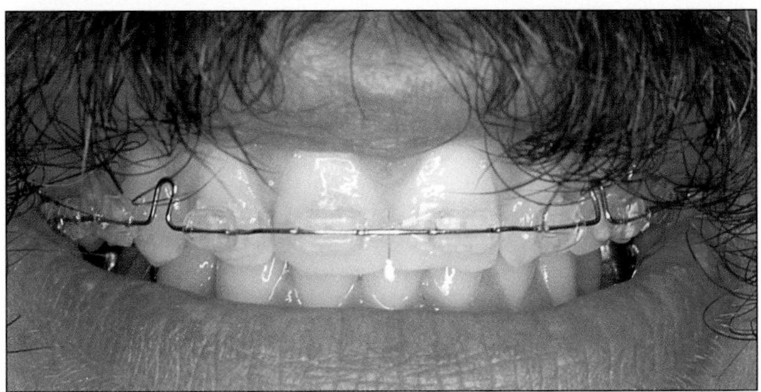

This patient felt that tooth-colored brackets were much less noticeable than the metal brackets, and so did not mind wearing them. The small amount of wire showing was not objectionable, and it only took fourteen months to help reposition this patient's teeth.

After

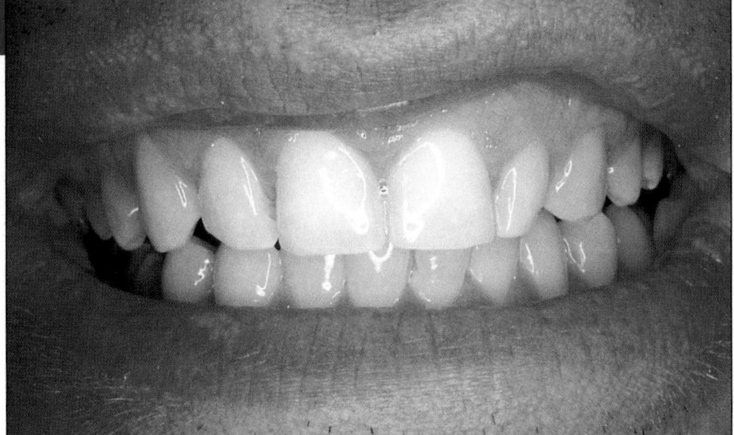

Orthodontic Treatment

This final result shows a much improved smile that involved a small amount of cosmetic contouring on the upper and lower front teeth following orthodontic treatment. While the patient must wear a retainer during sleep, the result will be permanent. Adults make up approximately one quarter of orthodontic patients today.

TREATMENT SUMMARY

ORTHODONTICS

Treatment Time Six to twenty-four months for most patients.

Patient Maintenance Special care by the patient by cleaning daily and checkups on a scheduled basis. Retainers frequently have to be worn at night for many years, at least a few nights a week, possibly indefinitely, to maintain tooth alignment. A water-powered cleaning device is also helpful if used daily.

Results of Treatment Spaces between teeth are closed.

Average Range of Treatment Life Expectancy Generally permanent. (See footnote on p. 50.)

Cost $1550 to $7500, depending on number of teeth involved and what appliance therapy is chosen. (See footnote on p. 50.)

ADVANTAGES

1. Closes space between teeth
2. Permanent solution for most individuals
3. No tooth reduction required
4. May be the least expensive treatment (compared to crowning or bonding replacement)

DISADVANTAGES

1. Time-consuming (six to twenty-four months)
2. Teeth may return to original position if retainers are not worn
3. It is more difficult to clean teeth during treatment

THE BEAUTY OF BONDING

Bonding falls under the second category of the three Rs—restoration. In recent years, it has proved to be a highly effective treatment for closing spaces between the teeth.

Composite resin, a plastic material, is applied to the teeth to make them wider in areas where gaps exist. Bonding also may be used to close a space temporarily, until crowns are made, for example. On the other hand, if you are having your spaces closed through orthodontics, even if some of your teeth are too dark, bonding can be used to lighten them while the spaces are being closed. The procedure can be performed without anesthesia in one office visit.

If you are closing gaps with bonding, also consider taking care of any other visible defects such as rotated or broken teeth at the same time. As in most esthetic problems, computer imaging can help show you how many teeth will need treatment. Also remember that gum disease or bone loss must be treated before bonding takes place. The only exception to this rule is when your dentist believes that the loose teeth need to be splinted together.

Before

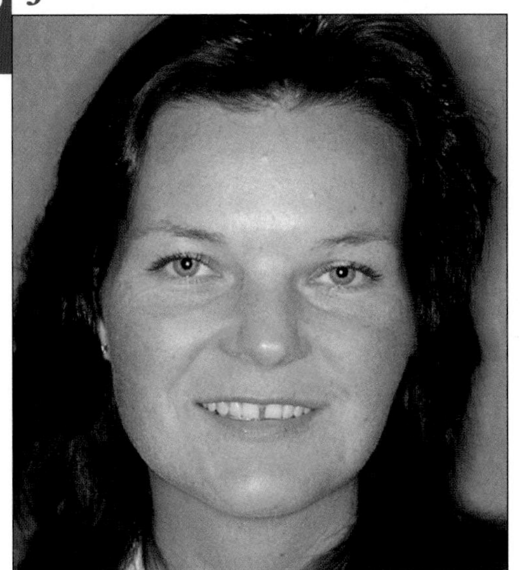

DIASTEMA

This 29-year-old teacher wanted to improve her appearance. She was especially concerned about the space between her front teeth. When looking at her whole face, you can see how the squareness of her face is accentuated by the squareness of the teeth and the wide space. Also, notice how the hair away from the brows emphasizes the square frame of the face. Thus, shapes of teeth, hairstyle and a space between the teeth all help reinforce the squareness.

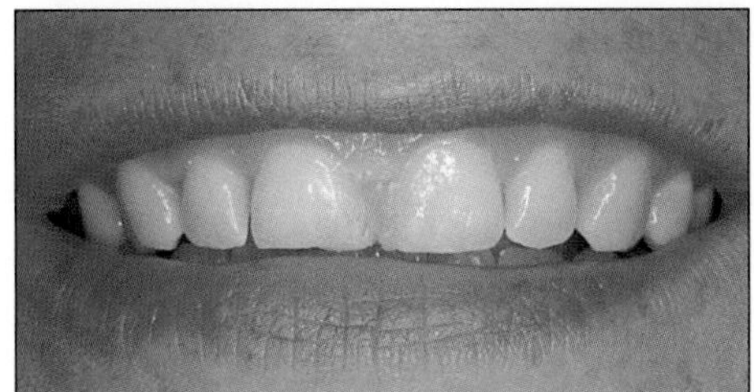

Soft tooth-colored wax was added between the two front teeth to show the patient the approximate result of treatment. The end result will look better since the teeth will be cosmetically contoured before the spaces are closed with composite resin.

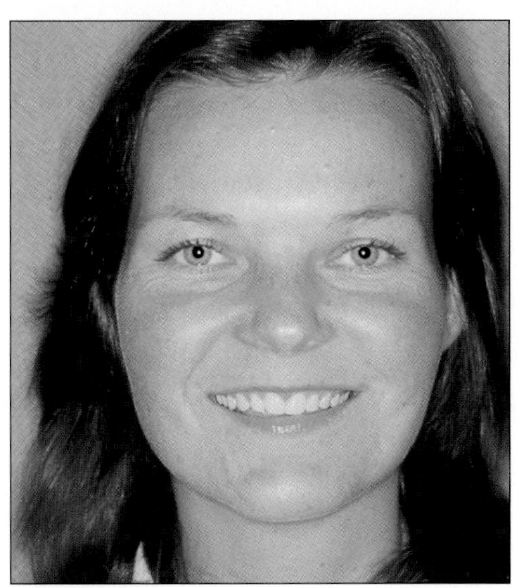

Composite resin bonding and cosmetic contouring were used to close the space and reproportion the four front teeth. However, if the patient had left it at this, only her smile would have been improved and her overall facial appearance, although prettier, is certainly not much less square.

After

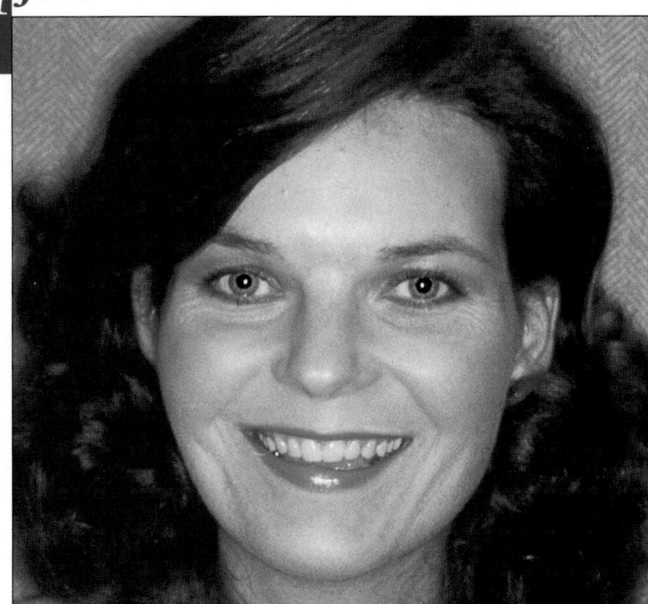

COMPOSITE RESIN BONDING, PLUS COSMETOLOGY

A new hairstyle and makeup are combined with a new smile, and the final result is striking. Notice how her face looks more oval and more feminine. Combining cosmetology with cosmetic dentistry can do wonders to change appearance.

Before

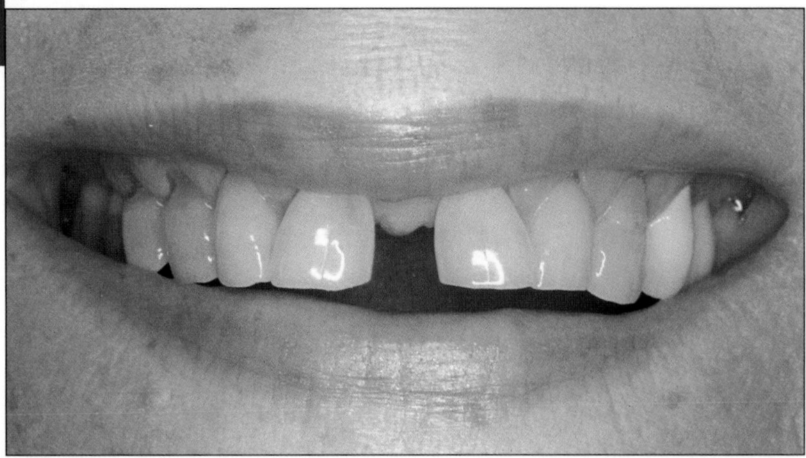

Large space plus erosion

This 60-year-old airline reservationist had an extremely large space between her two front teeth. She also had an advanced erosion that can be seen as a "ditching in" at the necks of the teeth on the upper right side.

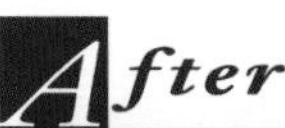

After

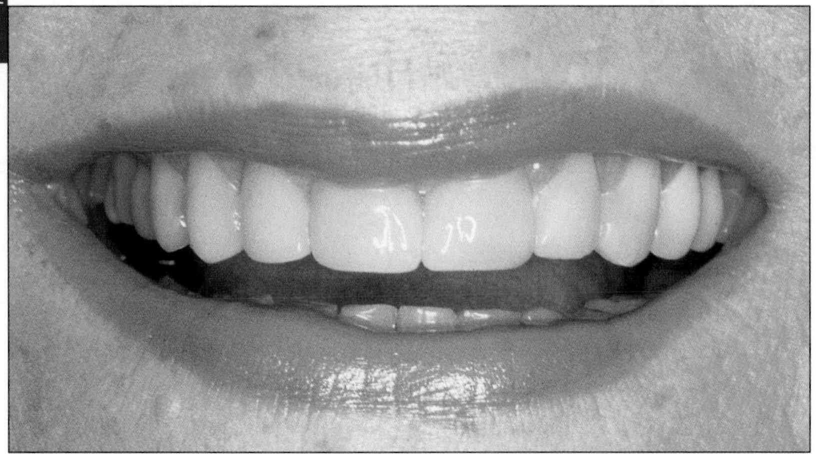

Bonding six teeth to close spaces

Although orthodontics is the best treatment for patients with large spaces, sometimes a compromise plan can be achieved. Success was accomplished for this patient by creating spaces between the adjacent teeth through cosmetic contouring and then closing the spaces with composite resin. The result is a totally new smile with well-proportioned teeth rather than two oversized front teeth closing the space. This procedure was accomplished in one appointment for approximately one third the cost of crowning. The fact that the teeth did not have to be reduced for crowns, and that the erosion was also corrected with a more conservative procedure, was very important to this patient.

Before

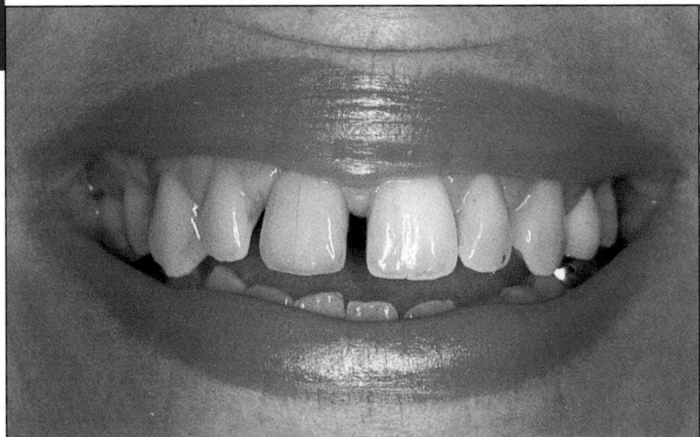

Multiple spaces, discoloration and reverse smileline

This newspaper columnist and author had large spaces between her front teeth to the extent that her teeth were "flaring out." This caused a reversed smileline in that the bottom of her cuspids were lower than her central incisors. The teeth were different colors; many of them were too yellow and stained. Finally, the protruding upper right cuspid overlapped the tooth behind it (first bicuspid).

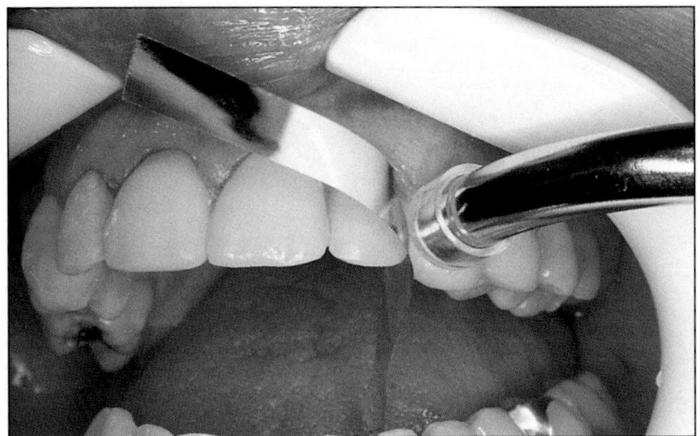

Each tooth is individually bonded by first etching the teeth and then building up layers of composite resin until all the teeth are coated. The resin is hardened (polymerized) by high-intensity light. This figure shows one of the side teeth being polymerized by the high-intensity light.

After

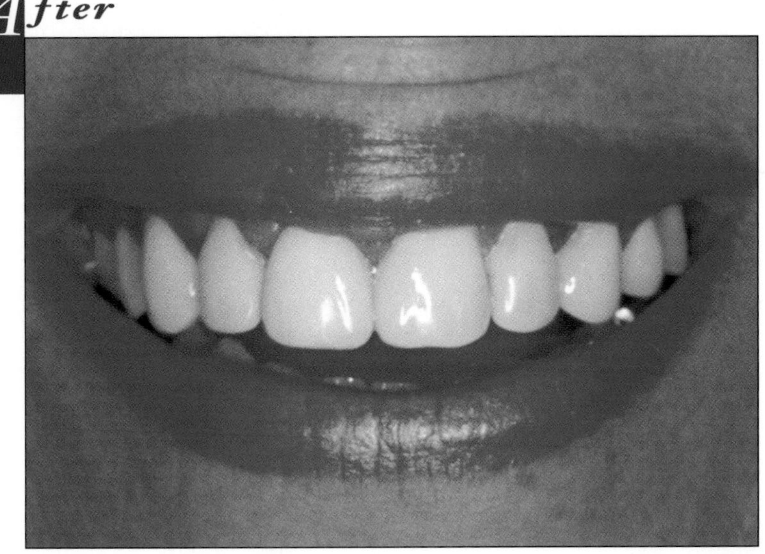

Composite resin bonding and cosmetic contouring

All the front teeth have now been bonded with composite resin to lighten as well as close the spaces between the teeth. The teeth were also lengthened to improve the smileline. Cosmetic contouring helped to blend in the fronts of the teeth to help create a more harmonious relationship between the teeth. The right cuspid doesn't protrude or drop down, but blends in with the other teeth just as the contoured lower teeth do. The right lower incisor doesn't stick up and call attention to a fang-like projection as it did before. The entire treatment was done in one long appointment.

Closing Spaces Caused by Small Teeth

In cases where there are only two or four small front teeth, bonding may be the ideal solution. However, treatment may require bonding more teeth than the ones actually affected in order to keep them in proportion. Otherwise, teeth may appear too bulky. This effect can be minimized if teeth are lengthened slightly and the edges are not perfectly even.

If computer imaging does not provide enough information for you (it illustrates only two dimensions), ask your dentist to add white wax to a model of your teeth so that you can get a better idea of the end result. Although there is a distinct difference between waxing and bonding because of the way light is reflected, this "mock-up" will give you some idea of what the final result will look like. You can also have your dentist use a temporary bonding directly on your teeth to get a good idea of how your smile will change.

Before

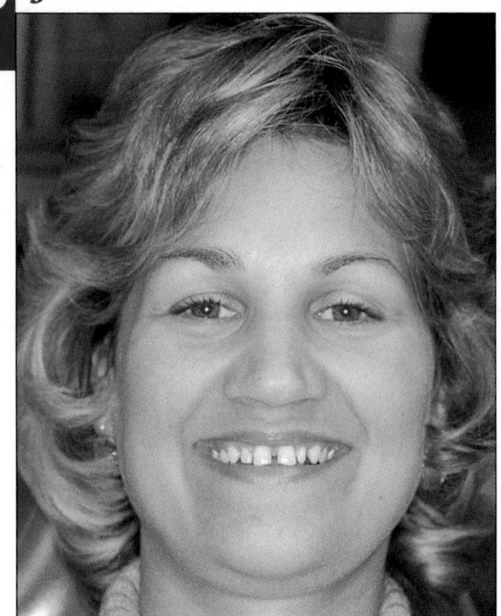

MULTIPLE SPACES—TEETH TOO SMALL FOR FACE

Although orthodontic treatment could have been used to close the spaces for this patient, the result would not have been ideal since her teeth were too small for her face.

After

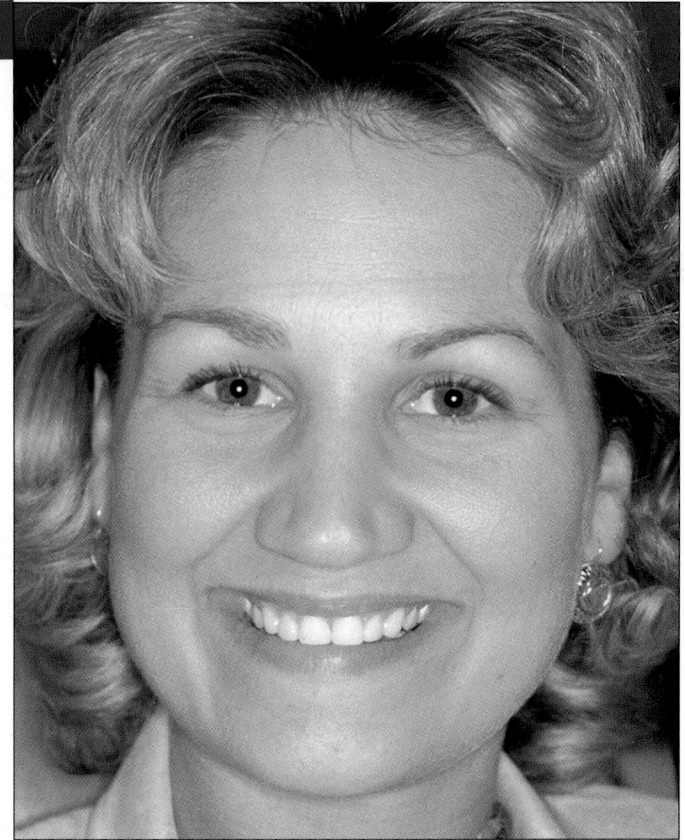

COMPOSITE RESIN BONDING

A one-appointment procedure closed the spaces with more proportionate teeth, giving this patient a more attractive smile.

Before

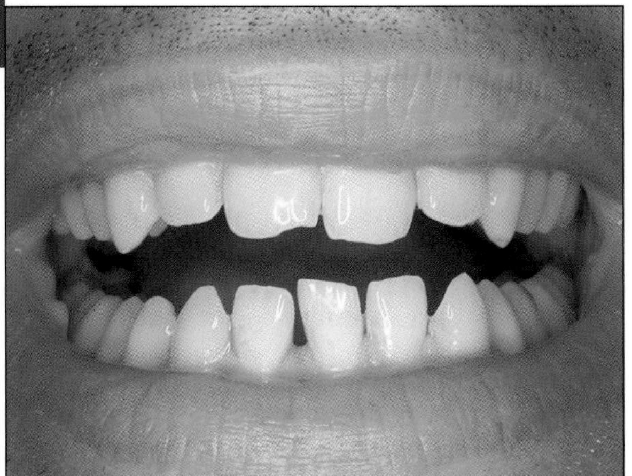

Uneven teeth with lower spacing

This 29-year-old food sales executive had lost a lower tooth and the teeth shifted, causing unattractive spaces to show when he talked or smiled. The upper incisors were uneven due to chipping.

After

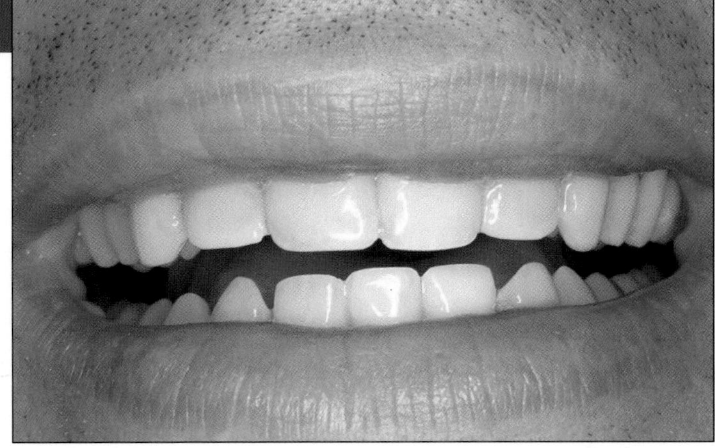

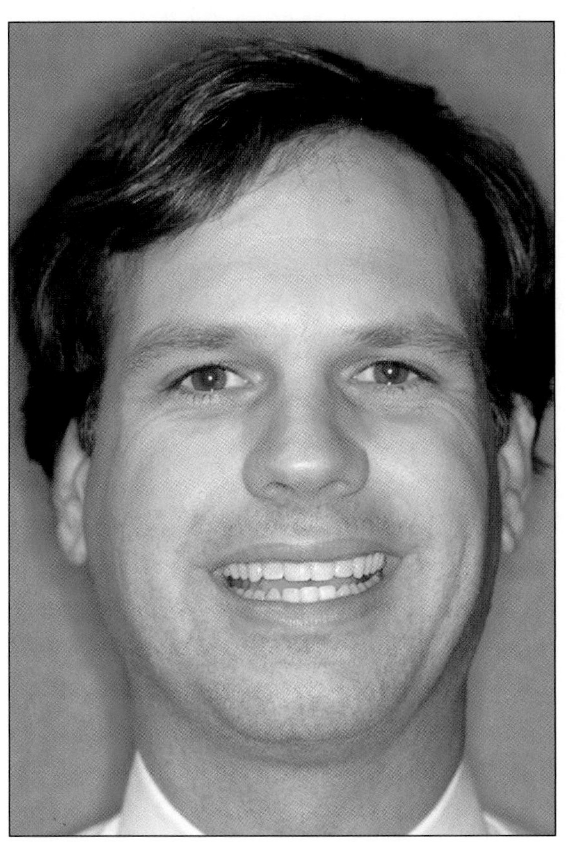

Composite resin bonding and cosmetic contouring

After a one-appointment procedure with composite resin bonding and cosmetic contouring of the upper and lower front teeth, this man's smile is much improved. See how good even three, instead of the usual four, lower front teeth can look when they are in proper balance with the rest of the mouth? The same relative position of the upper central incisors, slightly longer than the laterals, helps keep a more youthful smileline. His new smile helped improve his life through a better job. Considerable research has shown that when people feel confident, their ability and outlook on life tends to improve.

Before

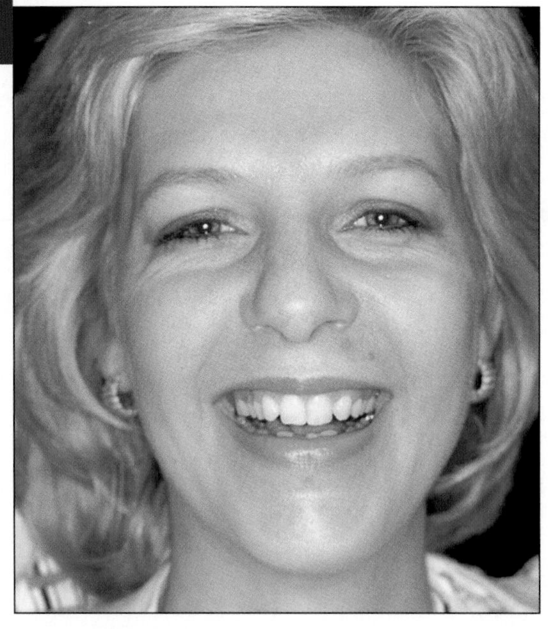

Spaces caused by missing lateral incisors

This television news anchor was missing the two teeth on either side of her front teeth. Her cuspids moved into these positions, leaving slight gaps that showed up on video during close-ups.

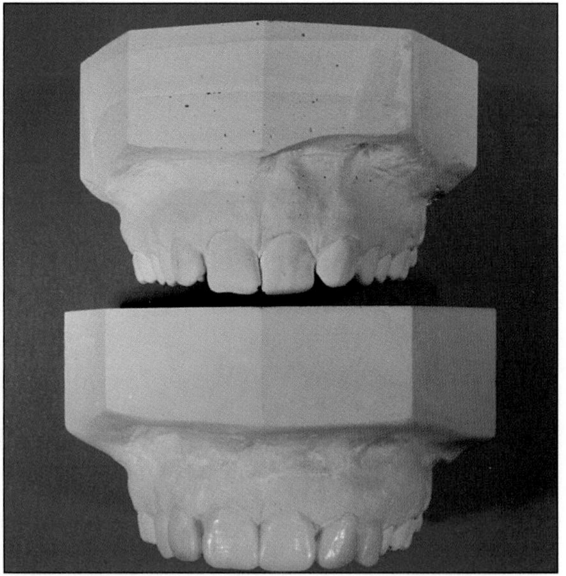

In addition to computer imaging, another way to preview the final result is to ask your dentist to make two study casts in which the teeth are reshaped and waxed to look exactly as they will in the mouth. This before-and-after wax-up showed the patient how the new bonding procedure would look.

After

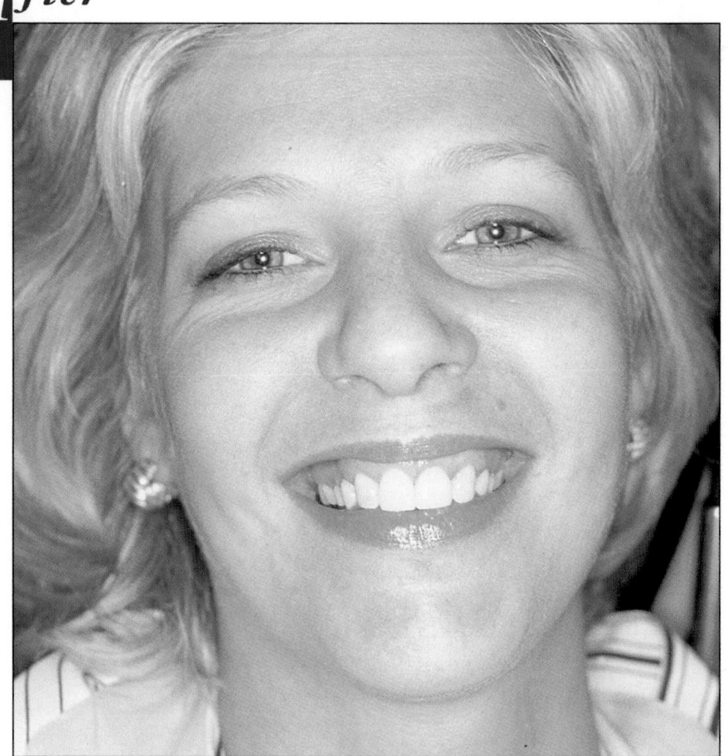

Composite resin bonding and cosmetic contouring

A one-appointment procedure that consisted of composite resin bonding and cosmetic contouring of the upper and lower front teeth helped improve this woman's smile. Her cuspids were reshaped and filled out with bonding to make them look like the missing teeth. The molars behind them were then made to look like cuspids so that it appears as if she has a full complement of teeth.

TREATMENT SUMMARY

BONDING

Treatment Time One to two hours per tooth.

Patient Maintenance Professional cleaning three or four times yearly. Avoid hard foods on front teeth. Bonding to fill in a space is more susceptible to chipping. Proper use of floss daily is required. One problem with most direct bonded restorations is that they can stain or chip. Expect to have some repolishing or repair as necessary.

Results of Treatment Most spaces can be filled in to look very natural.

Average Range of Treatment Life Expectancy Five to eight years. Professional refinishing once every year or so. (See footnote on p. 50.)

Cost Approximately $225 to $950 per tooth. (See footnote on p. 50.)

ADVANTAGES

1. Little or no reduction of tooth structure
2. No anesthesia required
3. Reversible procedure
4. Economical, more so than crowning
5. Teeth can also be lightened

DISADVANTAGES

1. Can chip or stain more easily than crowns
2. Has limited esthetic life
3. Treatment may involve extra teeth to obtain proportionate space closing
4. Teeth may appear somewhat thicker

Problems with Bonding

Bonding can be used successfully on both upper and lower teeth. However, bonded teeth are more likely to chip, crack and stain than natural teeth, particularly the lower front teeth, which are more susceptible to forces from chewing. This also means that some repairs to the bonding are considered normal maintenance during its life expectancy. If you have bonded teeth, professional cleanings several times a year are a must. And even then, the bonding may need to be replaced in 5 to 8 years.

Before

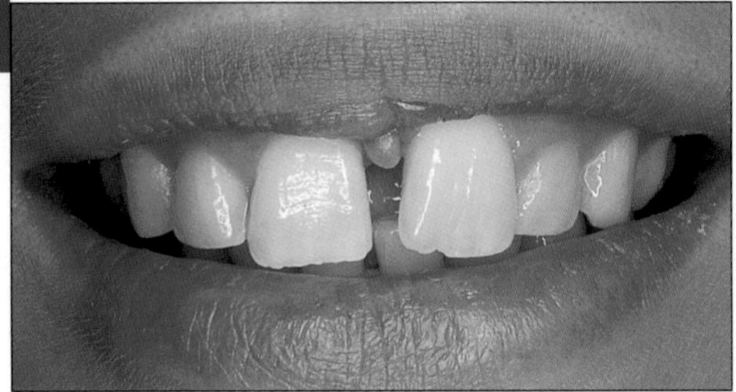

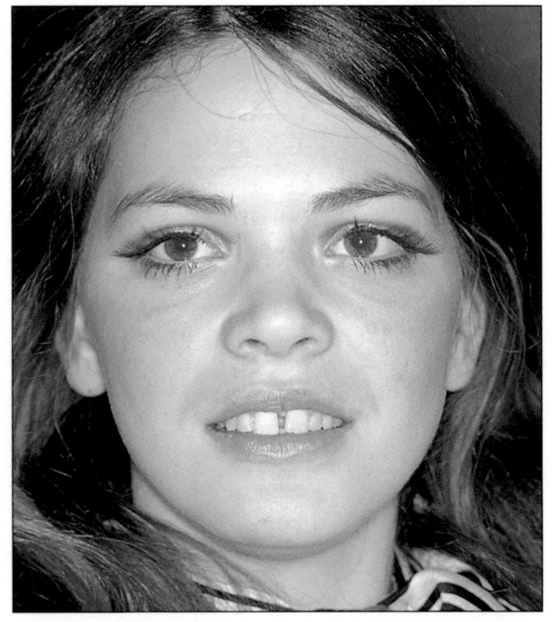

SPACED AND PROTRUDED TEETH

This 21-year-old woman was embarrassed to smile due to the spaces between her front teeth. She did not want to have orthodontic treatment because of her objection to the typical metal bands she thought she would have to wear.

After

ORTHODONTICS, GUM SURGERY, COMPOSITE RESIN BONDING AND COSMETIC CONTOURING

Removable appliances with Teflon-coated wire helped straighten the teeth and close the spaces. Cosmetic surgery to her gums was also performed to remove tissue between the upper two front teeth. Closing the spaces took only three and a half months because the patient found she did not mind wearing the appliances full time. Composite resin bonding and cosmetic contouring were also done to close minor spaces in between the teeth at the gumline.

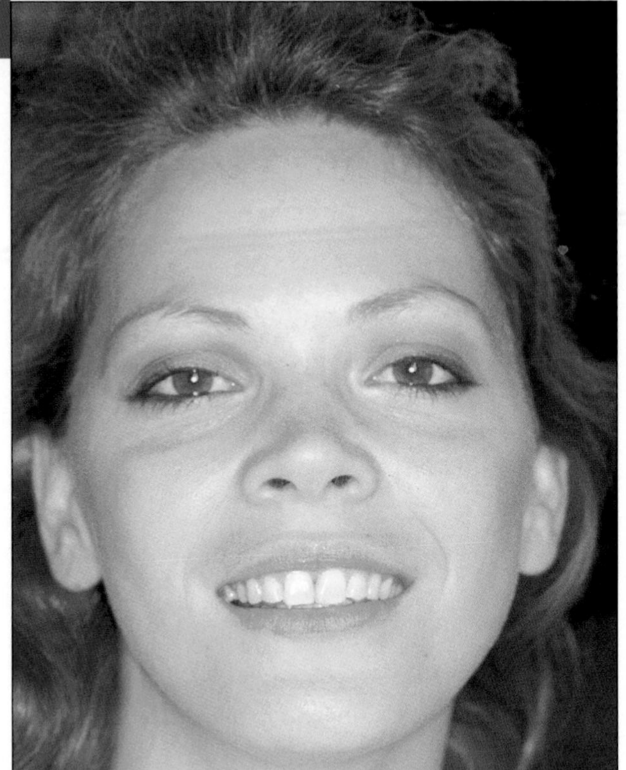

Cosmetic dentistry helped make it possible for this young lady to become a fashion and photographic model due to new self-confidence and an improved smile. Total treatment time was approximately four and a half months.

Before

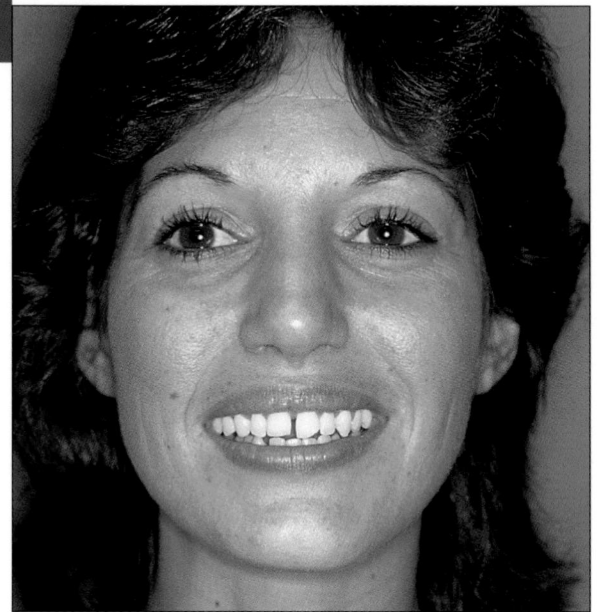

PROTRUDED TEETH CAUSING SPACE BETWEEN CENTRAL INCISORS

This thirty-three-year-old cosmetologist was concerned about her protrusion and the space between her front teeth.

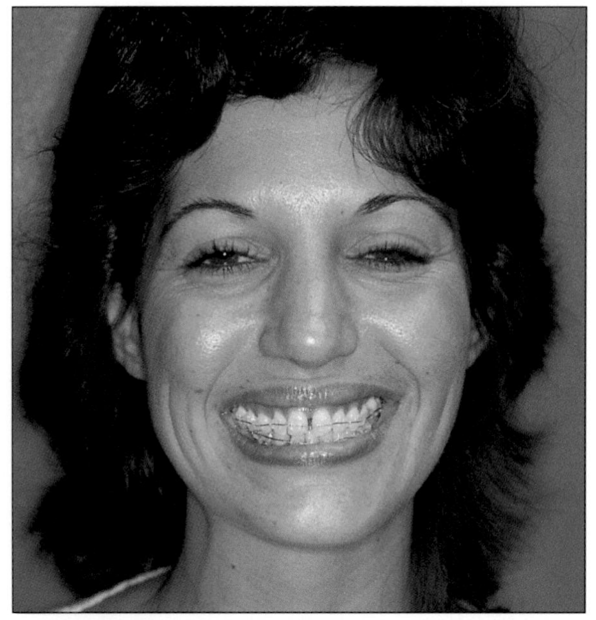

ORTHODONTIC TREATMENT

Orthodontic treatment using plastic brackets successfully retracted the teeth and closed the space.

After

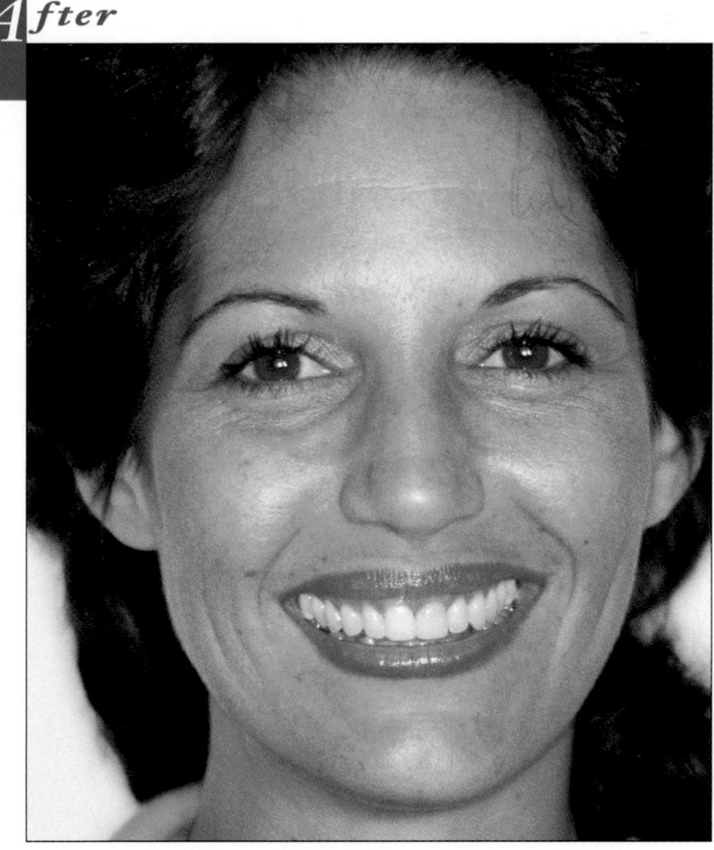

ORTHODONTICS, COSMETIC CONTOURING AND COMPOSITE RESIN BONDING

Although orthodontic treatment alone made her smile more attractive, a combination of cosmetic contouring and composite resin bonding further enhanced it. Looking your best can sometimes mean a combination of several treatments.

Laminating Provides Perfect Proportion

Although bonding is the quickest way to close spaces between the teeth, laminating with either laboratory-made composite resin or porcelain is also an option.

Although laminating takes at least two appointments and typically costs much more than bonding, a major advantage is the proportional accuracy that it provides. This technique is especially effective when spaces are not uniform.

Before

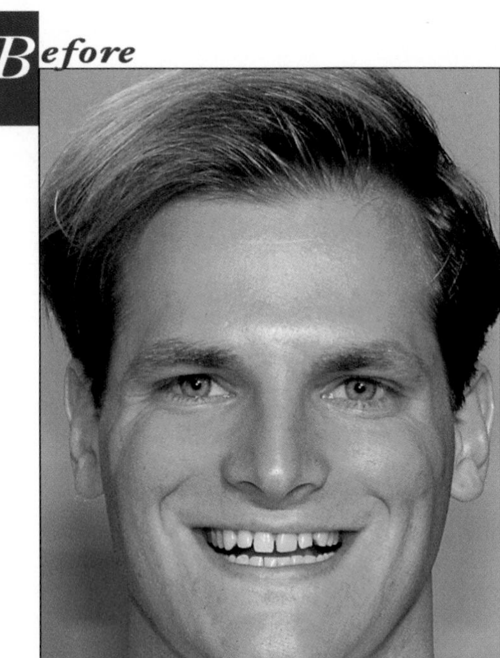

Multiple diastemas

This twenty-one-year-old male model was able to photograph perfectly without smiling but wanted to improve his marketability by enhancing his smile.

After

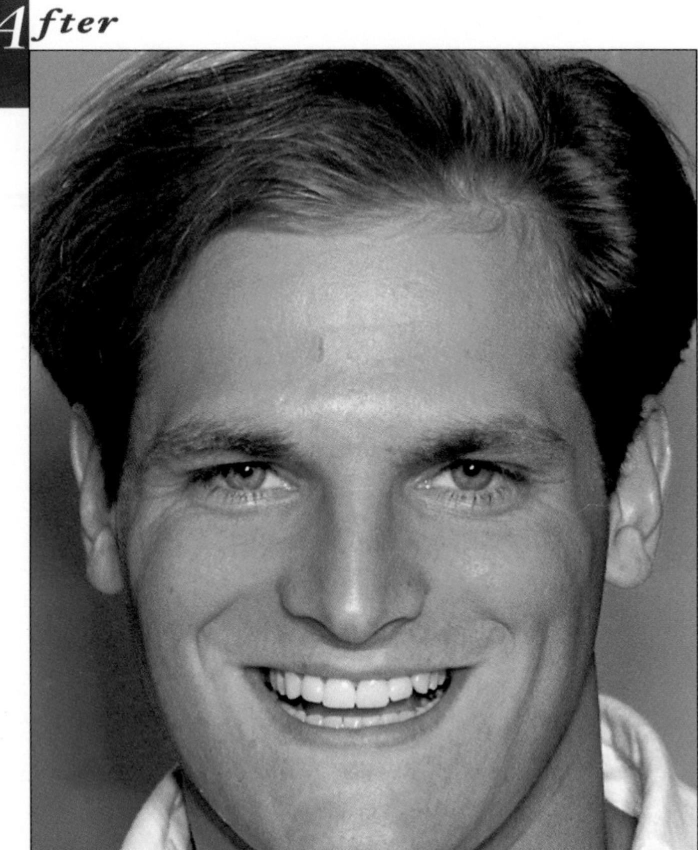

Porcelain laminate veneers

Four laminate veneers eliminated the dark spaces between his teeth when he smiled. The treatment enhanced the total facial look of this model.

TREATMENT SUMMARY

PORCELAIN LAMINATES

Treatment Time Two office visits. The teeth will be prepared and an impression made during the first visit, which can take from one to four hours. The laminates will be fitted and inserted during the second visit, which may also take the same amount of time. Expect to spend more time for more extensive treatment.

Patient Maintenance The teeth should be professionally cleaned about three to four times yearly. Some precautions on eating habits: as with bonding and crowning, take special care when biting into or chewing hard foods with your laminated teeth, since they will not be as strong as enamel.

Results of Treatment A polished, natural-appearing result that effectively closes spaces.

Average Range of Treatment Life Expectancy Four to twelve years. (See footnote on p. 50.)

Cost Approximately $450 to $2500 per tooth. (See footnote on p. 50.)

ADVANTAGES

1. Easier to obtain proportionate closure of spaces
2. Less chipping than bonded restorations
3. Etched porcelain provides an extremely good bond to enamel
4. Wears less than the composite resin laminate
5. Less stain—less chance of color or luster loss
6. More conservative—less tooth reduction than crowning
7. Lasts four to twelve years as compared to plastics (three to eight years)
8. Gum tissue tolerates porcelain well
9. No anesthetic usually required
10. Color change possible
11. Less expensive than crowning

DISADVANTAGES

1. More costly than conventional bonding
2. More difficult for dentist to produce a polished surface after contouring in the mouth
3. More difficult to repair if the laminate cracks or chips
4. Can be an irreversible procedure if much enamel is removed

Crowning to Close the Gap

Although crowning can provide beautiful results—filling gaps and lightening color just like bonding—it typically is not the treatment of choice for spaces between the teeth because it requires considerable reduction of natural tooth structure. However, in cases where teeth are badly damaged, these finely sculptured look-alikes are often appropriate.

Like laminating, crowning is a more time-consuming and costly procedure than bonding. Unlike bonded or laminated teeth, crowned teeth are not as likely to chip. However, replacement is typically required within five to fifteen years.

Occasionally, a space is so large that a patient prefers that a slight gap be left intentionally in the crowns for a more natural appearance.

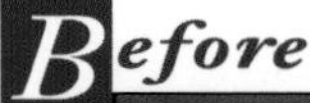

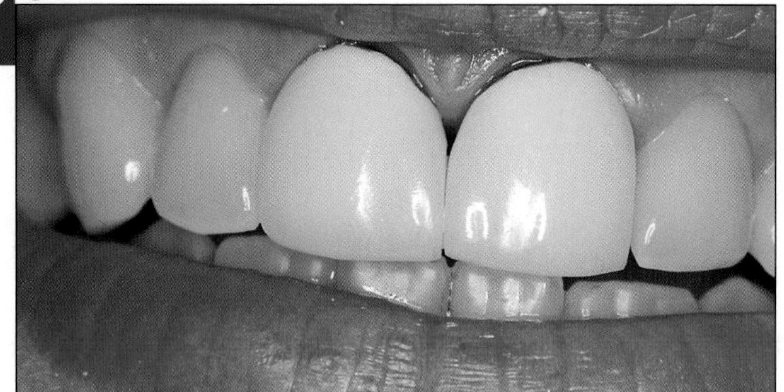

Central crowns too wide for face

When this young lady smiled, she revealed two large crowns that were placed to mask a large gap between her two front teeth.

After

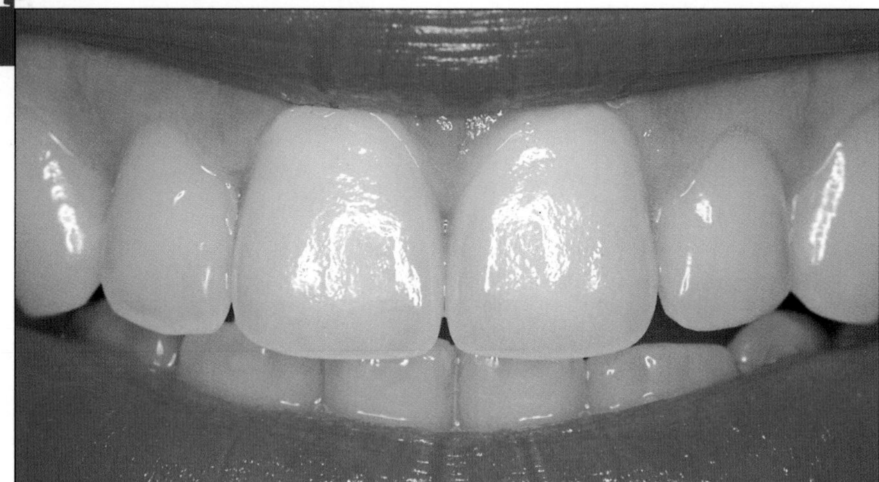

Orthodontics plus new crowns

The existing crowns were made thinner, and orthodontic treatment closed the newly formed spaces. Finally two new porcelain crowns were made to enhance the smile.

Before

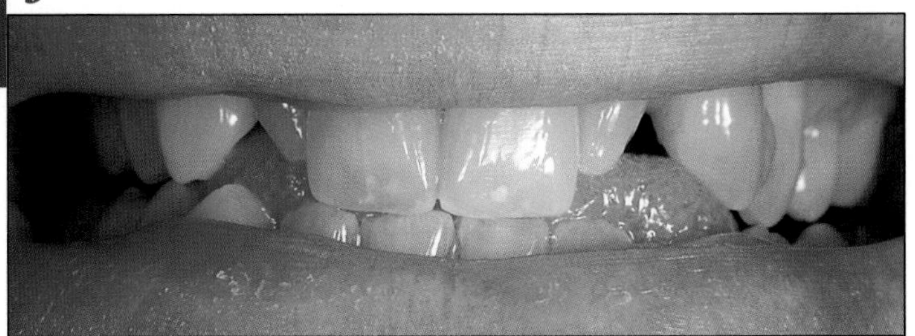

PEG-SHAPED LATERAL INCISORS

This thirty-five-year-old salesman was so ashamed of his appearance he avoided smiling.

After

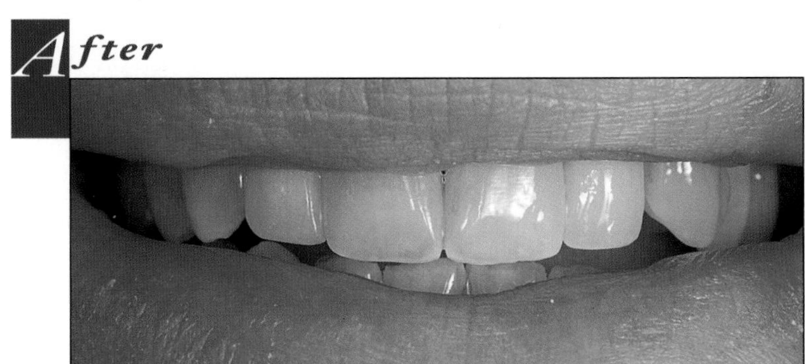

FULL CROWNS

Both lateral incisors were crowned to help improve the smileline. In many instances, porcelain laminates or even composite resin bonding can be used as a more conservative means of altering tooth shape.

TREATMENT SUMMARY

CROWNING

Treatment Time Usually two appointments of approximately one to four hours on up to four teeth. Expect to spend more time as more teeth are treated or more extensive treatment is performed.

Patient Maintenance Crowns are designed to look and feel like real teeth, but extra care must be taken to avoid tooth fractures in order to protect the remaining natural tooth root. Fluoride treatments should be given once a year. Flossing every day is essential with crowns.

Results of Treatment Crowning can achieve the ultimate in shaping teeth to fill spaces.

Average Range of Treatment Life Expectancy Five to fifteen years. Life expectancy is directly proportional to problems with tissues, fractures and recurrent decay. (See footnote on p. 50.)

Cost Approximately $550 to $3000 per tooth. (See footnote on p. 50.)

When to Crown When tooth enamel is insufficient to bond.

ADVANTAGES

1. Crowns can be shaped to esthetically fill gaps
2. Teeth can be lightened to any shade
3. Some realignment or straightening of the teeth is possible
4. Should last about twice as long as bonding

DISADVANTAGES

1. Can fracture
2. Requires anesthesia
3. Original tooth form is altered
4. May need to be replaced after five to fifteen years
5. More costly than bonding

Temporary Stand-In: Removable Acrylic Overlay

The removable acrylic overlay is a device formed from thin acrylic or plastic made to fit into the space and blend with adjacent teeth. The intimate fit of the appliance to the teeth holds it in place.

Removable acrylic overlays were more commonly used before the advent of composite resin bonding. Often worn by models, actors and actresses, the appliance was requested by people who didn't want to crown their teeth just to close a space.

While these overlays may look attractive from a distance, they often don't bear up as well under close scrutiny. They generally add bulk to the natural teeth. It also can be difficult to obtain a realistic-looking tooth because the plastic is so thin. The overlays can fracture and discolor easily, and eating with them can be a problem.

In some cases, however, the removable acrylic overlay may still be a desirable alternative. On the positive side, it's inexpensive. And it hides spaces well, particularly for photographic purposes.

Before

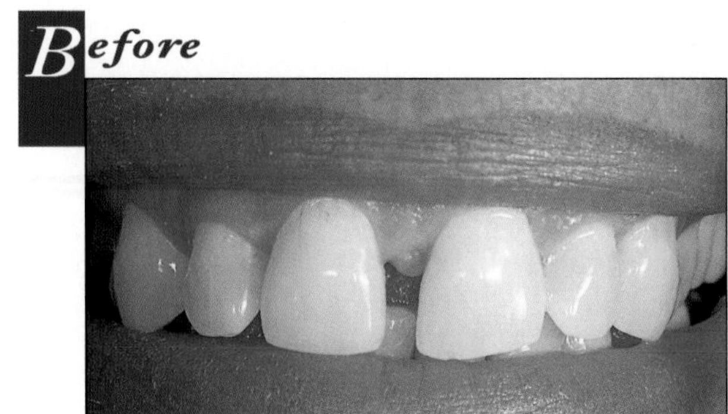

Diastema

This 52-year-old woman wanted to have her spaces closed for certain occasions, such as when being photographed, but she did not want to have her teeth altered with restorations or orthodontic treatment, nor did she want to close the space permanently.

After

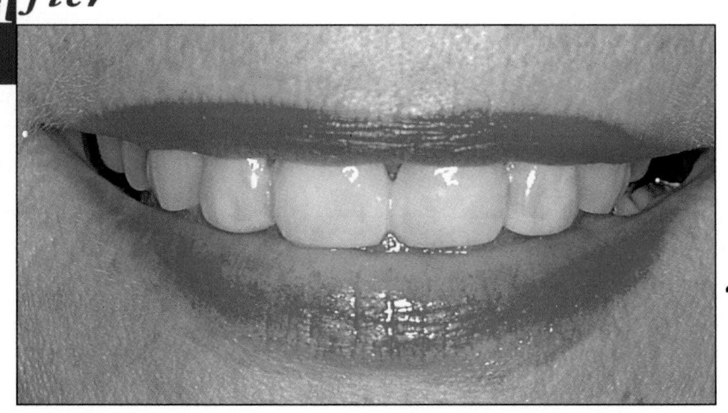

Removable acrylic overlay

A removable acrylic overlay was made to give the patient immediate results, without permanently altering her tooth structure. This allows the option of orthodontia or any other type of treatment later. The major problem with this type of removable appliance is that the plastic teeth are extremely thin and fragile and can easily fracture.

A Missing Tooth Can Spoil an Attractive Smile

Don't underestimate the value of every tooth in terms of beauty—even those in the back of the mouth. Although the spaces created by these missing teeth may not be visible, they can cause a variety of problems.

For example, chewing forces may shift to other surfaces, causing the front teeth to flare out and creating unwanted spaces. An altered bite can also cause the collapse of facial features. The more teeth that are lost and not replaced, the greater the odds that wrinkles and lines will form, causing premature, unnecessary aging.

Missing teeth should be replaced with a bridge, overdenture or implant. Only if the missing tooth is the last molar can it go unreplaced. If the corresponding tooth above or below it is also missing, a change in appearance generally does not occur.

If you are missing a tooth, there are three ways it can be replaced: a fixed bridge, a removable bridge, or an implant. Depending on your circumstances, each can be successful. Information on implants begins on p. 143.

How a Bridge Replaces a Missing Tooth

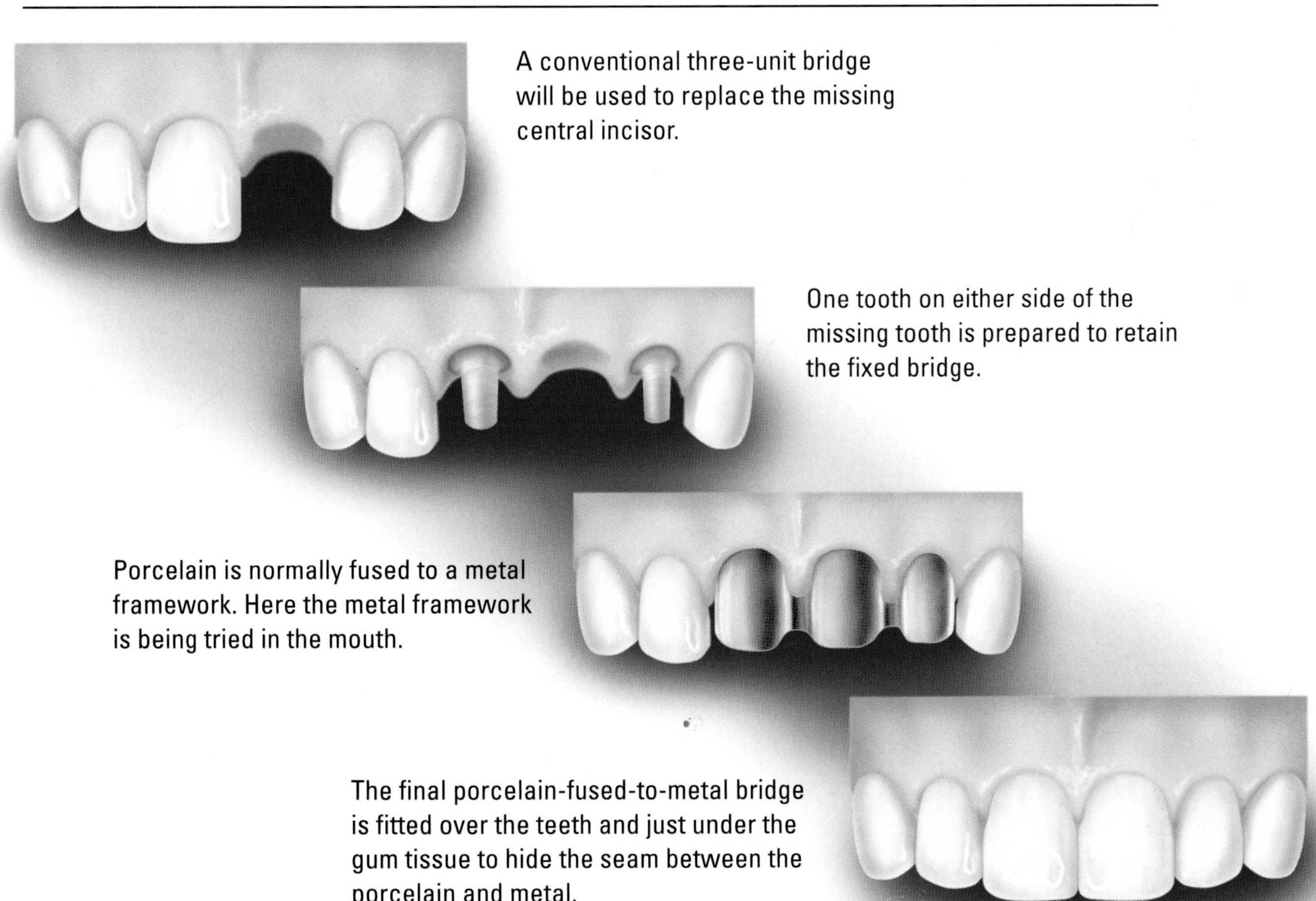

A conventional three-unit bridge will be used to replace the missing central incisor.

One tooth on either side of the missing tooth is prepared to retain the fixed bridge.

Porcelain is normally fused to a metal framework. Here the metal framework is being tried in the mouth.

The final porcelain-fused-to-metal bridge is fitted over the teeth and just under the gum tissue to hide the seam between the porcelain and metal.

Before

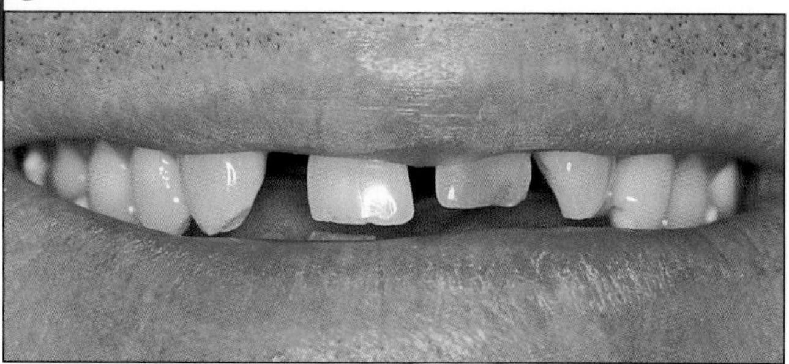

Missing lateral incisors

This fifty-year-old man wanted to enhance his appearance. Missing lateral incisors and irregular spacing created a problem too difficult to solve strictly through restorative therapy.

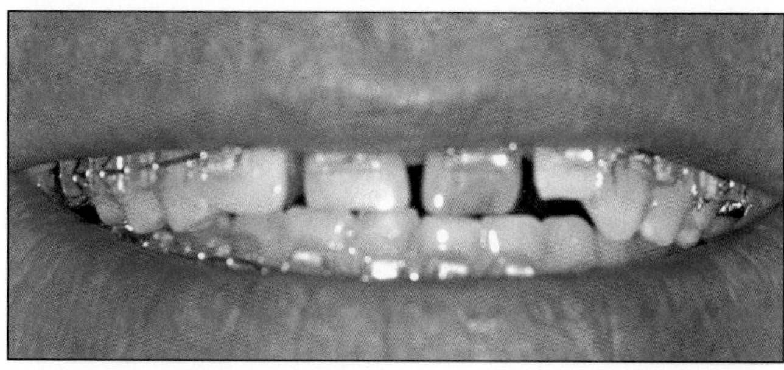

Orthodontics

The patient underwent sixteen months of orthodontic treatment with tooth-colored brackets.

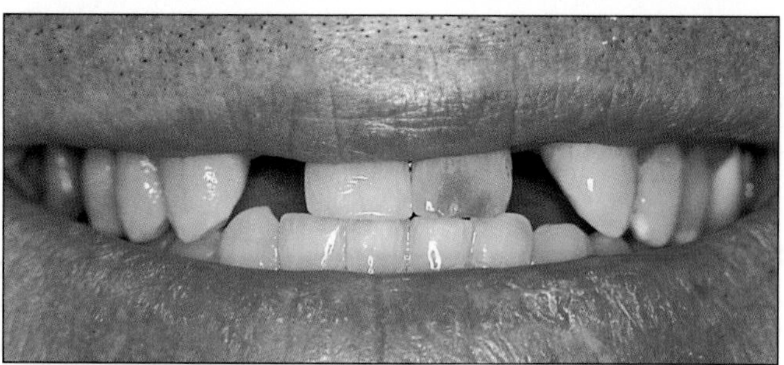

After orthodontic treatment. Adequate space allows proportionate restoration of his upper front teeth.

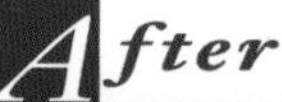

After

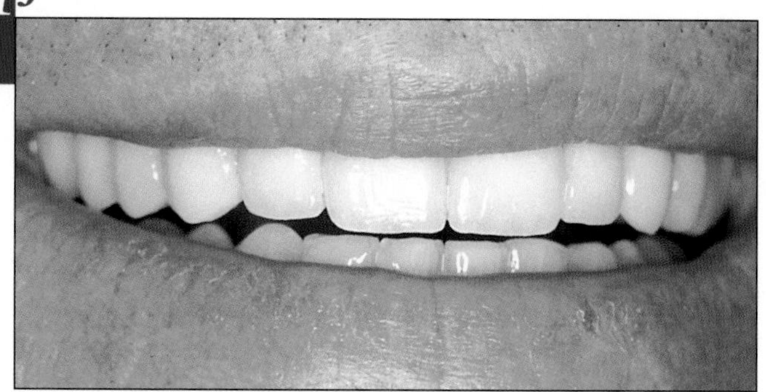

Final restorative treatment consisted of fixed bridges and porcelain laminates on the upper teeth and in-office bleaching for the lower teeth.

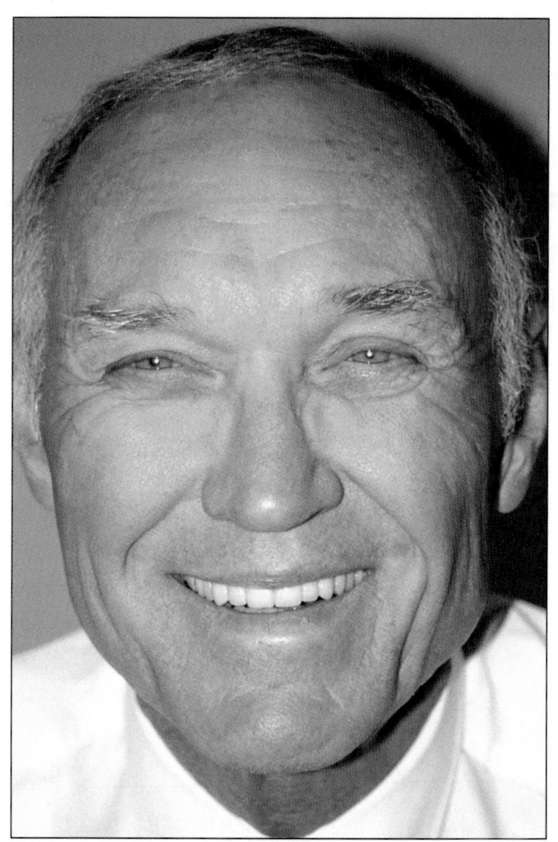

See just how important the smile can be to one's overall appearance. In this patient, combination therapy contributed to a proportionate, esthetic and functional result.

Fixed vs Removable Bridges

Bridges can either be cemented into place (fixed) or attached around adjacent teeth (removable). Either type can be used to replace missing teeth and to treat gum loss and spaces at the gumline.

Fixed bridges are typically made of porcelain. When additional strength is needed, this material is bonded to a precious or nonprecious metal. Although precious metals such as gold are generally more expensive, they are tarnish resistant. Some nonprecious metals can tarnish, leaving a slightly dark line at the gum unless porcelain encases the metal, hiding the metal from the front.

Selecting the removable bridge over the fixed bridge because it is less expensive initially may not be a wise decision

Fixed bridges usually last longer than removable appliances. They also look and feel better. However, they typically require that adjacent teeth be crowned to provide an anchor. If there is no tooth to which the fixed bridge can be attached, then a removable appliance can be used.

The framework for most removable bridges is made of a white nonprecious metal that has high strength and is tarnish resistant. Acrylic or porcelain teeth are then attached to this framework with gum-colored plastic so that the restoration looks as natural as possible.

Although patients often select the removable bridge over the fixed bridge because it is less expensive initially, this may not be a wise decision. Removable bridges often cause unnecessary wear and tear on adjacent teeth. And the savings are questionable because removable bridges have shorter lifespans.

In the final analysis, many variables should be considered before any restorative treatment is undertaken, including the amount of remaining tooth structure surrounding the missing tooth or teeth, your individual esthetic needs and your financial resources.

Also consider your height. If you're short, and you need to replace a tooth in the lower jaw, you should realize that the metal on a bridge or crown may be visible to others even though it is on the inside of your mouth. If you're tall, and you need to replace a tooth in the upper jaw, the same applies. If you are concerned about either of these possibilities, consult with your dentist before treatment begins. There are ways to alleviate this problem.

Conventional fixed bridge

A beautiful esthetic result can be achieved with a conventional fixed bridge because the teeth needed to anchor the bridge on either side of the missing teeth are made into crowns and no metal shows. However, you need to realize that the three or more units (each tooth, including the missing tooth, is considered a unit) will be joined so you will have to change the way you floss. No longer will you be able to floss through the teeth, but rather you will need a "floss threader" that allows you to floss under or between the teeth.

In addition, there must be sufficient room for porcelain between upper and lower teeth when replacing a missing tooth with a fixed bridge. If not, either a crown-lengthening surgical procedure or orthodontic treatment can usually help create the needed room.

TREATMENT SUMMARY

CONVENTIONAL FIXED BRIDGE

Treatment Time Two to four weeks.

Patient Maintenance Daily cleaning under bridge with floss threaders.

Results of Treatment Esthetic replacement of lost tooth or teeth.

Average Range of Treatment Life Expectancy Five to fifteen years. (See footnote on p. 50.)

Cost $475 to $3000 per tooth unit. (See footnote on p. 50.)

ADVANTAGES

1. Longest life
2. Easy to clean
3. Improves your bite
4. Helps prevent movement of adjacent and opposing teeth

DISADVANTAGES

1. Difficult to match shade of porcelain
2. Costs more than cantilever (see next)
3. More tooth reduction than cantilever or resin-bonded bridge
4. May be difficult to make look natural in cases of ridge or gum loss

Cantilever fixed bridge

If an anchor can be provided by only one tooth, a cantilever restoration may provide a pleasing esthetic effect at less expense than a conventional bridge. It requires anchoring the tooth to only one side and using one, two or more teeth to suspend the replacement tooth or teeth. However, life expectancy is usually not as long with this type of bridge.

The cantilever fixed bridge may be considered a more conservative treatment because fewer teeth are reduced, and the esthetic results can be as good as or better than those obtained with a conventional bridge.

TREATMENT SUMMARY

CANTILEVER FIXED BRIDGE

Treatment Time Two to four weeks.

Patient Maintenance Must clean under bridge. Easier to use floss threaders.

Results of Treatment Esthetic tooth replacement.

Average Range of Treatment Life Expectancy Five to fifteen years average life. (See footnote on p. 50.)

Cost $475 to $1850 per tooth unit. (See footnote on p. 50.)

ADVANTAGES

1. Less tooth structure reduced because fewer teeth required
2. Less expensive than conventional bridge
3. More natural separation possible between teeth

DISADVANTAGES

1. Less structural support
2. Unless the bite is perfectly balanced, too much torque can damage the replacement tooth

Resin-bonded fixed bridge

Another type of fixed bridge with esthetic appeal is the resin-bonded bridge or "Maryland bridge." It costs about one half to one third as much as a conventional fixed bridge.

The primary advantage of the resin-bonded bridge is that it requires little or no tooth reduction. Nor does it require full crowns on either side of the missing tooth. Instead, the metal framework is bonded to the tooth with resin cement. This also means a small amount of metal will probably show on the tops of the teeth where it is bonded. If the teeth adjacent to the missing tooth are intact and in good condition, this type of restoration may be the best choice. If there are cosmetic problems with the adjacent teeth, however, a conventional bridge should be considered.

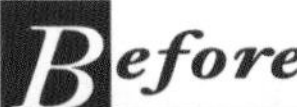

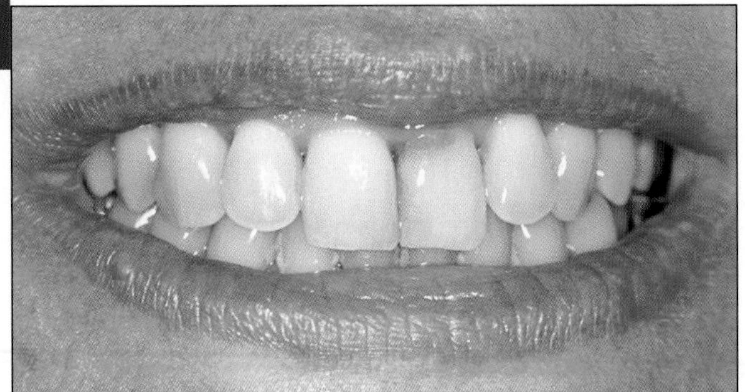

Internal resorption

This woman had an uncommon condition that caused the inside of the tooth to erode away.

After

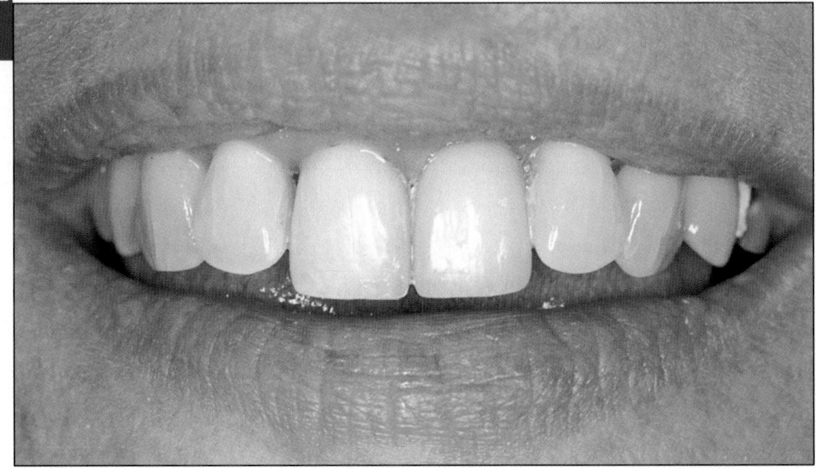

Resin-bonded bridge

During the three months it took for the gum tissue to heal, a removable bridge served as a temporary for the missing tooth. The final replacement was a resin-bonded fixed bridge.

How a Resin-Bonded Bridge Is Attached

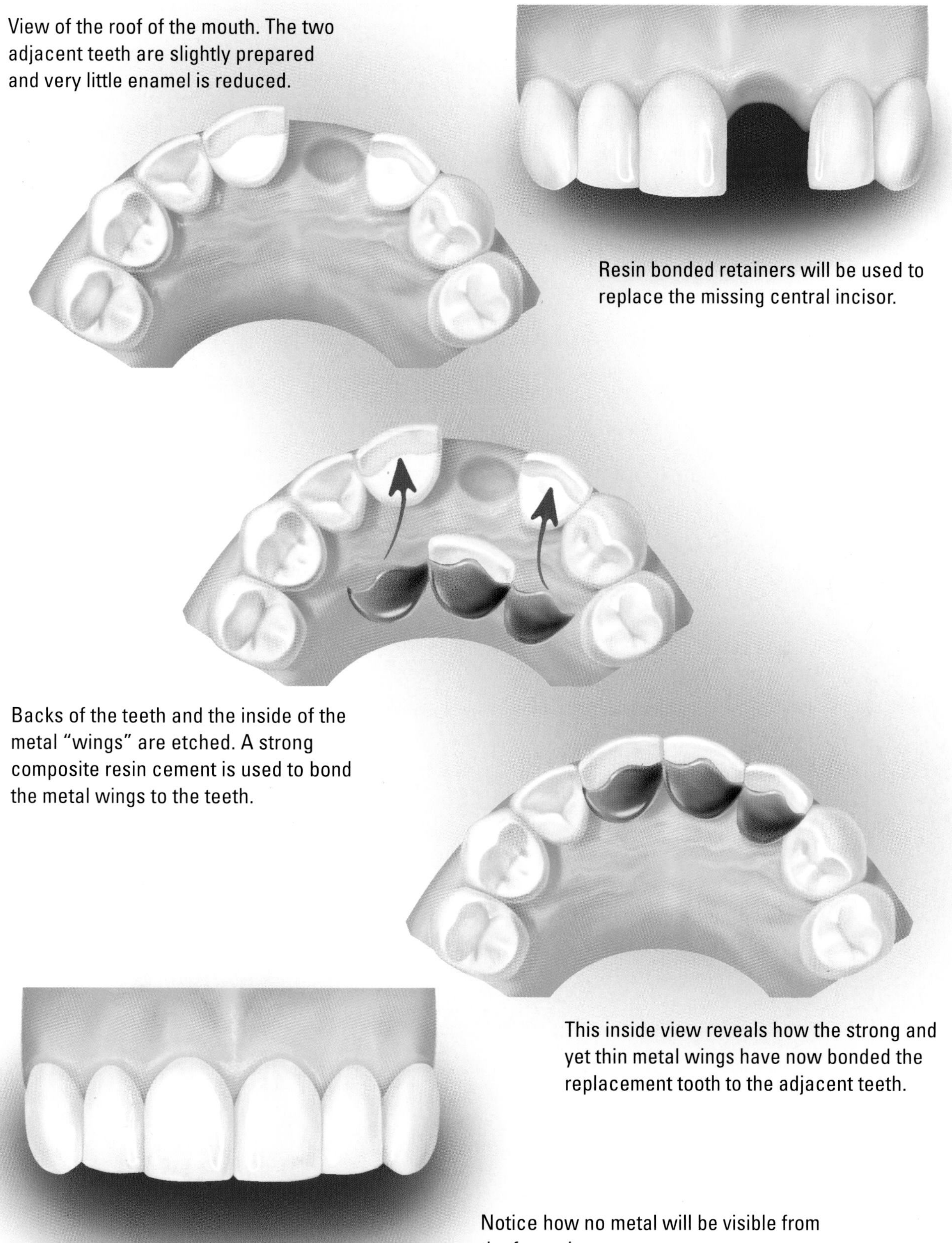

View of the roof of the mouth. The two adjacent teeth are slightly prepared and very little enamel is reduced.

Resin bonded retainers will be used to replace the missing central incisor.

Backs of the teeth and the inside of the metal "wings" are etched. A strong composite resin cement is used to bond the metal wings to the teeth.

This inside view reveals how the strong and yet thin metal wings have now bonded the replacement tooth to the adjacent teeth.

Notice how no metal will be visible from the front view.

TREATMENT SUMMARY

RESIN-BONDED FIXED BRIDGE

Treatment Time Two to four weeks.

Patient Maintenance Same as for conventional bridge. Daily cleaning under bridge with floss threaders.

Results of Treatment Tooth replacement without reducing other teeth.

Average Range of Treatment Life Expectancy Five to ten years. (See footnote on p. 50.)

Cost $500 to $1850 per unit, about one third to one half as much as similar conventional bridge. (See footnote on p. 50.)

ADVANTAGES

1. Less expensive than conventional bridge
2. No anesthesia required
3. Less tooth reduction

DISADVANTAGES

1. Less ability to alter shape and sizes of teeth
2. Tissue can shrink around gum, leaving spaces between teeth
3. Metal backing may show through if the teeth are thin
4. Teeth to which the bridge is attached must be in excellent condition
5. May not last as long as a conventional bridge

Conventional removable bridge

The conventional removable bridge attaches to adjacent teeth with metal clasps. If these clasps show when you smile, the result can be esthetically displeasing. In such cases, the precision-attachment removable bridge described next should be considered.

If you can't afford the precision-attachment method of hiding clasps, then a removable bridge with a tooth-colored flexible clasp can be made to replace the missing teeth. Keep in mind, however, that this restoration doesn't offer the support or the stability of the conventional metal-clasp bridge. It may also need to be replaced every few years.

Before

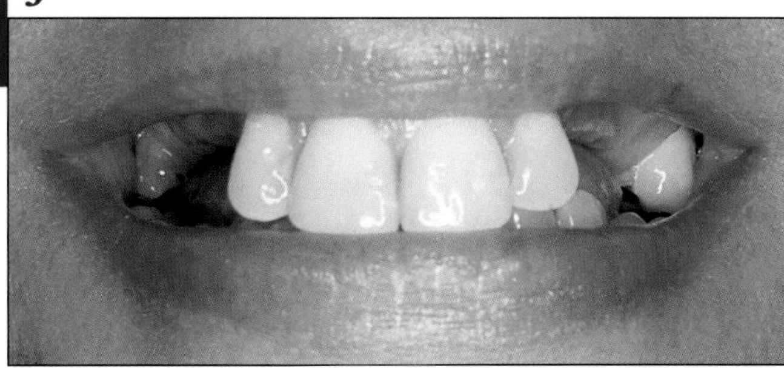

MISSING TEETH

This woman had lost many of her upper back teeth. At the time, she could not afford fixed bridgework and did not want to show the metal clasps from a removable bridge. She avoided smiling in order to hide these back spaces.

After

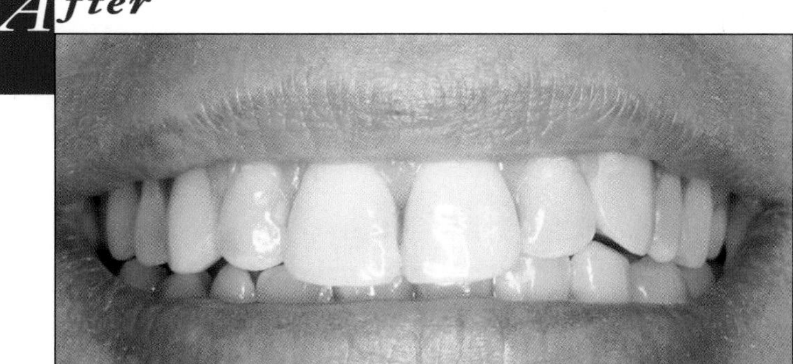

TOOTH-COLORED CLASP REMOVABLE BRIDGE

A flexible removable bridge provided an interim solution for this patient. The tooth-colored clasps conceal the nature of the appliance, providing a more esthetic smile. These appliances, however, do not last as long as a metal removable bridge, and they need to be remade more frequently. For the most esthetic and long-lasting result, implants or fixed bridges should eventually be constructed.

TREATMENT SUMMARY

CONVENTIONAL REMOVABLE BRIDGE

Treatment Time Four to eight weeks.

Patient Maintenance Must remove bridge and clean after eating.

Results of Treatment Least expensive way to replace missing teeth.

Average Range of Treatment Life Expectancy Five to ten years. (See footnote on p. 50.)

Cost $495 to $2500 depending on design and material used. (See footnote on p. 50.)

ADVANTAGES

1. Less expensive than fixed bridges
2. Helps to balance bite and increases chewing efficiency by replacing missing teeth
3. Prevents movements of adjacent and opposing teeth

DISADVANTAGES

1. Attachment may create possible wear and stress on supporting teeth
2. May not be as esthetic as a fixed bridge

Precision-attachment removable bridge

If you object to the metal clasps found in the conventional removable bridge, you will probably like the precision-attachment restoration. It involves placing a crown on the adjacent tooth or teeth with a place for the attachment in the back so that the clasp becomes invisible. Removable bridges that contain precision attachments are usually made of gold-containing alloys combined with porcelain or plastic teeth.

Although much more costly, precision-attachment removable bridges offer a superior and almost invisible method of restoring the teeth.

TREATMENT SUMMARY

PRECISION-ATTACHMENT REMOVABLE BRIDGE

Treatment Time Four to eight weeks.

Patient Maintenance Requires regular cleaning and adjustments.

Results of Treatment Removable bridge is less obvious.

Average Range of Treatment Life Expectancy Five to ten years. (See footnote on p. 50.)

Cost $950 to $5000 for precision removable bridge. (See footnote on p. 50.)

ADVANTAGES

1. Clasps are hidden
2. Superior retention

DISADVANTAGES

1. More expensive than clasps
2. Attachments can break
3. Attachments can wear

Temporary Bridge

You never have to be without your teeth. Your dentist can make a natural-looking temporary bridge—even on the day you lose a tooth! However, the temporary bridge has a much shorter life expectancy and should be replaced with a final bridge as soon as healing takes place.

Esthetic Problems of Bridges

There are two basic esthetic problems dentists have when making fixed bridges. The first is making the attached artificial teeth look like individual teeth. The second is making the teeth look like they are actually emerging from your gums.

No matter how skilled dentists are, they will occasionally have difficulty in solving these two problems and will need your patience.

The Combination Approach to Closing Gaps

There may be no single best way to solve your space problem. Instead, a combination of orthodontics, bonding and even a cantilever or conventional fixed bridge may be the most economical and esthetic approach.

A COMBINATION OF TREATMENTS MAY PROVIDE THE MOST ECONOMICAL AND ESTHETIC APPROACH

Just remember that it's always best to align teeth properly before undergoing bonding or any other restorative procedure. Work closely with your dentist to ensure that you obtain the best treatment available for your unique situation.

Overdentures: An Alternative to Full Dentures

An overdenture is a removable bridge designed for patients who have experienced a great deal of bone loss, usually due to gum disease resulting in missing and loose teeth.

An esthetically pleasing bridge can be made by reducing the top portions of the remaining teeth and covering the root structure with individual restorations. These teeth, in turn, are covered by a removable plastic appliance—the overdenture—which they help support. Although this is a more expensive treatment than a conventional full denture, it provides a much stronger biting surface and considerable control over esthetics.

If you have lost most of your teeth and are thinking about having the rest extracted and obtaining a full denture, consider an overdenture. Even saving just a few good roots can make a big difference in the way you chew.

TREATMENT SUMMARY

OVERDENTURE

Treatment Time Four to eight weeks.

Patient Maintenance Requires daily cleaning and periodic adjustments.

Results of Treatment Hides the fact you are wearing a removable bridge.

Average Range of Treatment Life Expectancy Five to ten years. (See footnote on p. 50.)

Cost $900 to $5000. (See footnote on p. 50.)

ADVANTAGES

1. Saves roots
2. Improves chewing ability
3. Better fit and retention as compared to normal denture
4. Less stress to supporting ridge tissue
5. Provides a good transition to a full denture
6. Allows the patient to retain some tactile sensation

DISADVANTAGES

1. Attachment can break
2. More costly than conventional denture
3. May be slightly bulkier than fixed or removable partial dentures

Immediate Denture

If you've been advised to have all your teeth removed and replaced with a full denture, consider an immediate denture first. The advantage lies in never having to be seen without teeth.

The procedure requires a preliminary office visit to make records. The laboratory then constructs a preliminary full denture that duplicates the appearance of your natural teeth or, if you want, that improves them in color, form and position.

At the next appointment, your front teeth can be removed and the immediate denture inserted. Because gum tissue will eventually shrink, however, a reline or a new denture eventually will be required.

TREATMENT SUMMARY

IMMEDIATE DENTURE

Treatment Time Two visits over a two- to four-week period.

Patient Maintenance Cleaning after meals to remove and prevent stains on dentures. Check probable gum shrinkage with your dentist. Requires relining.

Results of Treatment Can duplicate or improve your tooth color, form and tooth arrangement.

Average Range of Treatment Life Expectancy Usually no more than six months, but with a reline at approximately three months, can last much longer. (See footnote on p. 50.)

Cost Estimated $575 to $2500. (See footnote on p. 50.)

ADVANTAGES

1. You do not have to be seen without teeth
2. Helps keep ridge protected during healing following extractions
3. Easier transition to final denture
4. Can act as final denture

DISADVANTAGES

1. May require a final denture to be made
2. Possible added expense
3. Requires relining
4. May require frequent adjustments

Full Denture

One of the primary advantages of the full denture is its ability to maintain or even recreate lip and cheek support. Without this support, facial tissue sinks in, giving an aged look.

Esthetically, however, the full denture is a mixed blessing. On the one hand, it allows the dentist to change almost anything you want in your smile. On the other hand, after you lose your teeth the normal "landmarks" are gone—and so is the memory of how the teeth used to look.

Be patient and work with a dentist who is willing to help you obtain the smile you desire. Also remember that dentures wear just as natural teeth do. If you want to keep your facial support in tone, your dentures will eventually need to be relined or remade.

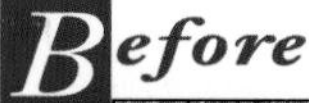

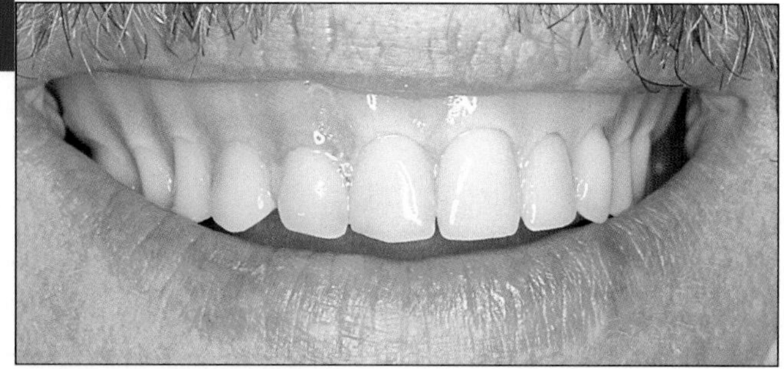

FALSE-LOOKING UPPER DENTURE

This 27-year-old physical education teacher was unhappy with his lipline, which exposed a considerable amount of gum. Although his bite was comfortable, he was displeased with the false appearance of his upper full denture.

After

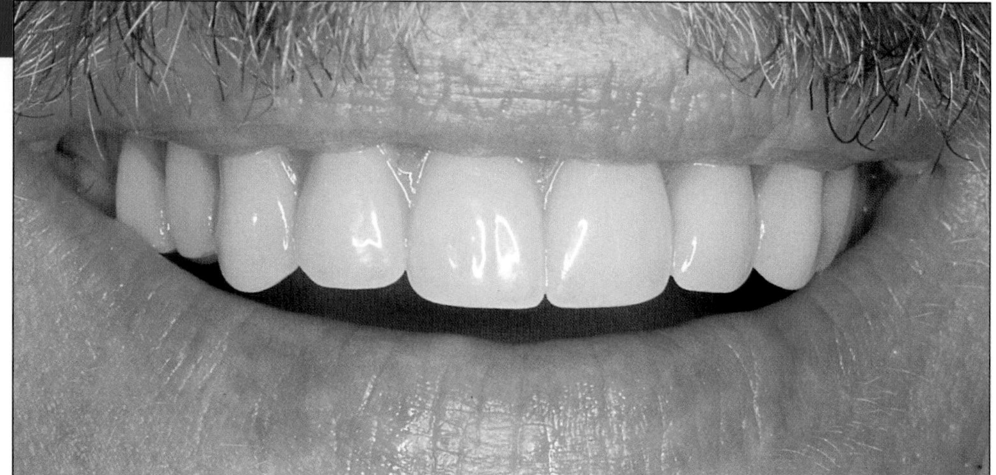

NEW DENTURE

A handsome smile resulted from a new full denture with larger teeth, which were repositioned so they could be inserted higher up into the arch. This dramatic change avoided so much show of gum.

Before

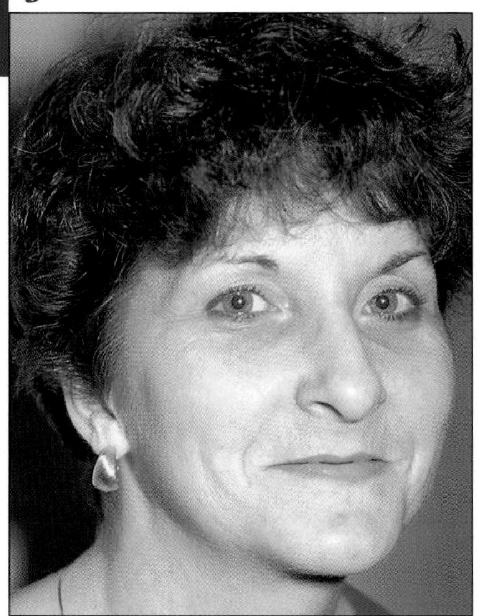

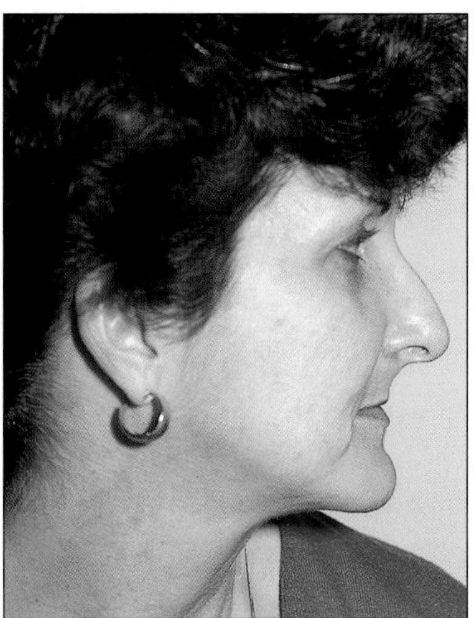

Missing teeth causing poor lip and cheek support

When teeth are present and in good position, the lips and cheeks are properly supported. If the teeth are lost and not replaced, part of the facial-tissue support is also lost.

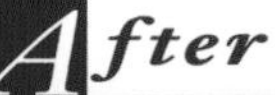

After

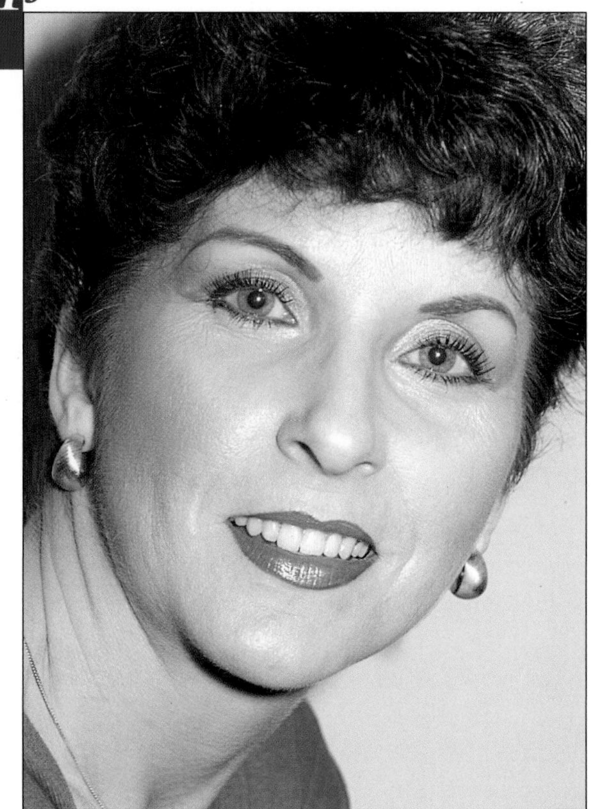

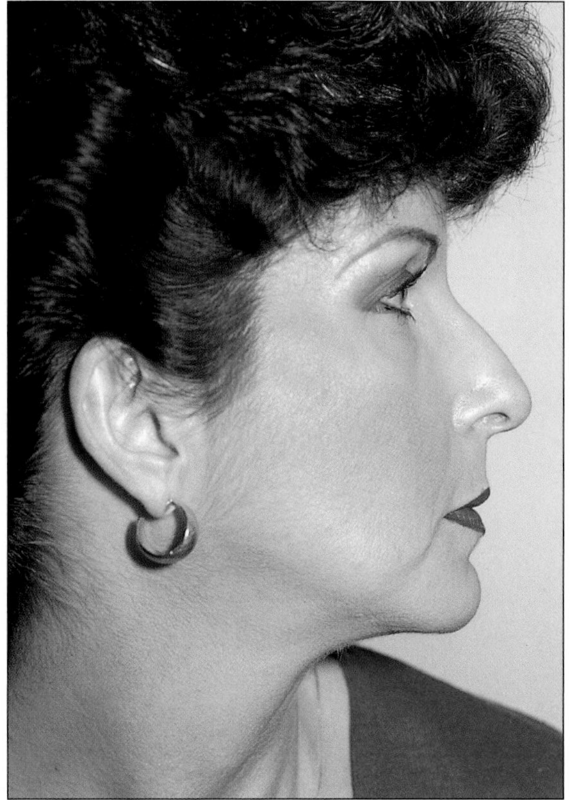

New full denture

A new full denture with properly positioned teeth can often restore missing facial support. Notice how much more youthful and attractive this woman's face is with a new lipline and makeup.

TREATMENT SUMMARY

FULL DENTURE

Treatment Time Two to four weeks.

Patient Maintenance Cleaning after meals to remove and prevent stains on denture.

Results of Treatment Esthetically pleasing results are possible.

Average Range of Treatment Life Expectancy Five to ten years. Tooth fracture may occur, and the need for relining may be necessary during this time. (See footnote on p. 50.)

Cost Estimated $525 to $4000 for upper and lower dentures (up to two to three times this amount for "special" cosmetic dentures).(See footnote on p. 50.)

ADVANTAGES

1. Maximum esthetics possible
2. More youthful appearance obtainable
3. Supports lips and cheeks
4. Can improve speech

DISADVANTAGES

1. Less chewing efficiency
2. Retention may be a problem
3. Needs maintenance
4. May need to be replaced every five to ten years
5. May impede speech in some instances

Tips for Denture Wearers

- Have a spare denture made in case of emergency.
- If you anticipate getting dentures, have your dentist make photographs and models of your teeth that can serve as a guide later.
- If you've lost all your teeth, make sure your full denture looks like natural teeth rather than a "perfect set." That way, no one will know you have dentures.
- Have your dentist check your gums regularly for proper fit. A denture that moves can affect speech and appearance and can make eating difficult.

5

Replacing Missing Teeth with Implants

For years, physicians have used various types of implants to replace missing body parts such as hip and shoulder joints. Today, dentists can replace missing teeth in much the same way. Dental implants have become a viable—and esthetic—dental replacement for thousands of patients.

What exactly is a dental implant? It is simply a metal or ceramic device that replaces the root of the natural tooth. After an implant is placed into the underlying bone, artificial teeth are attached to it, enabling normal function.

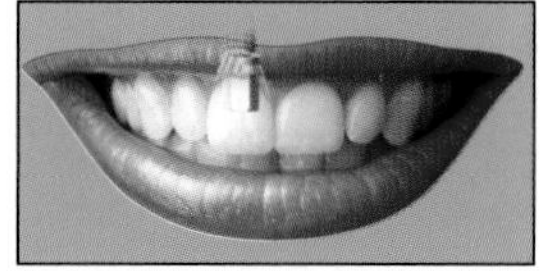

Whether an implant is right for you depends on where the implant will be placed, the kind and amount of bone available in the jaw, and the design of the tooth or teeth that will be placed on the implant. Your dentist can discuss the options with you and help you determine which is best for you.

Who Can Place Implants?

Implant treatment is usually provided by a team including a surgeon (a periodontist or an oral surgeon) to place the implant, and a technician and restorative dentist to fabricate the restoration and attach the tooth or teeth.

Although implant dentistry is not a formal dental specialty, many practitioners have undergone extensive implant training and some even limit their practices to implant treatment. In such cases, the implant dentist may perform both the surgical and the restorative phase of treatment.

If you are considering dental implants, discuss all of your options with your dentist. Don't be afraid to ask questions and to seek a second opinion. Implant treatment is complex, and not all dentists perform it. Choose someone with experience; you want to receive the best care possible.

The Stages of Treatment

Implants are not a quick fix. Treatment requires several months. First, your mouth will be examined thoroughly, and X-rays of your head, jaw and teeth will be taken. Impressions or molds of your teeth and jaws will also be made so that the dentist can determine exactly where the implants should be placed. The implant site is an important key to the success of the treatment. Additionally, you may also be required to undergo blood tests as well as a physical examination to determine your overall health status.

Once you and your dentist have decided which treatment option is right for you, surgery will be scheduled. The surgical phase of implant treatments is typically performed in two stages, although it can sometimes be done in one stage. During the first operation, an incision is made in the gums, the implants are placed beneath the tissue, and the gum is stitched back into place. This phase of surgery can be performed under local anesthesia in the dentist's office or under general anesthesia in a hospital or clinic.

THE SURGICAL PHASE OF IMPLANT TREATMENT IS TYPICALLY PERFORMED IN TWO STAGES

Following surgery, you will experience some swelling and discoloration of the gums as well as some discomfort, which can be relieved with medication. Within a few days, the gums should return to normal, and you will be able to resume most of your routine activities. To allow the implants to heal properly, a soft diet is recommended for four to six weeks.

The second stage of surgery is usually performed three to six months after the first in an outpatient setting. The dentist will numb the areas with local anesthetic and open the gum to expose the implants. He or she will then attach extension posts or "abutments" to the implants. The gums are then stitched into place around the abutments and a temporary restoration placed. At times, additional gum surgery may be required for esthetic reasons. If you are missing all of your teeth, a surgical pack or your old dentures (relined with a soft material) will be placed over the abutments to promote healing and reduce discomfort. Additional impressions may be taken of your mouth so that the dentist knows where to position your new teeth. You will also be taught how to keep the abutments clean.

About a month later, your new teeth will be fitted. In some cases, they will be attached to a metal framework. In other cases, the artificial teeth may be attached to natural teeth or stand alone

Several checkups will be scheduled during the following year so that your dentist can ensure that your implants are functioning properly. After that, you will need regular maintenance checkups with your dentist and hygienist team. Follow-up X-rays will be taken regularly.

Home Care Is Important

Just because implants are not "real" teeth does not mean oral hygiene is less important. Plaque accumulation on implants can cause inflammation of the gums, and eventually loss of bone surrounding the teeth. Therefore, thorough cleaning twice a day is critical. Your dentist will discuss the best method for taking care of your particular implant and may even recommend certain plaque-removal appliances that will help you maintain good oral health.

Before

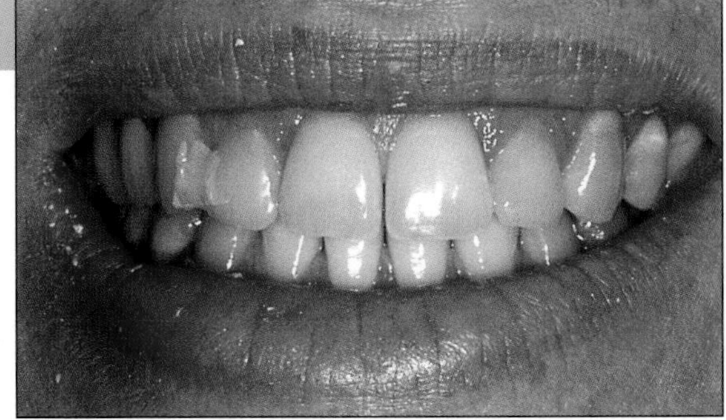

FRACTURED TOOTH IN PLACE

This lady fractured her upper left lateral incisor in an auto accident.

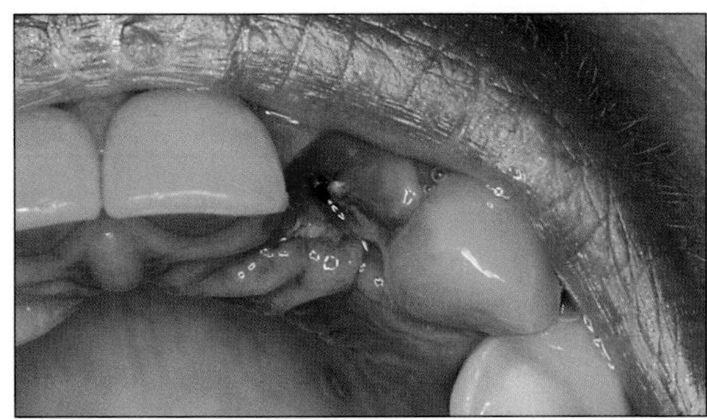

This photo shows the the remaining root.

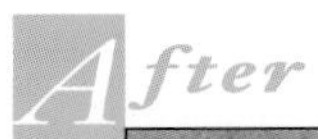

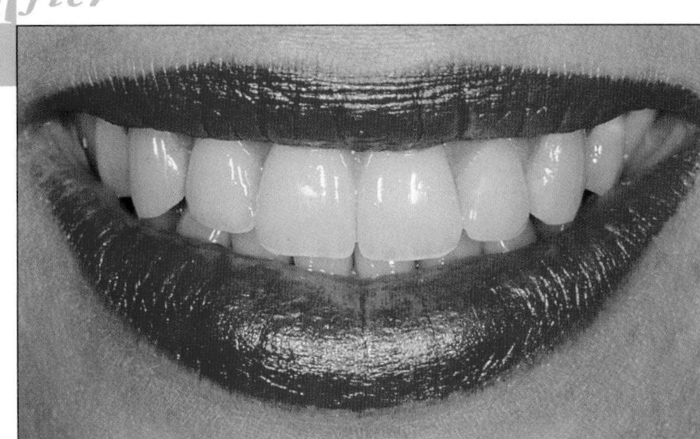

SINGLE-TOOTH IMPLANT AND CROWN

An implant restored the missing tooth with a porcelain-bonded-to-metal crown.

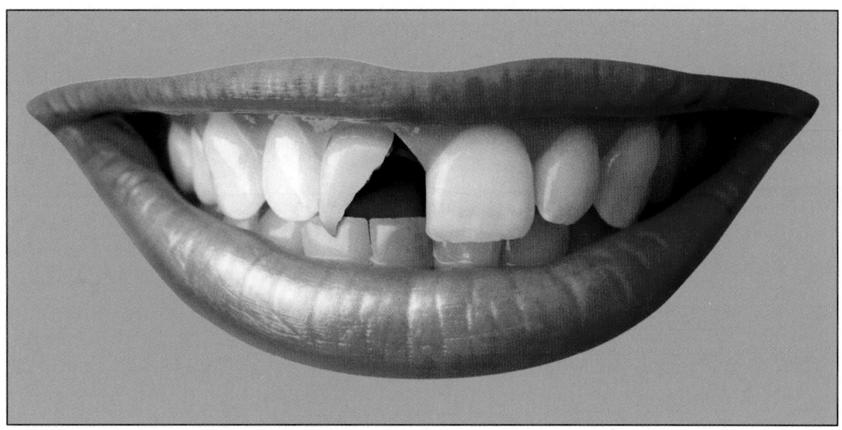

A fractured tooth that requires extraction.

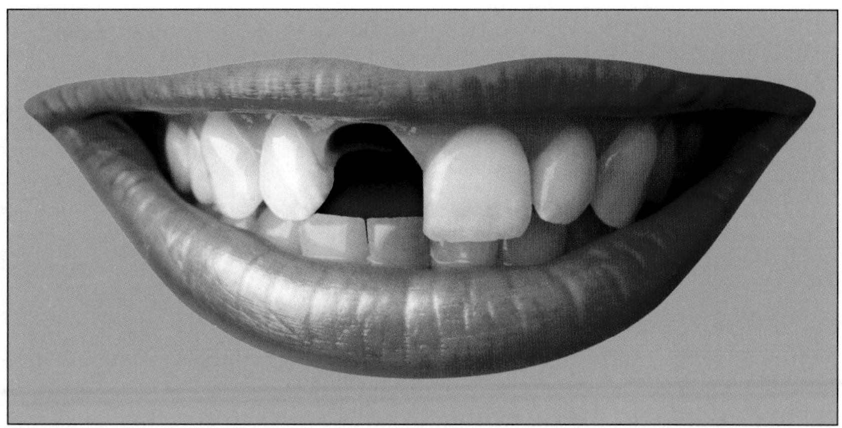

Appearance of the gum after the tooth extraction.

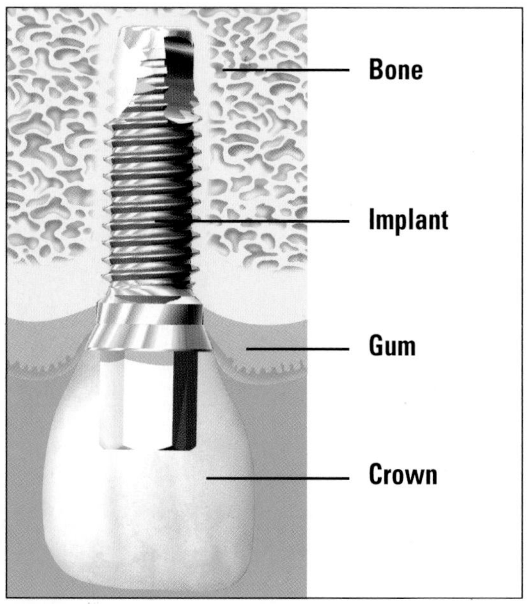

An implant has been surgically placed where the fractured tooth was extracted. A new crown will later be attached to the implant.

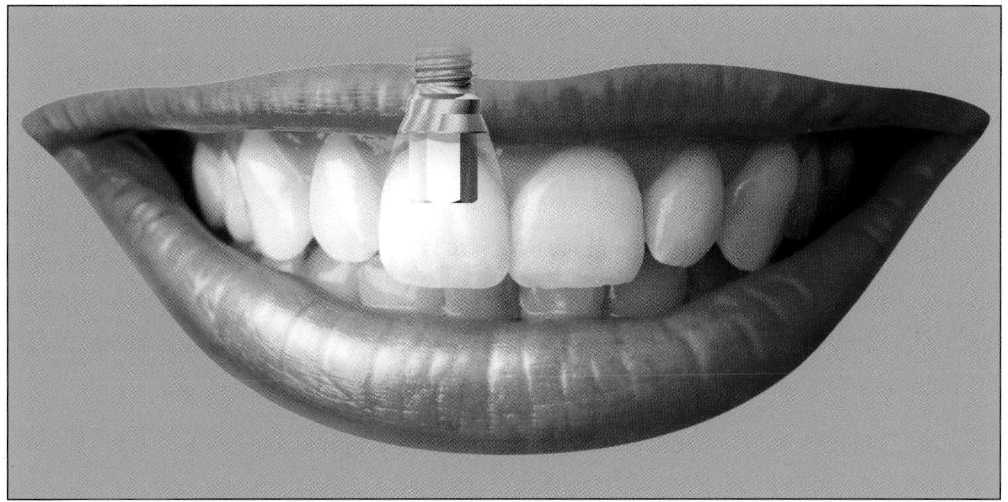

This cross-section shows how a ceramic crown is fitted to a bone-supported implant.

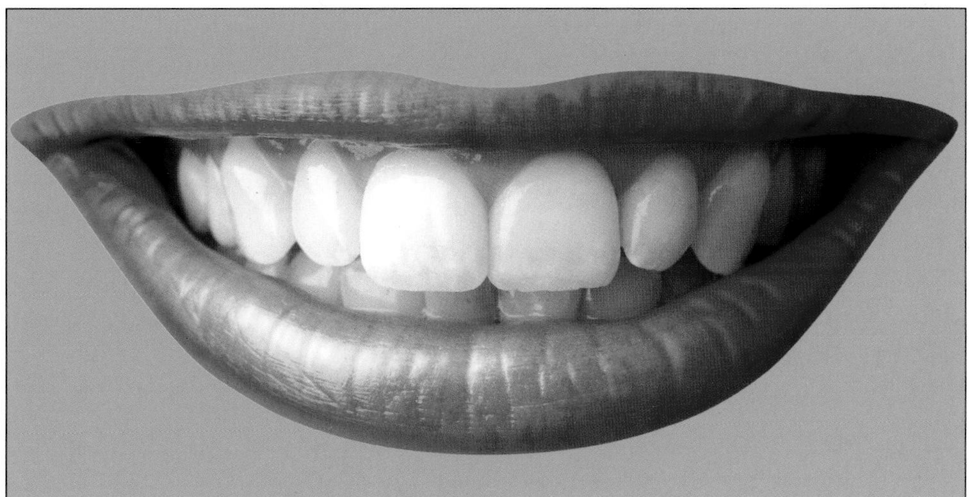

The final result after implant and crown placement is both functional and esthetic.

Not Just for Single Teeth

Patients with multiple missing teeth can also benefit from implant treatment. If sufficient bone is present, patients who have worn a fixed or removable bridge can opt for implant-supported bridges. This means that even if you have worn a fixed bridge, a removable partial denture or a full denture, you may still be a good candidate for implant dentistry. Implants also act as an excellent source of anchorage for patients with loose or ill-fitting dentures.

There is also good news for patients who have been told previously that they do not have sufficient bone for implant placement. If the surgeon, after evaluating your bone quantity or quality on special radiographs (X-rays), or even a CAT scan, believes there is not enough bone for implant placement, he or she may recommend a bone graft. A bone graft involves taking a small amount of bone from another part of your body (such as your hip) to replace lost bone elsewhere. After a period of healing, sufficient bone should be available for implant placement.

Implant therapy has been tremendously beneficial to patients who have been unable to wear, or do not want to wear, removable or fixed bridges.

Implants Are Not for Everyone

Dental implants are not the right restorative choice for every patient. First, you must have enough healthy jawbone to support an implant, or you may require a bone graft. Gum tissues should be disease-free. Patients with medical conditions that affect the body's ability to heal and repair itself, such as diabetes and cancer, as well as patients with conditions affecting ability to use the hands and arms, are usually not good implant candidates. Likewise, patients who are not committed to thorough home care are better off with other restorative options.

Treatment Summary

Implants

Treatment Time Surgical placement time per implant is approximately one hour depending on the complexity of the procedure. Healing is approximately three months in the lower jaw and six months in the upper jaw while the implant permanently attaches to the bone. After healing, another appointment may be necessary to uncover the implant and place a healing cap so your dentist can construct a final crown.

Patient Maintenance Daily flossing and home care as instructed by your dentist. Professional cleanings four times per year. Exam by restorative dentist at least once a year.

Results of Treatment Best approximates having your own natural tooth (or teeth). Provides tooth that is natural appearing and individually functioning. Avoids unnecessary tooth structure removal on natural adjacent teeth.

Average Range of Treatment Life Expectancy Once successfully integrated into the bone, the implant can last indefinitely, barring infection. The life expectancy of the restoration will be the same as described elsewhere in this book (for a crown, five to fifteen years). (See footnote on p. 50.)

Cost $985 to $2800 per implant. (See footnote on p. 50.)

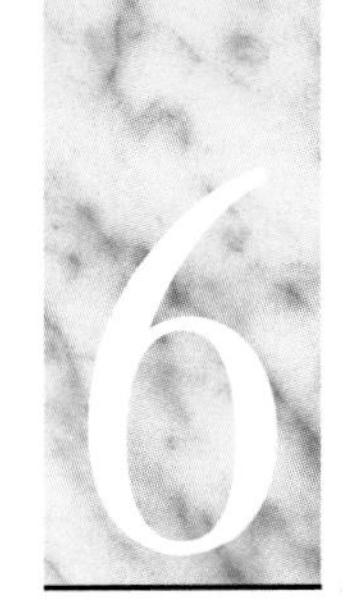

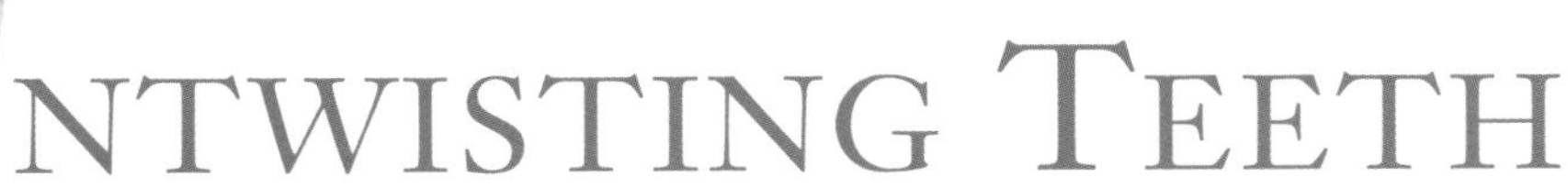

Untwisting Teeth

Living with anything less than beautiful, straight white teeth can be a source of great unhappiness. If you have crowded or crooked teeth that overlap, protrude or recede in a haphazard fashion, it may be perceived as a personal disfigurement. It is, however, possible to remedy this situation. This chapter will tell you how it's done.

There's More Than One Way

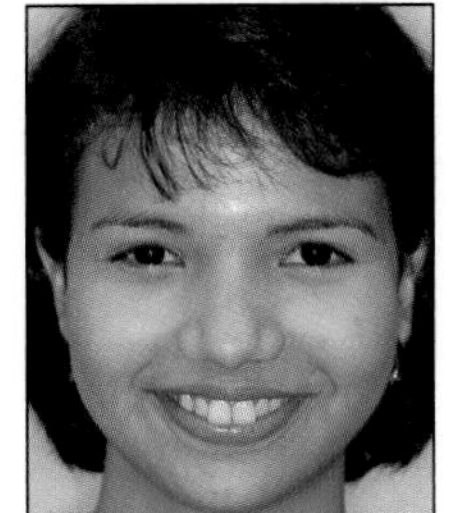

Contrary to popular belief, orthodontic straightening is not the only way to treat crowded teeth. Less expensive and less time-consuming methods may be used if the problem is not too severe. The objective of esthetic treatment is to give an illusion of straight teeth. Although the teeth may not be in perfect alignment, if they give the impression that they are, the esthetic goal will have been reached.

Such an illusion can sometimes be achieved with cosmetic contouring, a simple and painless reshaping procedure performed by reducing some of the tooth structure with finely ground diamonds. If cosmetic contouring isn't a viable solution, composite resin bonding may be an effective alternative because the fronts or backs of the teeth involved can be "built out" to fall in line with neighboring teeth. This procedure is usually performed in conjunction with cosmetic contouring.

Crowning has limited use for crowded and crooked teeth because the orientation of the tooth to be crowned must be aligned compatibly with the surrounding teeth. If it isn't, the crown won't be able to compensate for the difference. In other words, the same problem that existed with the natural tooth will also exist with the crown.

If orthodontics is performed, the teeth eventually will become aligned compatibly. Sometimes this is the only solution for extremely malpositioned teeth. If you have crowded teeth, chances are orthodontic treatment will be your best bet for the longest-lasting, most economical and best-looking solution.

CROWDED OR CROOKED TEETH MAY REQUIRE A COMBINATION OF TECHNIQUES

Crowded or crooked teeth may require a combination of techniques described in this chapter. Your ideal treatment, for example, may include orthodontics to reposition the teeth followed by bonding or crowning to improve esthetics. Although models can be used to show projected results, the choice of treatment ultimately depends upon your commitment of time and money, as well as your dental and esthetic needs.

Cosmetic Contouring: An Esthetic Compromise

Cosmetic contouring of the natural teeth has long been used for esthetic purposes. In fact, there is evidence that it is one of the oldest dental procedures known to man. A two thousand-year-old Mayan skull shows teeth contoured into points for cosmetic purposes. Even today, the Waiwire men of Central Africa point their teeth for esthetic reasons. If they don't, they may not be able to find a wife!

In modern dentistry, cosmetic contouring is used to improve the appearance of the teeth by giving the illusion of uniformity and alignment. When performed successfully, it is generally the most preferred therapy because no anesthesia is required, it is relatively inexpensive, and it takes less time than most other procedures. Moreover, function is often improved through cosmetic contouring. Reshaping and polishing malpositioned teeth make them easy to clean and reduce the likelihood of fracture.

Where other procedures are too expensive, cosmetic contouring provides a good compromise. In fact, in a two-year study of fifty beauty contestants, cosmetic contouring could have improved the smiles of more than 95 percent of the women. Perhaps even more startling is the fact that cosmetic contouring alone was indicated as the ideal treatment in 40 percent of the cases! If you have slightly crowded teeth, cosmetic contouring may provide an excellent solution to your problem as well.

Before

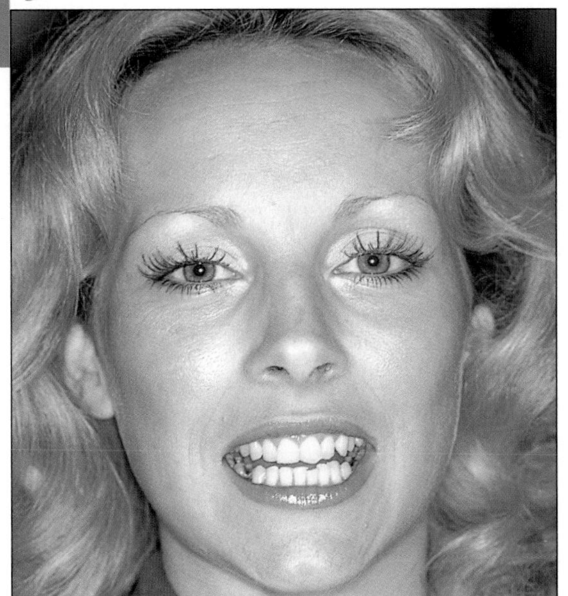

Overlapping, crowded front teeth

This 29-year-old model and actress had overlapping, crowded front teeth. She was naturally concerned about being restricted from making close-up photographs, but ruled out orthodontics as a means of treatment because she wanted immediate results. She was also reluctant to have her teeth reduced for crowning.

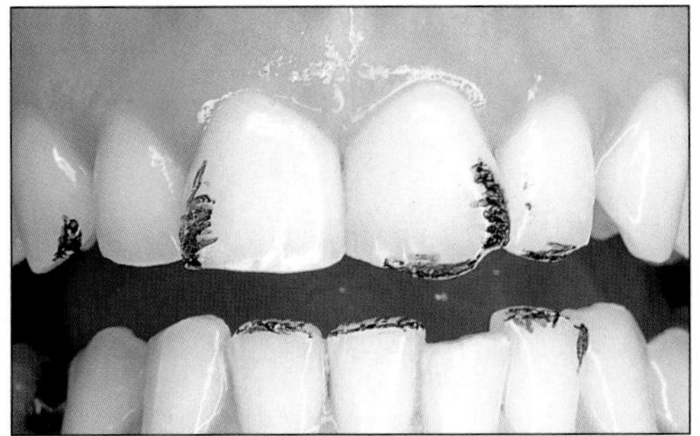

Since cosmetic contouring was decided upon as the restorative treatment, the teeth were marked to show the patient approximately where they would be reshaped.

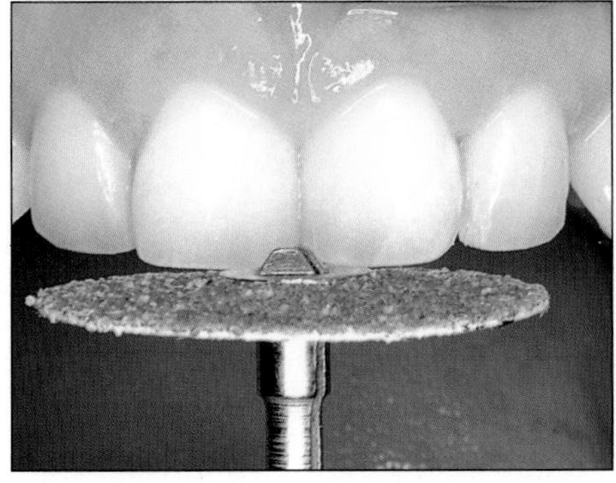

No anesthetic was required for cosmetic contouring. Here a rotary sandpaper disk is being used to level the teeth followed by repolishing.

After

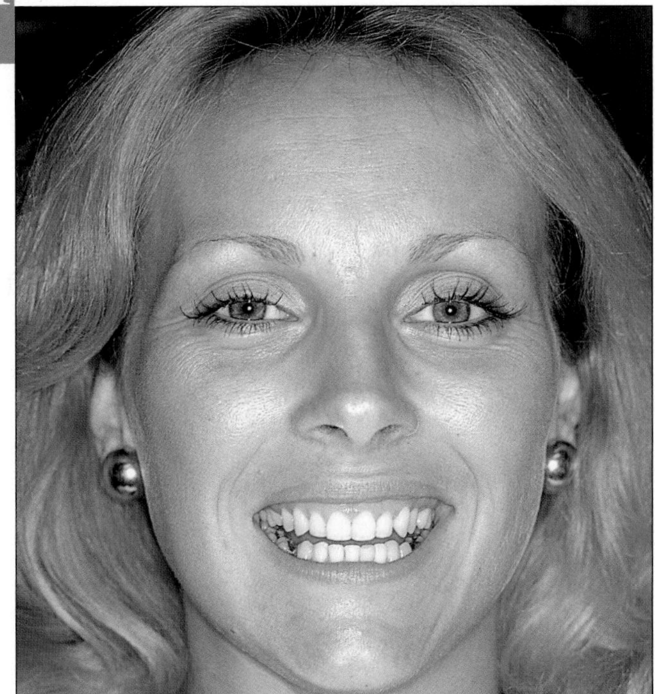

Cosmetic contouring

It took approximately one hour to cosmetically contour these teeth. The fractured lower tooth was later bonded with composite resin. You can see how an illusion of straightness was accomplished by recontouring the overlapping areas of these teeth. This is the most economical of all cosmetic procedures and in situations like this it can give dramatic results.

Before

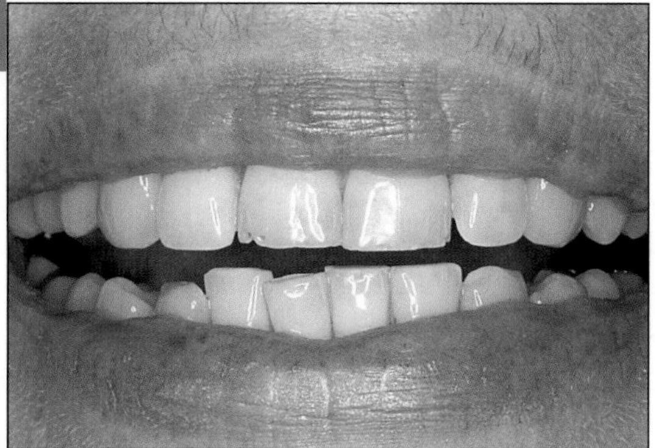

Crowded and worn dentition

This lady was displeased that her crowded and worn teeth were aging her smileline.

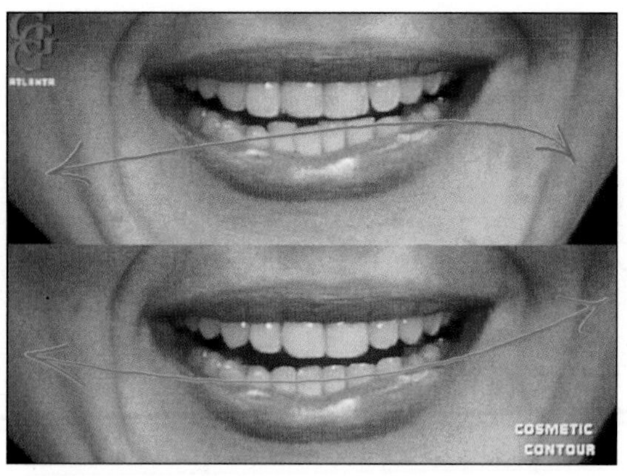

Computer imaging shows how her elongated lateral incisors helped to create a reverse smileline. The bottom image shows the ideal curve created by cosmetic contouring.

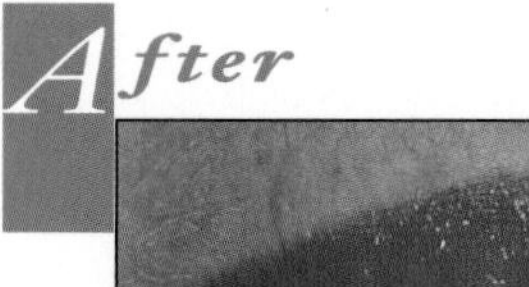

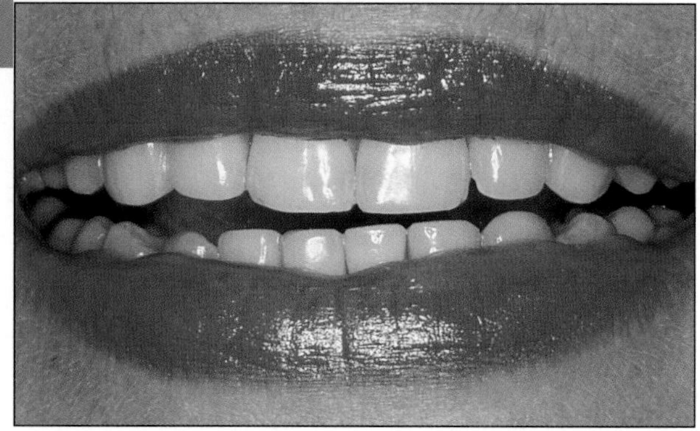

Cosmetic contouring

The corrected smile closely resembles the anticipated result.

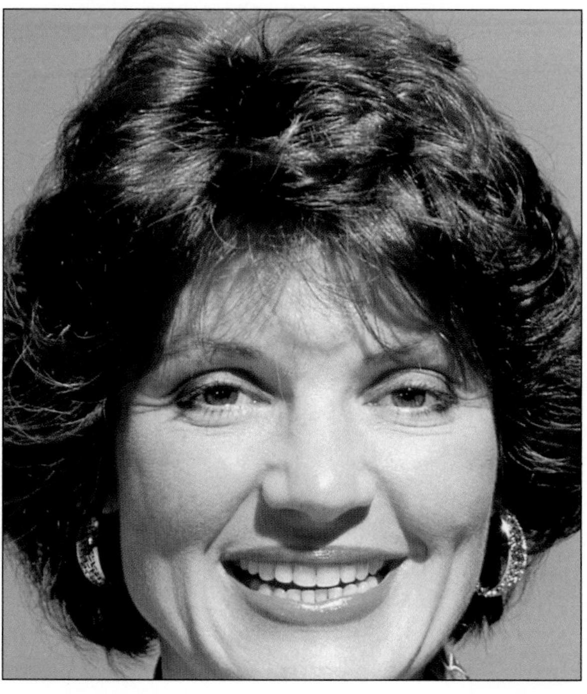

Correcting distractions such as a crooked nose or a tooth defect make it much easier to focus on the entire face rather than the esthetic problem.

Before

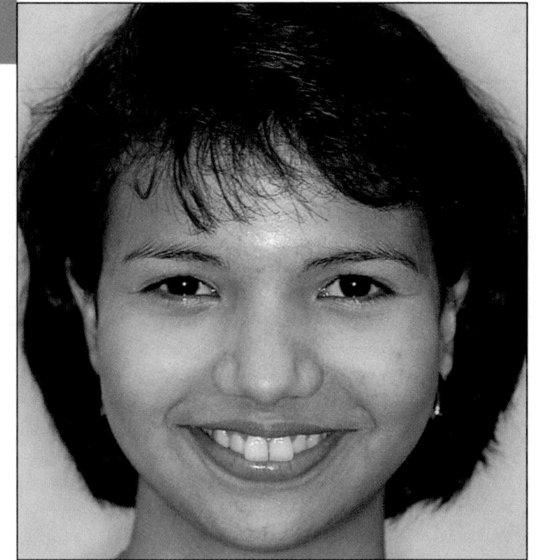

PROTRUDING CENTRAL INCISORS

This young woman had protruding front teeth that she wanted corrected without orthodontics.

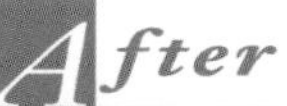

After

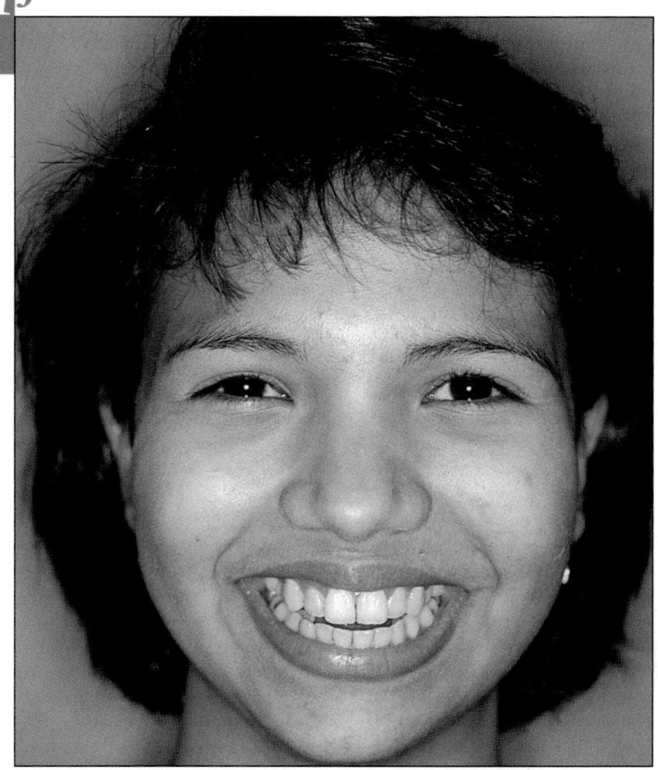

COSMETIC CONTOURING

Although repositioning of the front teeth would have been the ideal treatment, the patient preferred a compromise therapy. Cosmetic contouring was elected to help create the illusion of straighter teeth in one appointment.

Factors to Consider

Several factors should be considered before cosmetic contouring is begun. First, your dentist should evaluate your natural teeth and the effect that contouring may have on them. The bite must be correct if the health of the teeth, as well as the proper distribution of pressure during normal oral functioning, is to be maintained.

Second, the thickness of the tooth enamel must be checked. The removal of too much enamel can expose the underlying dentin, resulting in discoloration. This, of course, would defeat the esthetic objective. Removal of too much enamel may also cause the tooth to weaken and fracture or to become more susceptible to decay.

Occasionally, a conflict arises between maintaining maximum function and achieving maximum esthetics. In these cases, the final decision should be based on a trade-off among esthetics, the degree of bite change that will occur and the future health of the tooth. A plaster model cast also should be constructed so that you can see the limitations in your particular case.

COSMETIC CONTOURING IS NOT RECOMMENDED FOR YOUNG CHILDREN

Finally, cosmetic contouring is not recommended for young children. Because children have a large amount of sensitive pulp tissue in their tooth structure, cosmetic contouring can cause them discomfort—not only during the procedure, but afterward. Therefore, it is best to delay cosmetic contouring until after the formative growth years.

TREATMENT SUMMARY

COSMETIC CONTOURING

Treatment Time About one hour.

Patient Maintenance Normal brushing and flossing.

Results of Treatment Immediate reshaping of tooth structure makes crowded teeth appear the appropriate size.

Average Range of Treatment Life Expectancy Indefinite. (See footnote on p. 50.)

Cost $100 to $950. (See footnote on p. 50.)

ADVANTAGES

1. Less expensive than other forms of esthetic treatment
2. Permanent results
3. Immediate problem correction
4. Minimum treatment time
5. Generally painless; requires no anesthesia

DISADVANTAGES

1. Teeth are not repositioned
2. Improvement may be limited by functional consideration
3. Possibly some discomfort for children with large pulp canals
4. No improvement in color

Bonding: A Quick Compromise

Composite resin bonding also can be useful in treating crooked teeth. The treatment is often combined with cosmetic contouring so that less bonding is required. For example, the crowded teeth may be "built out" with bonding, while the edges of the adjacent teeth are shaped with cosmetic contouring. The result is an illusion of straightness that can be quite pleasing.

Bonding may also be used to lighten crowded teeth if they are discolored. However, if not all of the teeth are to be bonded, the adjacent teeth should be bleached before bonding is performed. Otherwise, some teeth will be much lighter than others—not an esthetically pleasing result!

The bite is the limiting factor when bonding the lower front teeth. Bonding of these teeth may not be successful because of the way the upper teeth may contact them. However, it is sometimes possible to reduce the amount of stress on the lower teeth by altering the way in which the upper teeth contact them.

If your crowded teeth are causing a narrowed or constricted arch, consider orthodontics. If this isn't feasible, however, a combined treatment consisting of cosmetic contouring and bonding may help correct arch malalignment.

Before

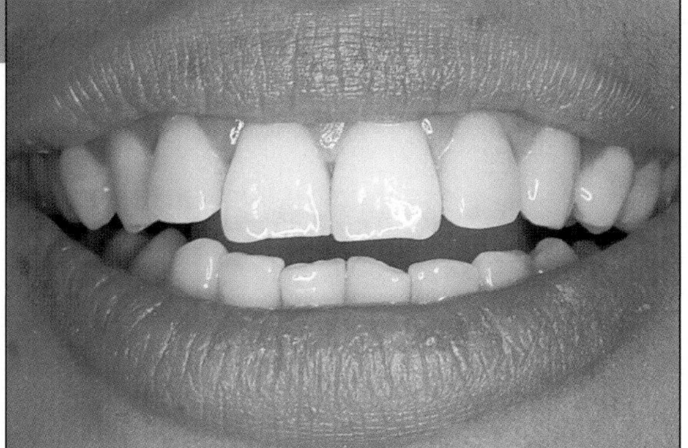

Crowded and worn upper and lower teeth

This television producer wanted to improve her smile without wearing braces if possible.

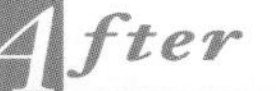

After

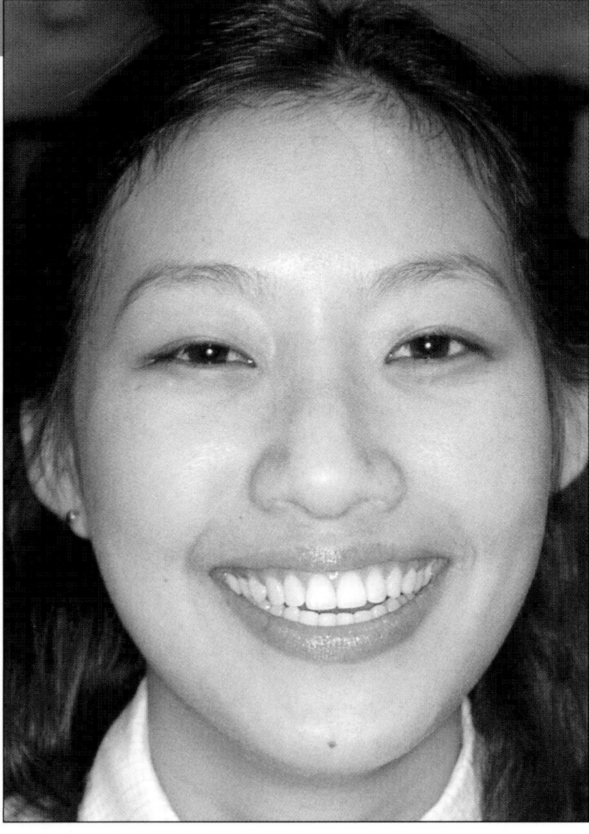

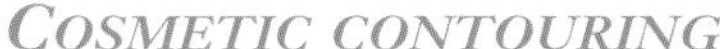

Cosmetic contouring

A one-hour appointment was all it took to help create an illusion of straight teeth and a new smile.

Before

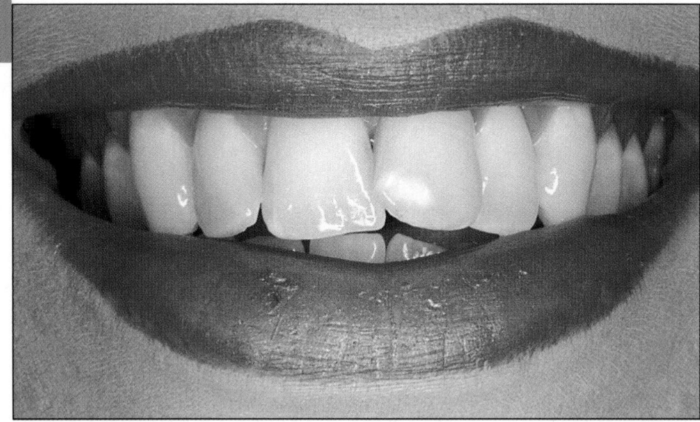

Crowded and Overlapping Front Teeth

This 28-year-old model had a beautiful face, but her crowded front teeth ruined her smile. As a compromise to orthodontic treatment, composite resin bonding was selected to help her teeth look straighter.

After

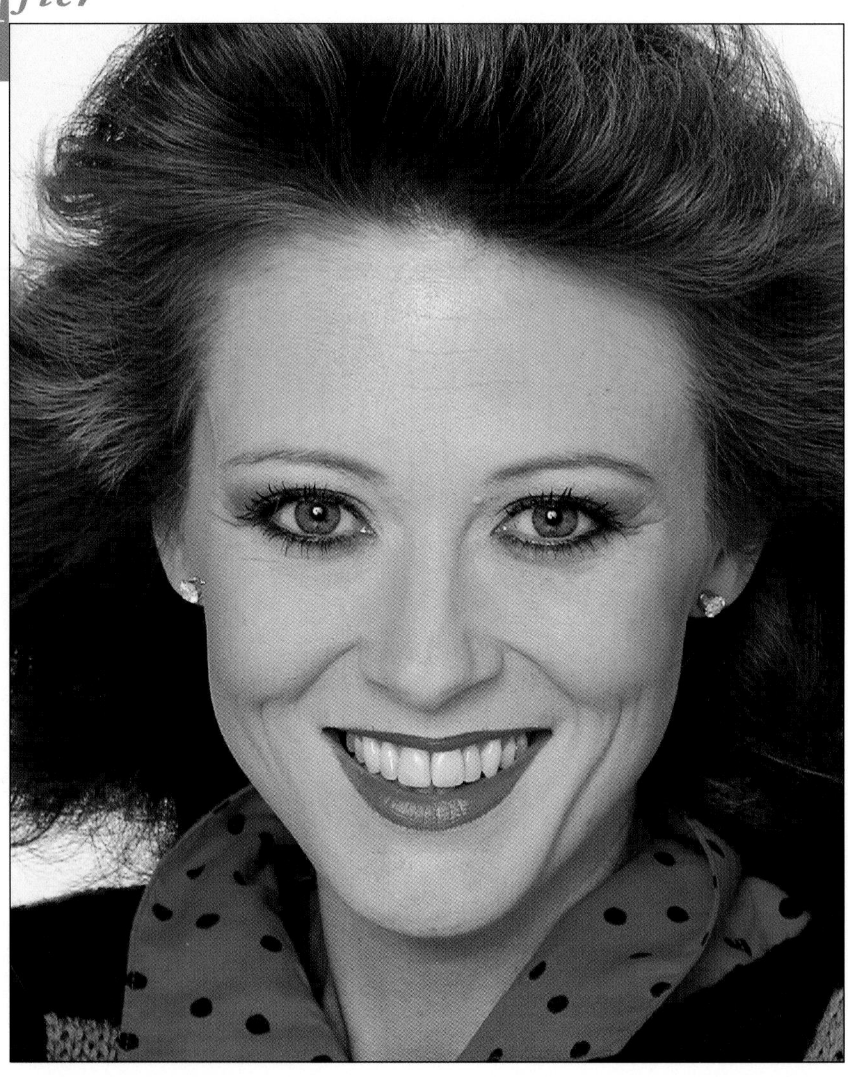

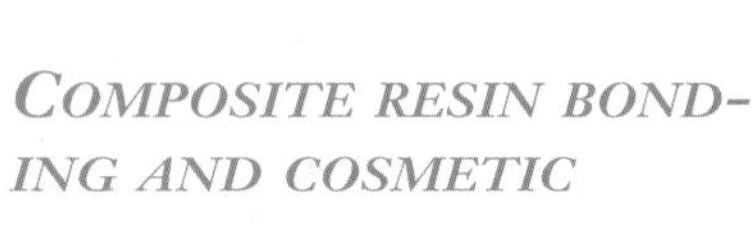

Composite Resin Bonding and Cosmetic Contouring

Three front teeth were bonded with an extremely fine composite resin to create a polished surface. Cosmetic contouring of both the upper and lower teeth helped attain an illusion of straightness. Notice how much straighter the smileline is after this one-appointment procedure.

Before

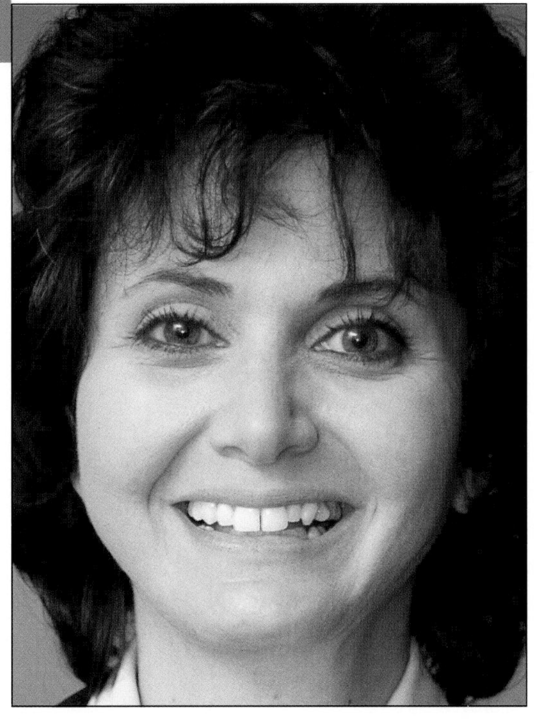

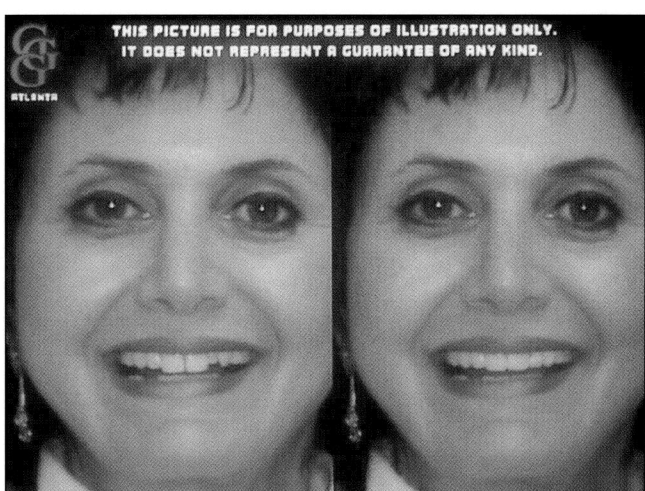

Computer imaging helps show both patient and doctor just how the final result can appear.

SMILE ASYMMETRY

This executive was dissatisfied with her asymmetrical smile and wanted to know if her teeth could be straightened without orthodontics.

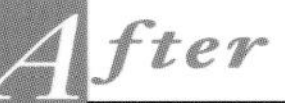

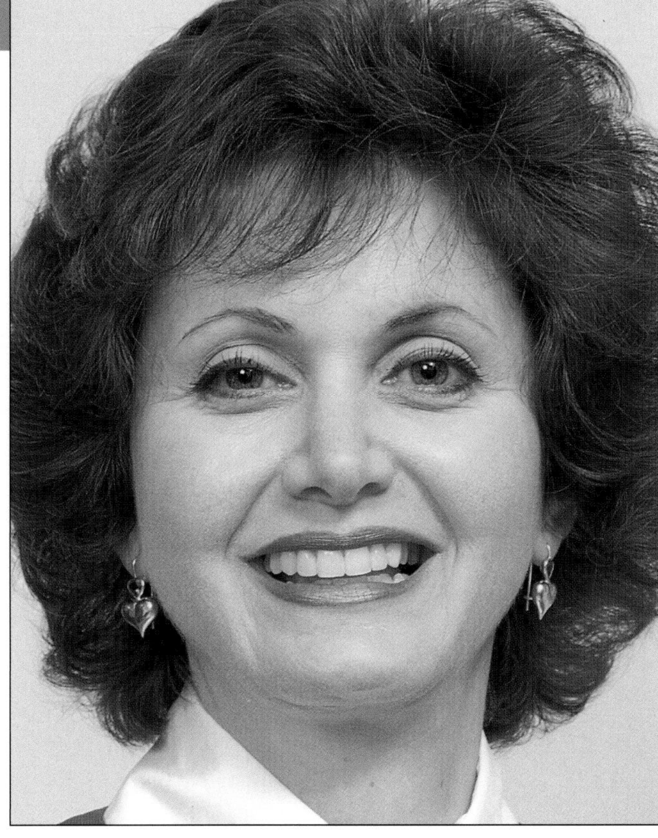

COMPOSITE RESIN BONDING, COSMETIC CONTOURING AND BLEACHING

A combination of treatments helped achieve the result seen here. Notice how much straighter and whiter-looking teeth can help brighten not only the smile but the entire face.

Before

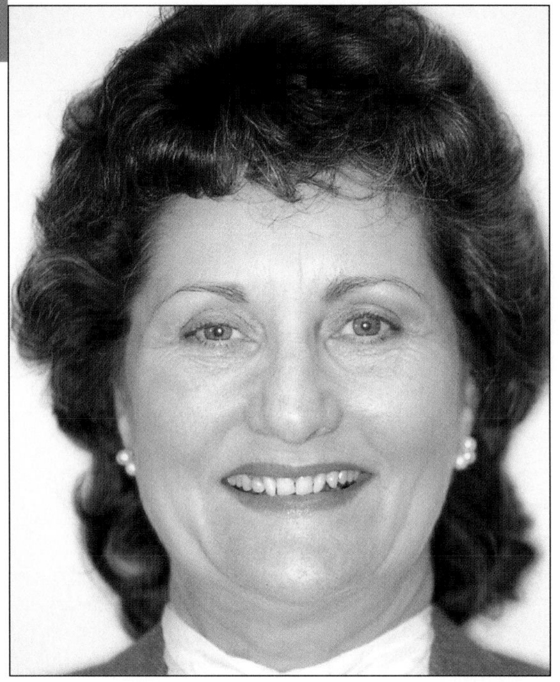

Overlapping lateral incisors

When the lateral incisors overlap the central incisors, they not only destroy proportion in the smile but create spaces as well. This lady also has a retained baby tooth.

After

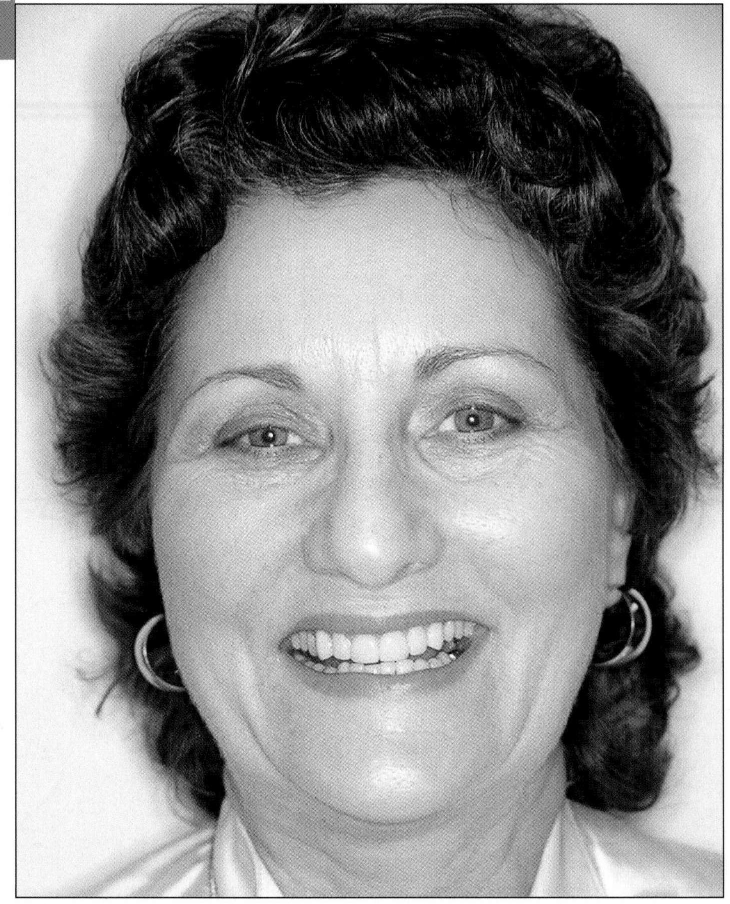

Composite resin bonding and cosmetic contouring

After slightly reproportioning the teeth, direct composite resin was placed on the front teeth. Note the improved proportion in size and form that occurred with this one-appointment procedure.

Before

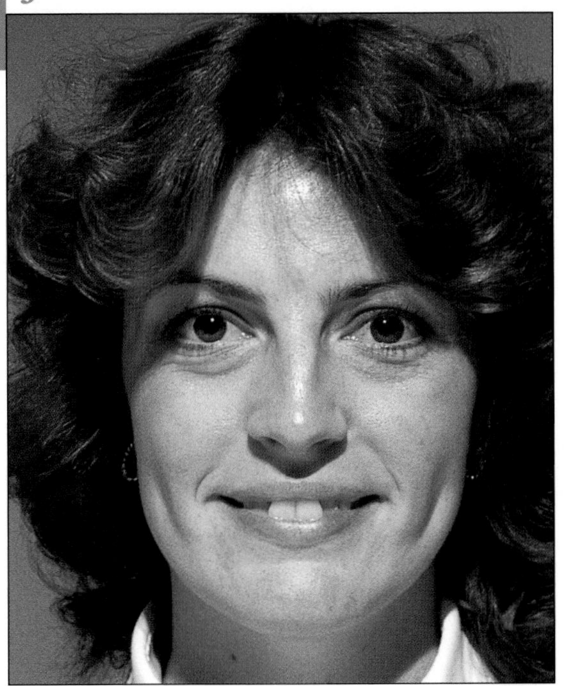

Overlapping front teeth

This 30-year-old horse trainer disliked her overlapping front teeth.

After

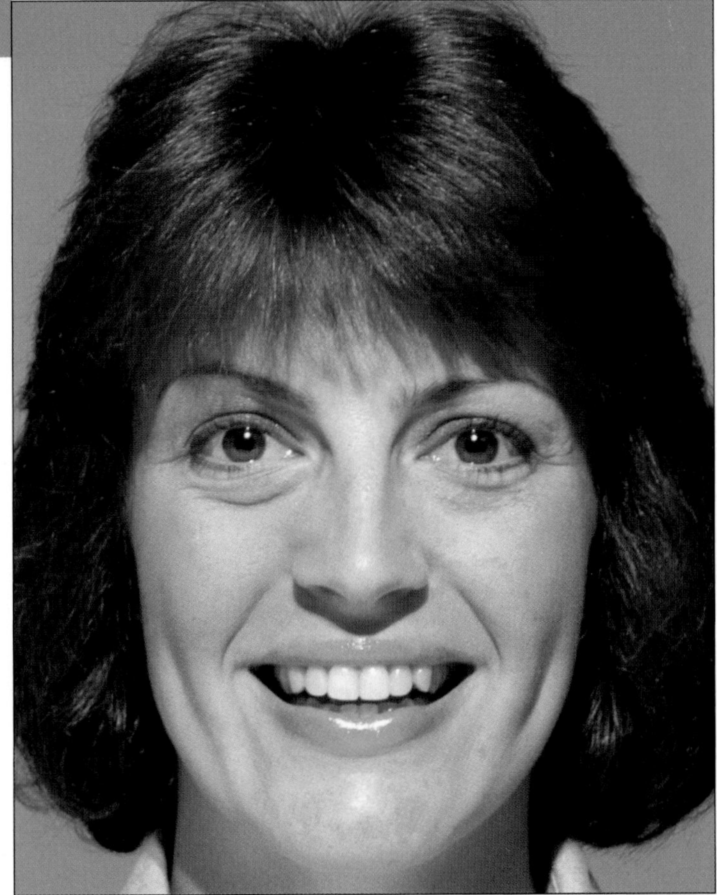

Composite resin bonding and cosmetic contouring

The upper two front teeth were cosmetically contoured to look narrower and to reduce some of the overlap. The adjacent lateral incisors were then built out with composite resin to blend in line with the newly contoured central incisors. This helped to round out the arch, making the teeth look much straighter. The entire procedure was done in one appointment without anesthesia. Notice how much more attractive the smile and face can be when improved teeth are combined with a new hairstyle.

Treatment Summary

Bonding

Treatment Time One to two hours per tooth.

Patient Maintenance Professional cleaning three to four times yearly. Eat wisely—these teeth can chip easily. Floss in and pull it through rather than popping the floss out. Expect some chipping or porosity to eventually occur requiring a repair.

Results of Treatment Straighter teeth in one appointment.

Average Range of Treatment Life Expectancy Five to eight years. (See footnote on p. 50.)

Cost $175 to $950 per tooth; repairs can run $65 to $285. (See footnote on p. 50.)

Advantages

1. Conservative because there is little or no reduction of tooth structure
2. Reversible procedure
3. More economical than laminating or crowning
4. No anesthesia required
5. Teeth appear straighter

Disadvantages

1. Does not reposition the tooth
2. The gums can become inflamed because of the crowding; in this case the basic problem is not corrected
3. Needs to be redone more often
4. Can stain or chip more than crowns
5. Teeth may appear somewhat thicker

Laminating: The Newest Solution

Laminating with composite resin or porcelain can also provide a reasonable compromise to orthodontic treatment in many cases. Esthetic improvement of overlapping or crowded teeth is first accomplished by cosmetic contouring. An impression is then taken of the prepared teeth, and a model is made. Using this model, the dentist constructs and arranges straighter-looking laminate veneers. In the case of porcelain veneers, the contoured teeth are etched with acid before the veneers are placed. A dentin bonding agent is then applied, which holds the veneer to the tooth.

In general, teeth that are oriented inward are built out. Although this technique creates the illusion of straightness, it also adds bulk to the teeth. It may take a week or two to relearn proper speech patterns due to the increased thickness. Fortunately, however, few people have any trouble with their laminate veneers.

Before

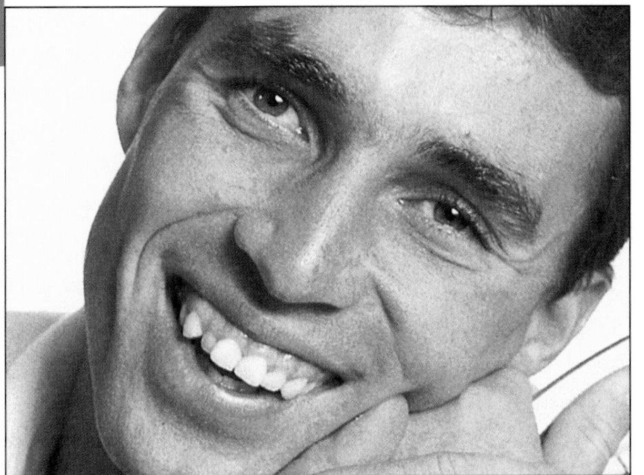

CROWDED TEETH, HIGH LIPLINE

This internationally known tennis personality wanted to improve his smile. This photo from a commercial advertisement shows not only a high lipline but tooth crowding with disproportionate teeth. (Photo courtesy of Swatch Inc.)

COMPUTER IMAGING

The patient had previously refused orthodontics, but computer imaging helped convince him that an esthetic compromise could be achieved through conservative gum surgery combined with porcelain laminates.

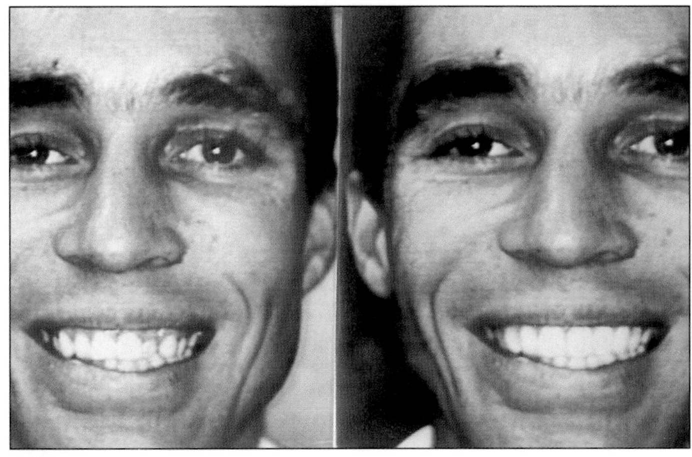

After

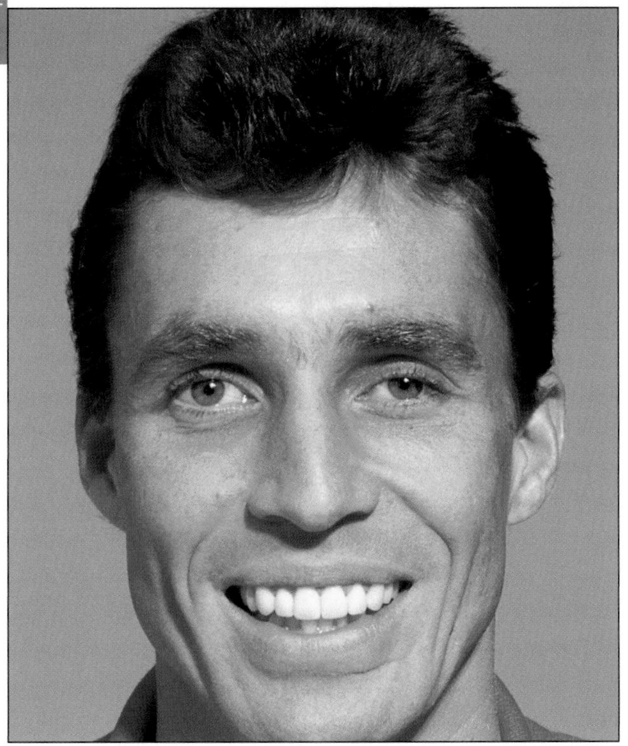

COSMETIC GUM SURGERY AND PORCELAIN LAMINATES

The final result shows a more handsome face with teeth that are more proportionate for his face.

TREATMENT SUMMARY

PORCELAIN LAMINATES

Treatment Time Two office visits. The teeth will be prepared and an impression made on the first visit, which can take from one to four hours. The laminates will be fitted and inserted at the second visit, which may take the same amount of time. Expect to spend more time for more extensive treatment.

Patient Maintenance The teeth should be professionally cleaned about three to four times yearly. Some precautions: as with bonding and crowning, take special care when chewing hard foods or biting into foods with your laminated teeth, to avoid chipping or potential fracture.

Results of Treatment A polished, natural-appearing result that can make teeth appear straighter.

Average Range of Treatment Life Expectancy Four to twelve years. (See footnote on p. 50).

Cost Approximately $450 to $2500 per tooth. (See footnote on p. 50.)

ADVANTAGES

1. Less chipping than with bonded restorations
2. Etched porcelain provides an extremely good bond to enamel
3. Wears less than the composite resin laminate
4. Less stain—does not lose color or luster
5. Can make more proportional results because they are constructed in lab
6. Lasts four to twelve years, as compared to plastics (three to ten years)
7. Gum tissue tolerates porcelain well
8. No anesthetic usually required

DISADVANTAGES

1. More costly than conventional bonding
2. More difficult to repair if the laminate cracks or chips
3. May eventually need repair or resealing of the margins if the cement washes out or debonds

Crowning: It Can Produce Dramatic Results

Crowning provides yet another way to correct the problem of crowded teeth. Although it is a much more involved treatment than cosmetic contouring or bonding, it may be a preferable alternative, particularly when teeth are erupting or when they recede at extreme angles from the root structure. In such cases, simply removing a little enamel does little or nothing to correct the problem.

Although crowning is more costly than the previously discussed cosmetic procedures (primarily because it must be performed during the course of several appointments), it can produce a more dramatic change. Adults who select orthodontic treatment for their children may choose crowning to treat their own overcrowding, especially if their teeth are damaged.

Tooth size is one of the major factors to consider when crowning because each tooth needs to be—or at least *appear* to be—proportional. The more teeth that are treated, the less obvious any distortions will be. If only one or two teeth are crowned, however, there may be a noticeable difference between the crowned teeth and the natural ones, depending on the space involved. Careful shaping through cosmetic contouring of both the teeth to be crowned, as well as the adjacent teeth, may make them appear more harmonious in size.

The more teeth that are treated, the less obvious any distortions will be

If you think you may want to crown your crooked teeth, it's wise to spend a little extra money for a wax-up. This will allow you to see the intended result before you reduce your natural teeth. *You can make a serious mistake by crowning a crooked tooth and thinking it is going to look terrific.* You may not be happy with the result. In such cases, you will not only have lost the money involved in getting crowns, but you will probably end up undergoing the treatment you should have gotten in the first place—orthodontics.

Before

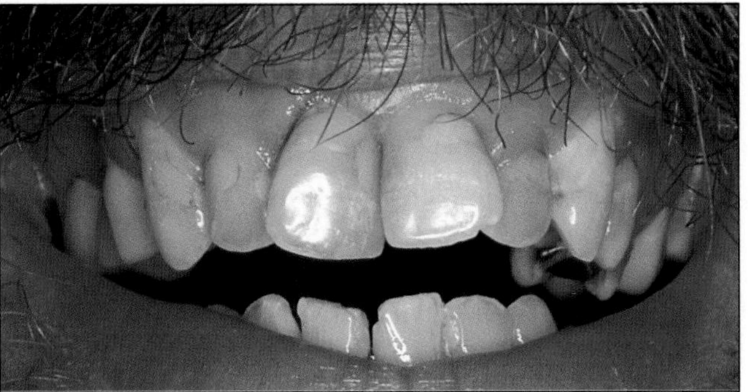

CROWDED AND DISCOLORED TEETH

Crowded and discolored upper teeth and spaces between the lower teeth spoiled the smile of this 38-year-old store owner. Although orthodontics was suggested as the ideal treatment, he chose a compromise that consisted of bonding the lower teeth and crowning the upper teeth.

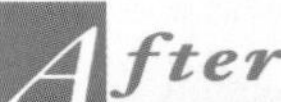
After

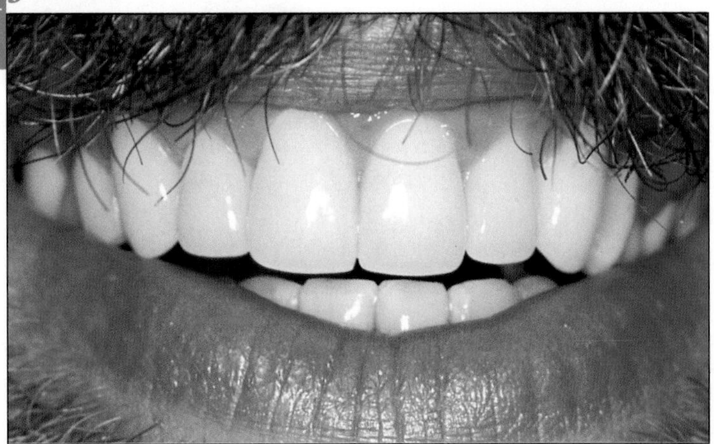

FULL CROWNS AND COMPOSITE RESIN BONDING

When teeth are as crowded as this, it is sometimes necessary to remove the nerves inside the teeth in order to prepare them for crowns with adequate porcelain thickness. Such a procedure was not necessary in this case, however, as full porcelain crowns improved the esthetics of the upper arch while the four lower teeth were bonded with composite resin to produce a handsome new smile.

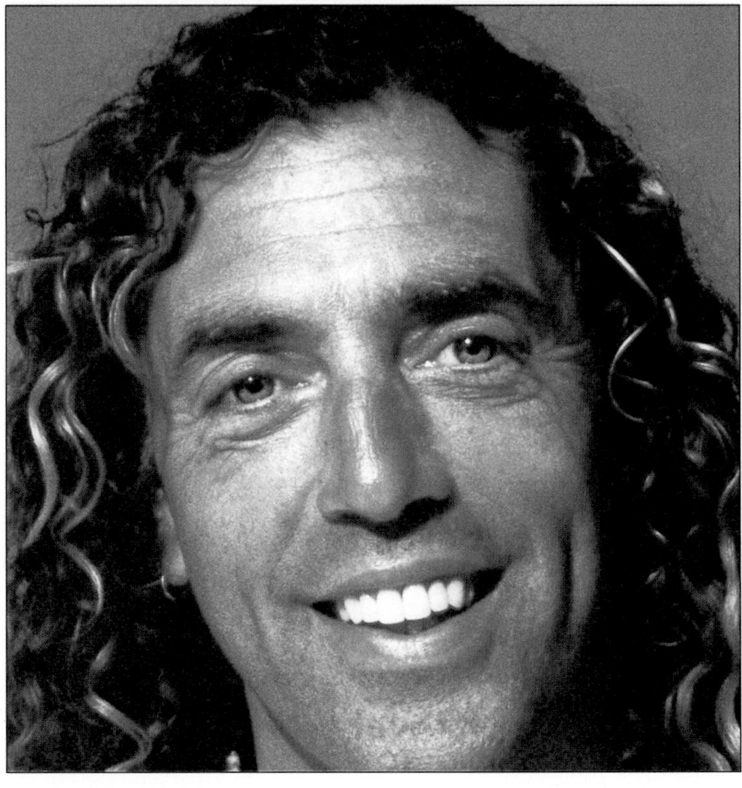

The final result pleased this patient so much that he no longer felt it necessary to hide his smile with facial hair.

Before

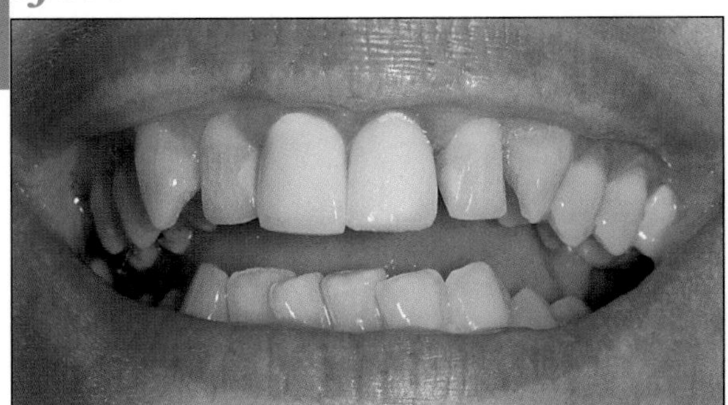

Insufficient Space for Properly Sized Teeth

A previous dentist had difficulty making appropriately sized crowns for this patient's front teeth due to crowding.

After

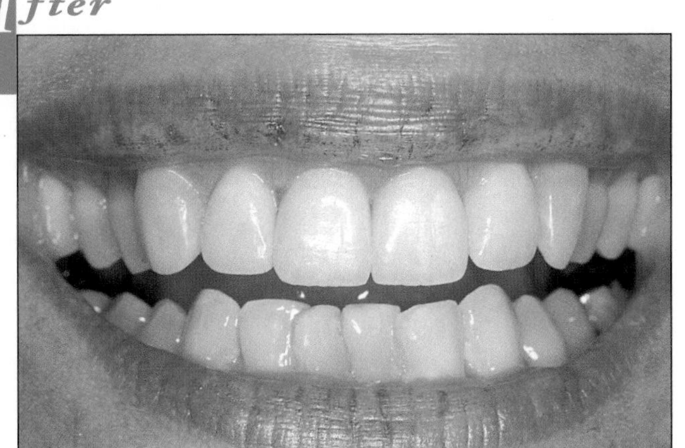

Integrated Therapy—Laminating, Bonding and Cosmetic Contouring

By reducing the adjacent teeth for porcelain laminates, plus slimming the width of the canines (cuspids or "eye teeth"), it was possible to crown only the two central incisors to improve the smileline. Porcelain laminate veneers were constructed for the two lateral incisors, and the cuspids were bonded with composite resin.

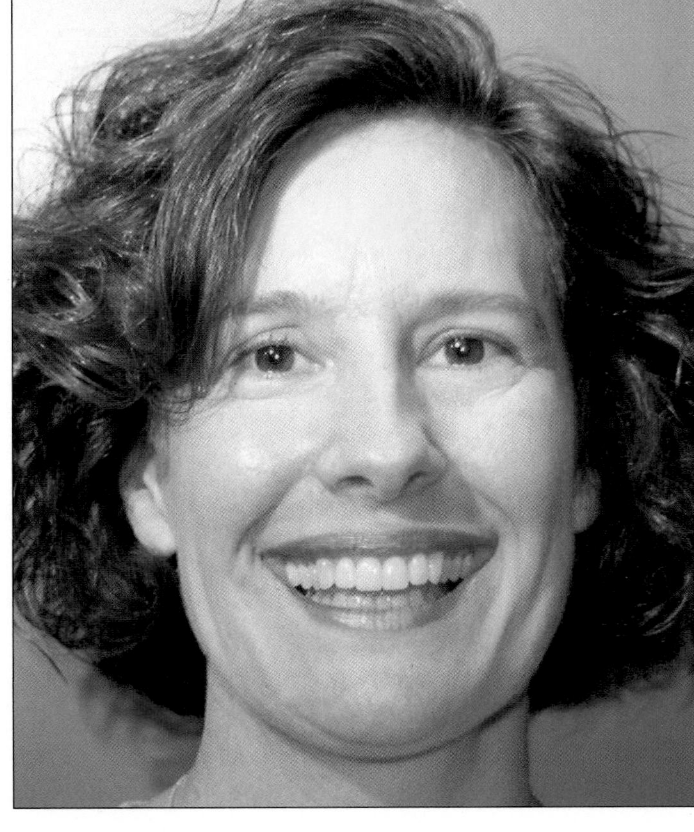

The final result shows a pretty smile that now complements the face.

TREATMENT SUMMARY

CROWNING

Treatment Time Usually two appointments of approximately one to four hours for up to four teeth. Expect to spend more time as additional teeth or more extensive treatment is included.

Patient Maintenance Care in biting hard objects to avoid fracturing the crowns. Fluoride treatments once yearly along with the use of fluoride toothpaste and flossing every day.

Results of Treatment Crowning can achieve the ultimate esthetic results in reshaping overly crowded teeth.

Average Range of Treatment Life Expectancy Five to fifteen years. Life expectancy is directly proportional to problems with tissue, fracture, and the danger of decay. (See footnote on p. 50.)

Cost $550 to $3000 per tooth. (See footnote on p. 50.)

ADVANTAGES

1. Teeth can be lightened to any shade
2. Takes less time than orthodontics
3. Crowned teeth stain less than bonded teeth
4. Longer life than composite resin bonding or porcelain laminates
5. Offers greatest latitude in improving tooth form

DISADVANTAGES

1. Can fracture
2. Requires anesthesia
3. Altered tooth form
4. Is not permanent; may need to be replaced after five to fifteen years
5. More costly than contouring or bonding
6. Is irreversible
7. May trigger pulp irritation in rare instances
8. May induce tooth sensitivity for a short time

ORTHODONTICS: IT'S REALLY THE BEST WAY

Orthodontics, or tooth straightening, is the treatment of choice when the top priority is keeping the natural, unaltered tooth. It is, without a doubt, the best way to correct malpositioned or crooked teeth, and it is also useful when the roots of adjacent teeth are impossible to separate for crowning. Occasionally, it is necessary to extract teeth in conjunction with repositioning, particularly in cases where crowding is causing bone loss.

In years past, orthodontics was shunned by many adults because treatment was lengthy and old-fashioned metal braces were conspicuous and unattractive.

Recently, however, dentistry has seen the advent of plastic or "invisible" braces, lingual or "behind the teeth" braces and removable appliances. Sometimes a combination of full metal bands on the lower arch and plastic brackets or lingual braces on the upper arch is preferred for more cost-effective, yet esthetic, tooth movement. So while orthodontic treatment may still take months or years to complete, it usually can be accomplished in a much more desirable manner. In fact, more than 25 percent of the patients now seen by orthodontists are adults, many of whom are more than 50 years old!

Before

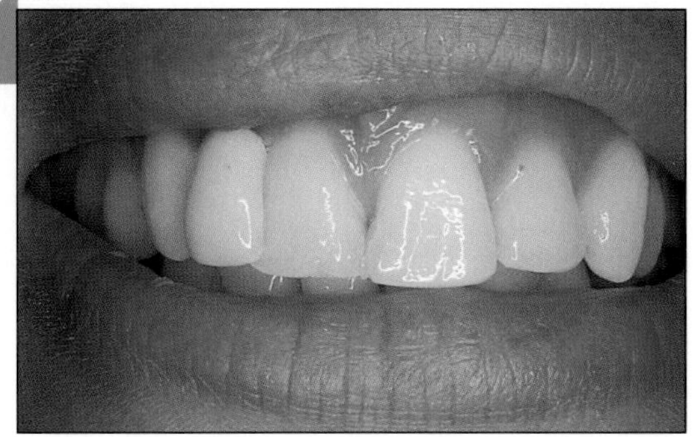

INSUFFICIENT SPACE FOR NORMAL-SIZED TEETH

This 27-year-old dental hygienist was missing a front tooth. Her right lateral incisor had been crowned previously, but the dentist had placed a tooth in front of the other teeth, complicating rather than alleviating her cosmetic problem. The left front tooth is larger than the right one and drops into the lower lip more than the right tooth does, reinforcing the imbalance in her smile.

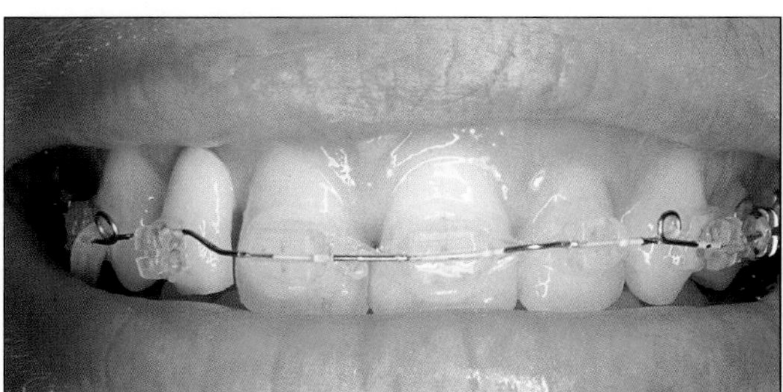

ORTHODONTIC TREATMENT

Tooth-colored brackets and coated white wire were used to help reposition the teeth. This type of fixed appliance is almost invisible from a distance. Although such appliances are not always appropriate, ask your general dentist or orthodontist if it is possible to use a more esthetic means of repositioning your teeth if the prospect of visible bands or brackets bothers you. The result of orthodontic treatment far outweighs the relatively short period of time that fixed appliances have to be worn.

After

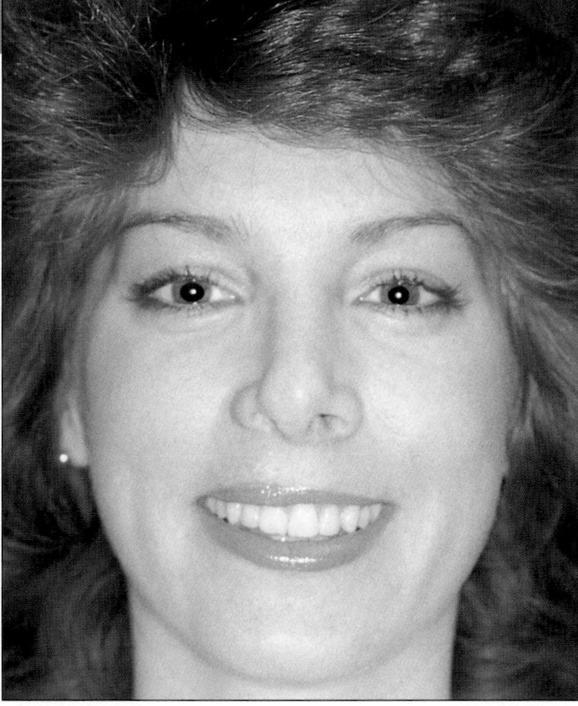

ORTHODONTICS AND FULL CROWN

Following orthodontic therapy, sufficient space existed to properly recrown the right lateral incisor, which helped produce a beautiful smile.

Before

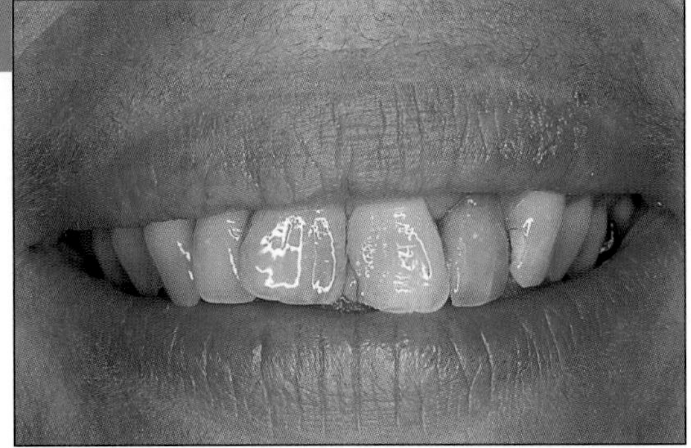

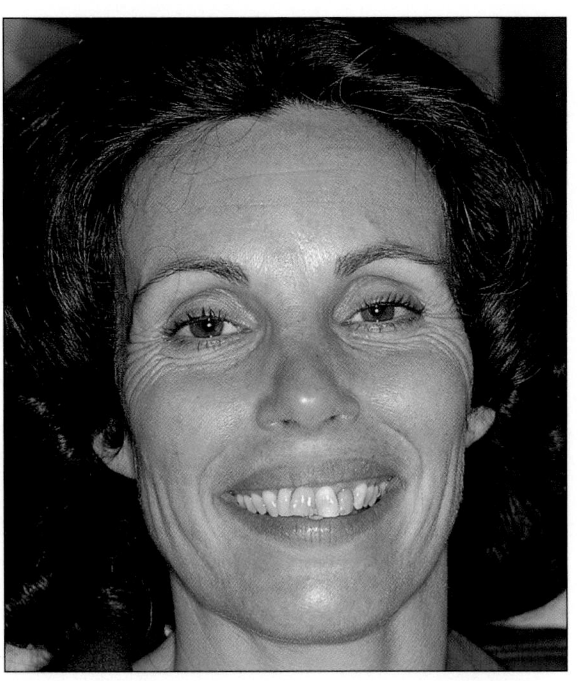

Protruded, Discolored and Crowded Teeth

Severe crowding of the discolored front teeth of this businesswoman ruined an otherwise attractive face. At first glance, one may think that crowning teeth produces an instant esthetic result. However, this procedure cannot correct the severity of the angle of protrusion. With crowning alone, the teeth would look better but would still stick out too far. Thus, orthodontics was the first step.

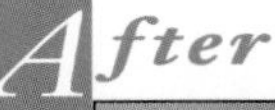

After

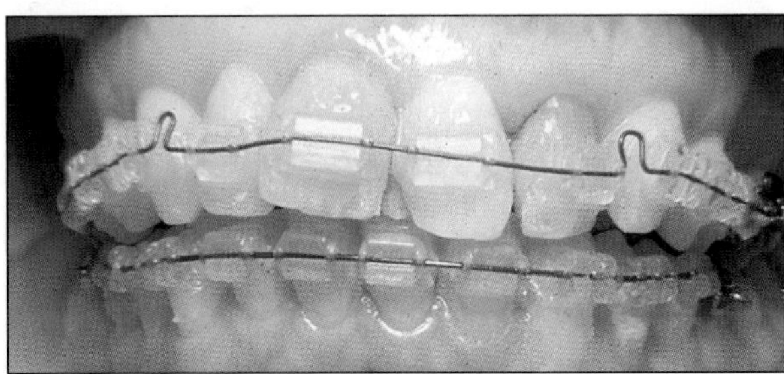

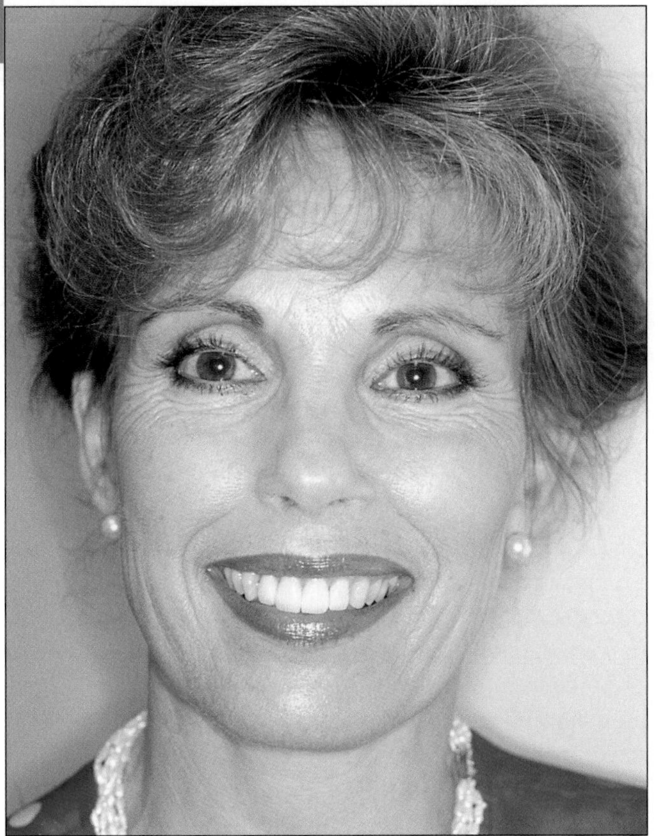

Orthodontics and Full Crowns

The teeth were first repositioned so that each would have proper space. Then four crowns were placed. Note the relaxed muscle tissue and especially the improvement in the upper lip in relation to the teeth. In these situations, it is preferable to correct the protrusion through repositioning the teeth and then, after orthodontics, either bonding, laminating or crowning. Worn and discolored teeth age a smile. Notice how much younger this woman looks with a brighter new smile plus new hairstyle and makeup.

Before

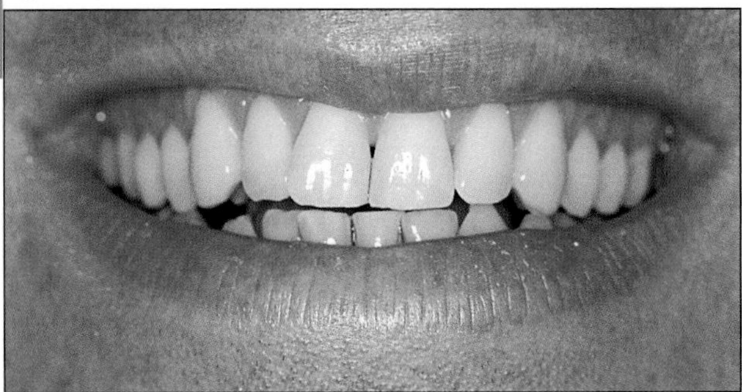

Crowded Front Teeth

This male model wanted to have his crowded front teeth corrected to both improve and maintain his smile.

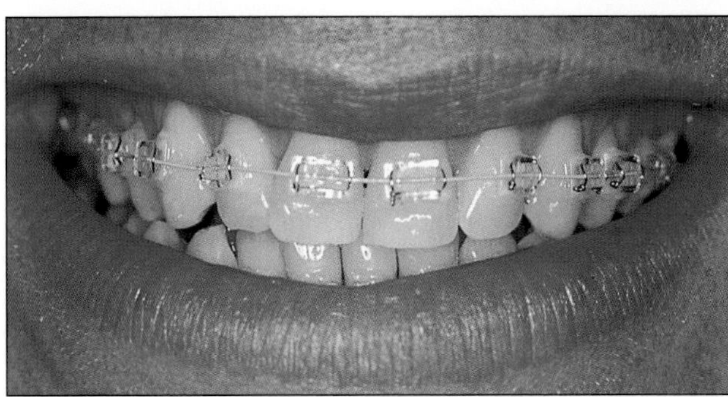

Orthodontics and Cosmetic Contouring

The patient opted for tooth-colored brackets, and orthodontic treatment straightened his teeth in less than six months.

After

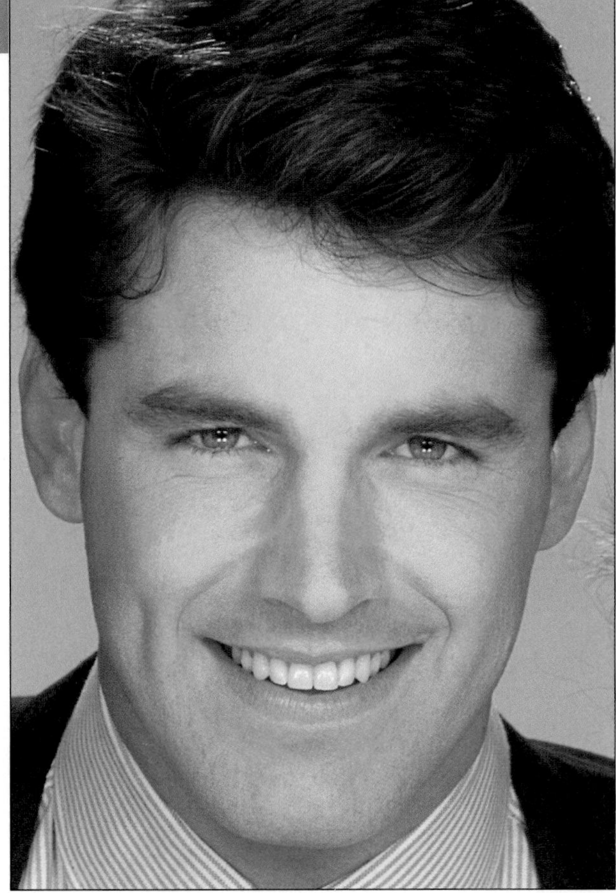

After orthodontic treatment, the teeth were cosmetically contoured to help perfect the smile of this young man. The final result was good enough to enable his smile to be used on a book cover.

Before

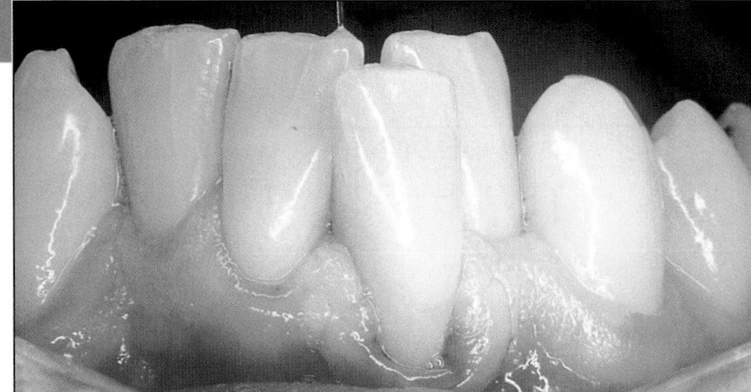

Extreme lower crowding

This 36-year-old salesman noticed his front teeth becoming much more crowded.

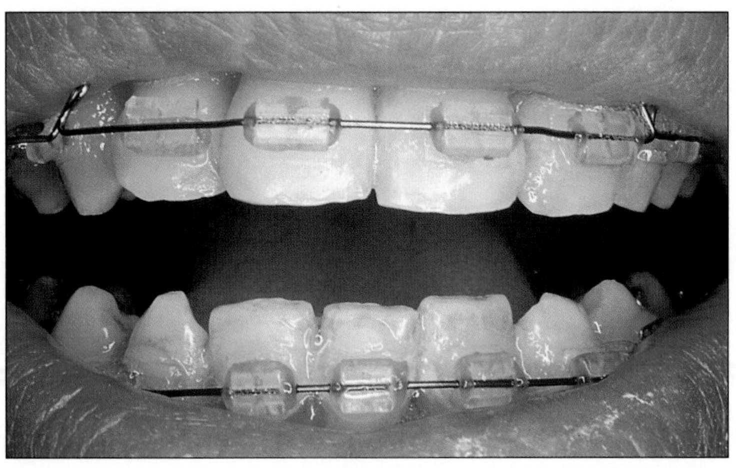

Orthodontics and extraction

With an extraction of the protruding front tooth and repositioning of the remaining teeth with tooth-colored brackets, it took less than twelve months to produce the results seen here.

After

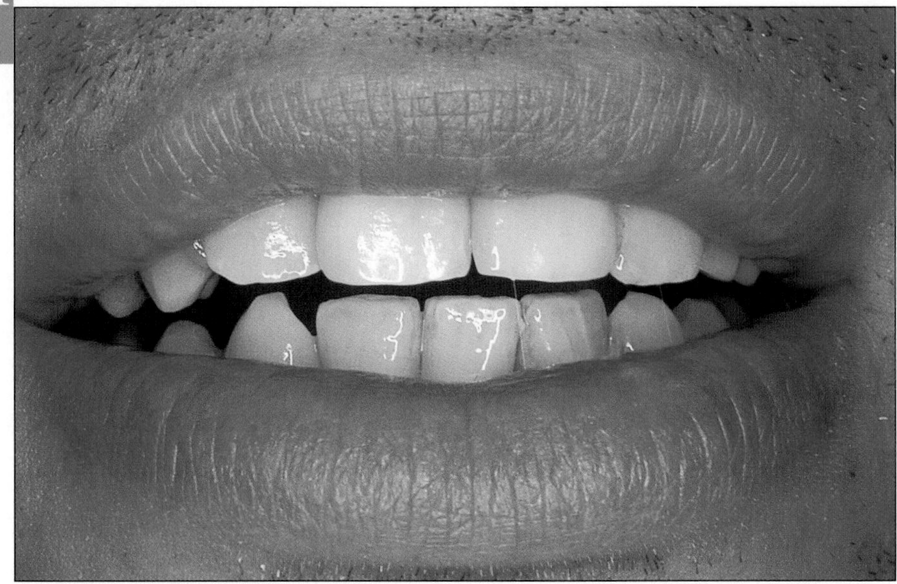

Before

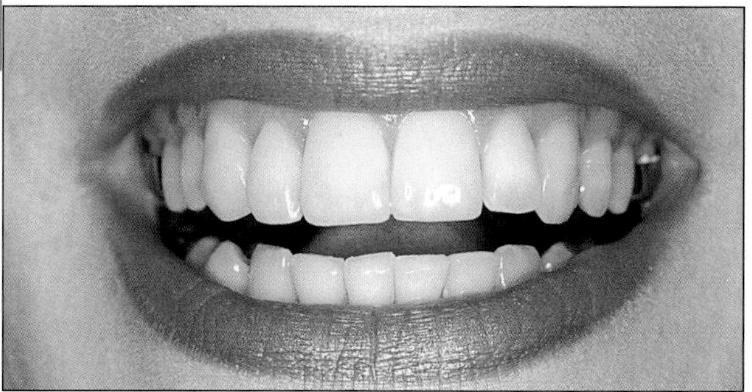

Mildly crowded teeth

While this smile may be acceptable for most people, this lady was concerned about the increasing crowding occurring in both her upper and lower arches. Teeth that get out of alignment can continue to crowd.

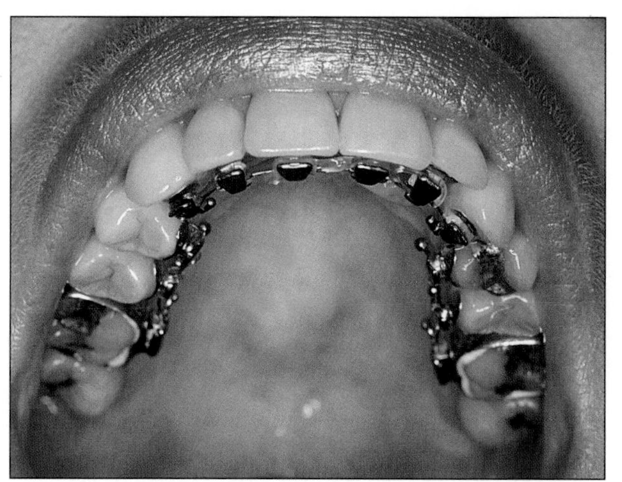

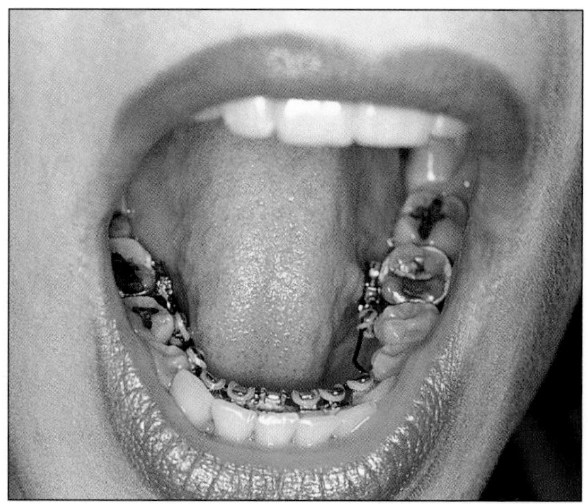

Hidden or lingual braces

Wanting to avoid visible orthodontic appliances, this patient opted for hidden or "lingual" braces. These cannot be seen unless you open your mouth wide and tilt your head back and down.

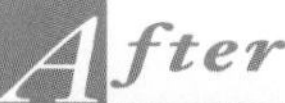

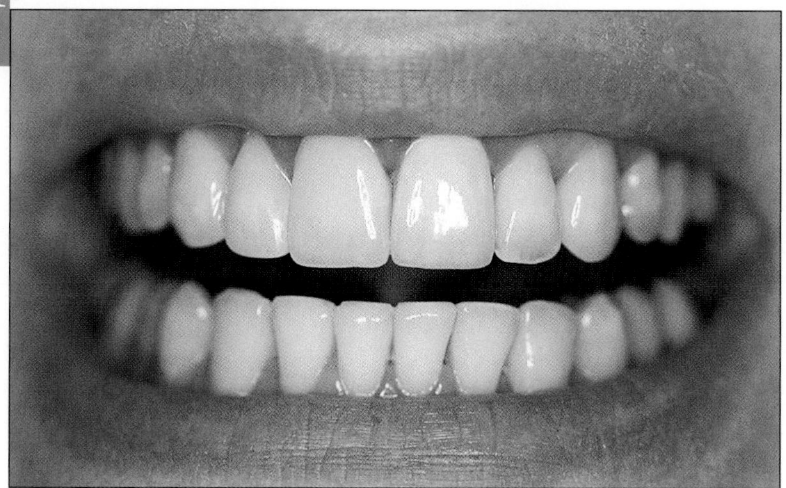

Note how the teeth are perfectly aligned after months of treatment. For lingual braces, expect to pay more per arch due to increased chair time and appliance cost. (See treatment summary on p. 173.)

Before

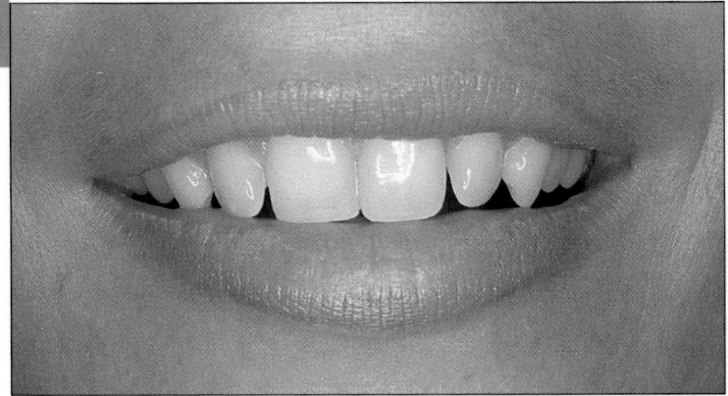

MINOR CROWDING

This popular model's slightly crowded front teeth kept her from having her best smile.

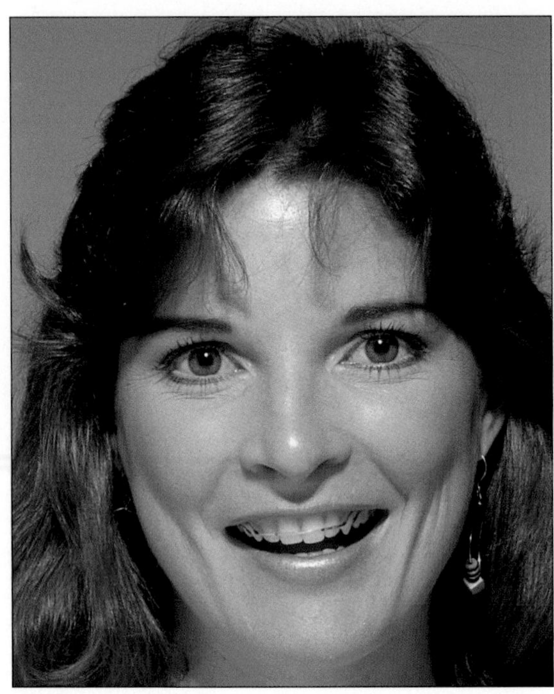

MINOR ORTHODONTICS

Less than six months of wearing a removable appliance was all it took to enhance this model's smile. The appliance can sometimes later be used as a retainer to help keep the teeth in their new positions.

After

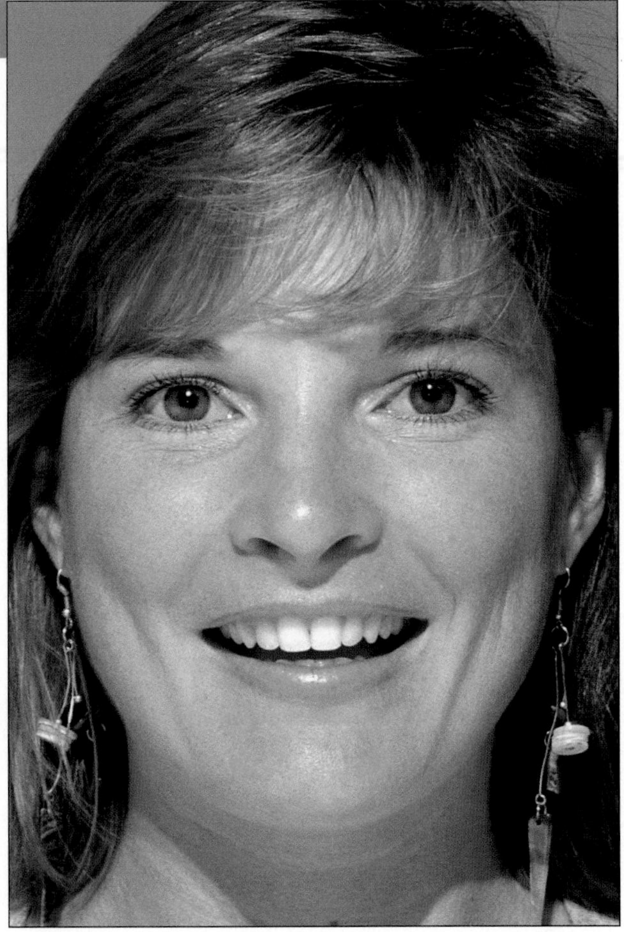

TREATMENT SUMMARY

ORTHODONTICS

Treatment Time Six to thirty-six months.

Patient Maintenance Special attention to daily cleaning; adjustment checkups every three to four weeks. Retainers will need to be worn at night indefinitely.

Results of Treatment Crowded and overlapped teeth can be straightened.

Average Range of Treatment Life Expectancy Generally a permanent treatment, but will usually require wearing a retainer at least a few nights weekly. (See footnote on p. 50.)

Cost $1500 to $7500, depending on number of teeth involved and appliance therapy chosen. Lingual or "behind the teeth" braces can cost up to $2000 per arch over normal fees. (See footnote on p. 50.)

ADVANTAGES

1. Can straighten misaligned teeth
2. Permanent solution for most individuals
3. Little or no tooth reduction required
4. May be less expensive than laminating, crowning or bonding, depending on the number of teeth involved
5. Improved tissue health due to better cleaning access

DISADVANTAGES

1. Time-consuming (six to thirty-six months)
2. Teeth may return to original position if retainers are not worn
3. May take a few weeks to get used to appliances

Best advice: With your dentist, develop a master treatment plan before starting orthodontic therapy. Be sure to include other treatment that may become necessary after orthodontic therapy is completed.

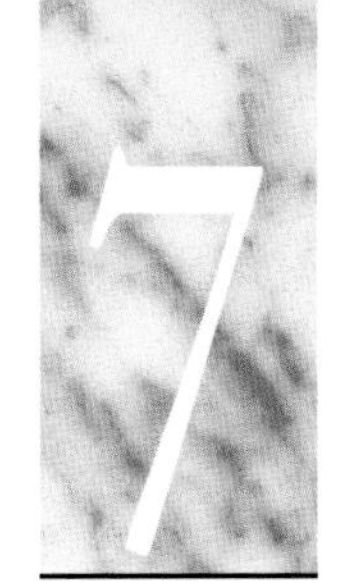

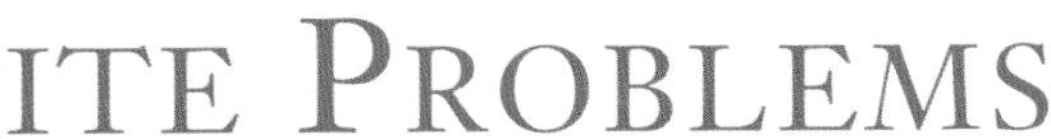

Bite Problems

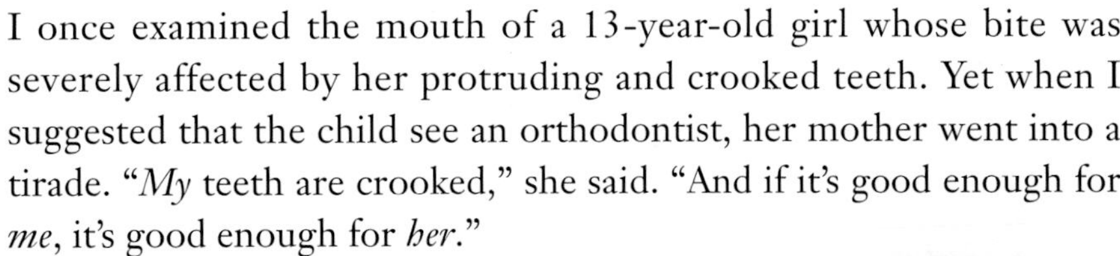

I once examined the mouth of a 13-year-old girl whose bite was severely affected by her protruding and crooked teeth. Yet when I suggested that the child see an orthodontist, her mother went into a tirade. "*My* teeth are crooked," she said. "And if it's good enough for *me*, it's good enough for *her*."

This response indicated a complete disregard for both the child's physical and psychological needs. And nothing I said about function, esthetics or the child's emotional welfare changed the mother's mind.

In more than 39 years of practicing dentistry, that mother is one of the few patients I have refused to treat. I couldn't bear the thought of her beautiful little girl suffering needlessly from problems that could have been easily corrected.

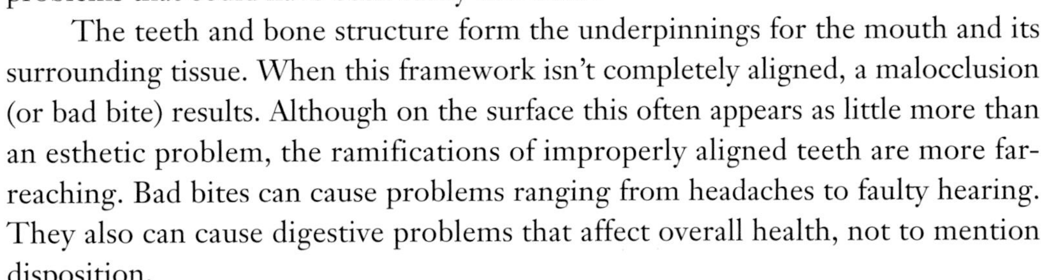

The teeth and bone structure form the underpinnings for the mouth and its surrounding tissue. When this framework isn't completely aligned, a malocclusion (or bad bite) results. Although on the surface this often appears as little more than an esthetic problem, the ramifications of improperly aligned teeth are more far-reaching. Bad bites can cause problems ranging from headaches to faulty hearing. They also can cause digestive problems that affect overall health, not to mention disposition.

Many adults, as well as children, suffer from bite disorders that affect their physical and social well-being. Fortunately, modern dentistry offers a variety of ways to treat improperly aligned bites—many of which are imperceptible to others. This chapter outlines various bite disorders and the options that are available to treat them.

Bad Bites: Inheritance or Habit?

A bad bite is typically caused by inheritance. Inherited bad bites result when the teeth do not fit in the jaws properly, or when the teeth are not in a correct relationship with the rest of the face. Although protruding upper and lower teeth are often inherited, they may not always cause bite problems.

Destructive personal habits also can cause bad bites, particularly when pressure on the bottom teeth causes them to move inward as is the case in lip or nail biting. Persistent thumb-sucking can also affect the bite and cause the permanent teeth to protrude. Although this habit stops voluntarily at about age six in most cases, consult with your child's dentist to determine if attempts should be made to break the habit earlier. Another major cause of bad bites is loss of teeth without proper replacement with implants or fixed or removable bridges. **Failure to replace missing teeth can cause the bite and the face to "collapse," resulting in an aged and unattractive appearance.**

Before

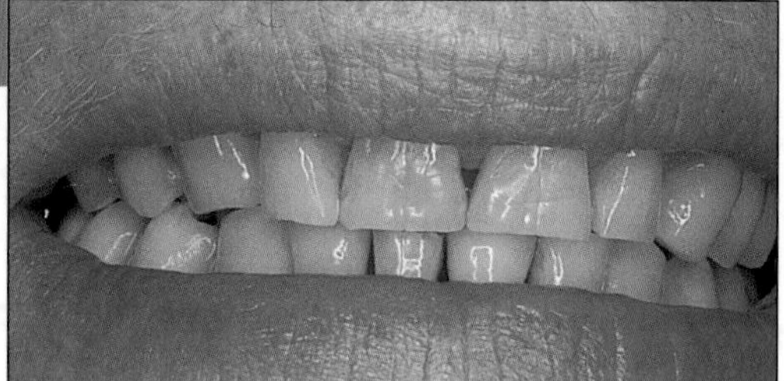

Worn teeth

This 57-year-old woman had worn her back teeth down so much that the front teeth also began to wear. Creating a removable appliance for the patient was the first step; it would help determine if the bite could be slightly opened and permit longer teeth in the front of the mouth. This new relationship might also allow the jaw muscles to relax and be more comfortable since the patient had lost so much of her biting surface. After approximately three months of wearing the plastic appliance, the teeth were ready to be rebuilt in a new relationship.

After

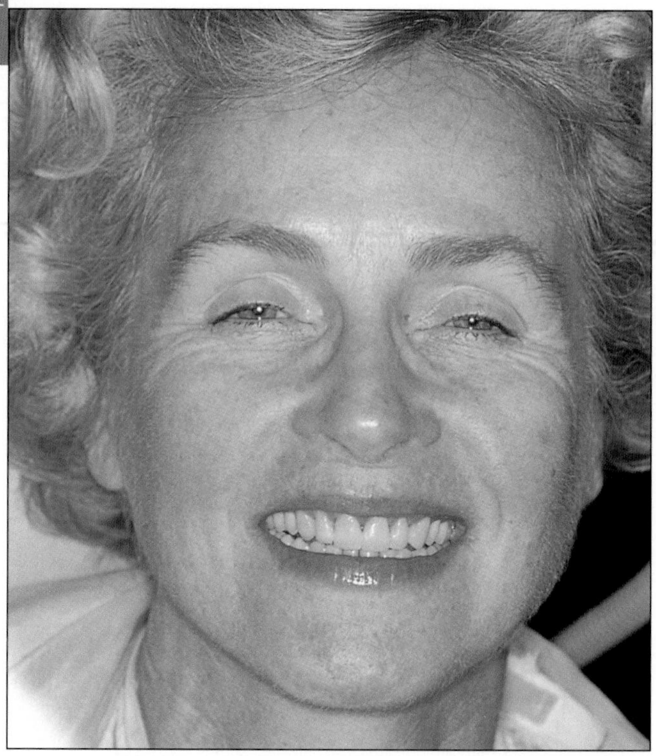

Crowns and composite resin bonding

All the back teeth were crowned with porcelain fused to metal. The front teeth were bonded with composite resin, which produced a prettier new color and shape, and lengthened the teeth as well. The combined approach greatly improved her smile as well as her appearance.

Before

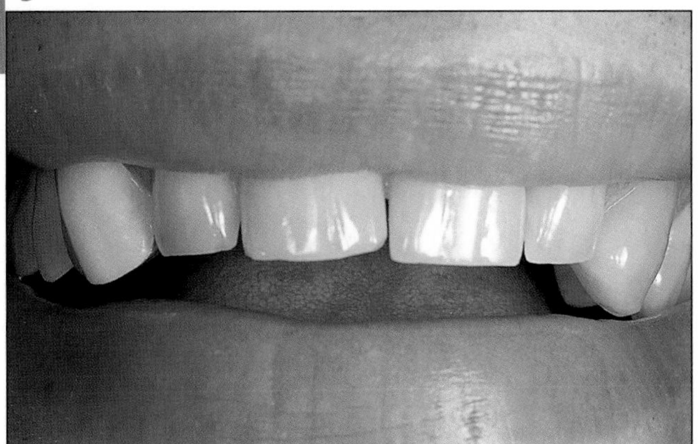

ACCELERATED WEAR OF UPPER FRONT TEETH CREATING AN OLDER SMILELINE

This 25-year-old male model had an older appearing smileline because his cuspids were longer than his other front teeth, which were worn, but not uniformly. A "Dracula look" resulted.

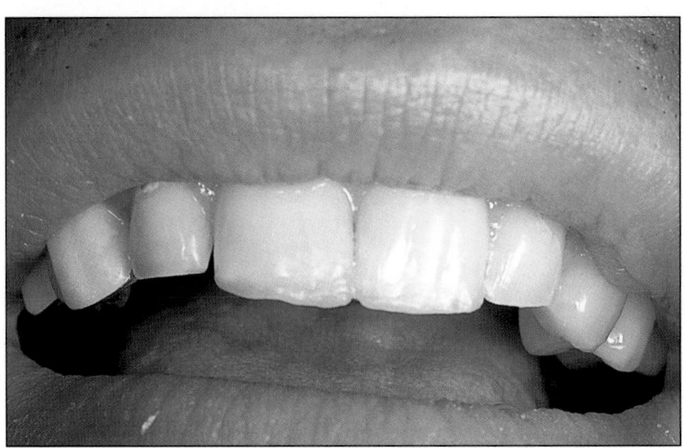

Wax was placed on the front teeth to show the patient what the final result would look like. This does not take much time and is painless. Computerized imaging can also be used to visualize the potential result.

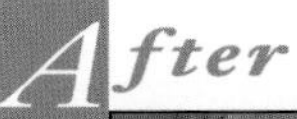

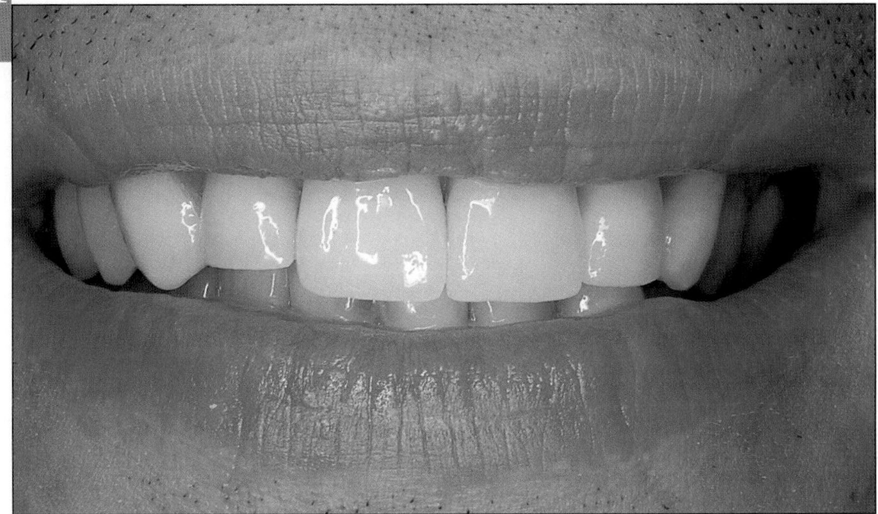

FULL CROWNS

The upper four teeth were crowned to make them longer and the back bridge was replaced. Notice how making the two front teeth longer helps create a more youthful and appealing smileline.

TMJ Disorder and Bruxism: Joint Problems Can Affect Your Bite

Five pairs of muscles control the movements of the mouth and lower jaw. When the teeth are out of alignment, these facial muscles may go into spasms, creating misalignment of the temporomandibular or jaw joints. This can lead to a problem known as temporomandibular joint (TMJ) disorder. Symptoms include headaches, neck pain, back pain and earaches. Unfortunately, patients often consult a number of medical specialists before discovering that their jaws are the source of their problem.

Treatment of TMJ disorder depends on the extent of facial disfigurement. Often, muscle relaxation therapy brings the face into alignment. Sometimes orthognathic (jaw) surgery is also required. However, no plastic surgery should be performed until the TMJ disorder is corrected.

Bruxism, or grinding the teeth, also can contribute to bite problems and TMJ disorder. Some clinicians believe that bruxism is caused by stress. Others believe it is an unconscious attempt to create a better bite by grinding down those teeth that do not meet properly. Regardless of the origin, bruxism can cause esthetic problems. Worn lower front teeth can result in tooth erosion and brown staining. Worn upper front teeth can result in an aging, drooping smile.

Before

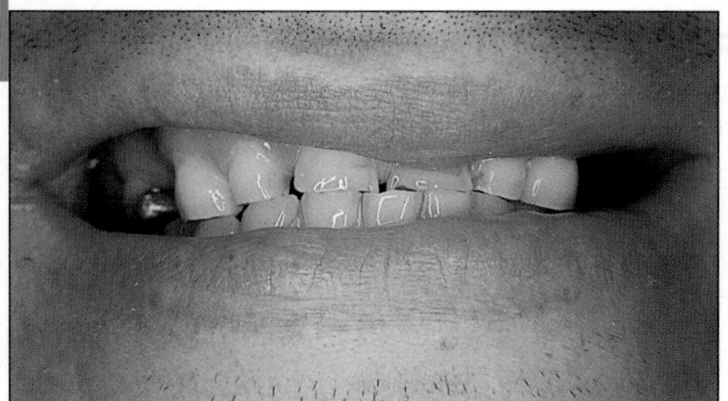

Closed bite due to extensive tooth wear

This 30-year-old salesman complained of unattractive teeth. His habits of clenching and bruxism had caused considerable tooth wear. He was also missing all the teeth behind the left cuspid, which helped cause bite collapse in the back, produced lip sag, and gave the face a tense look. Teeth wear slowly under normal conditions, but faster with bruxism or bite collapse. If patients lose their back teeth and do not have them replaced, the loss of vertical support can occur prematurely.

After

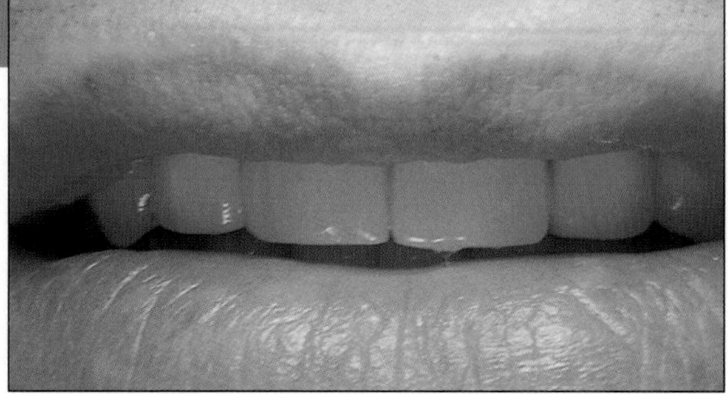

Full crowns, removable appliance and fixed bridges

Treatment for this patient consisted of a removable plastic bite appliance to open the jaws slightly to the original bite position he had before the teeth had worn down. It took about three months to make certain the temporomandibular joint (TMJ) and related facial muscles were relaxed. This was the ideal position for the new teeth to be rebuilt to. Note how the new crowns and improved bite relationship helped produce a more relaxed lipline.

Before

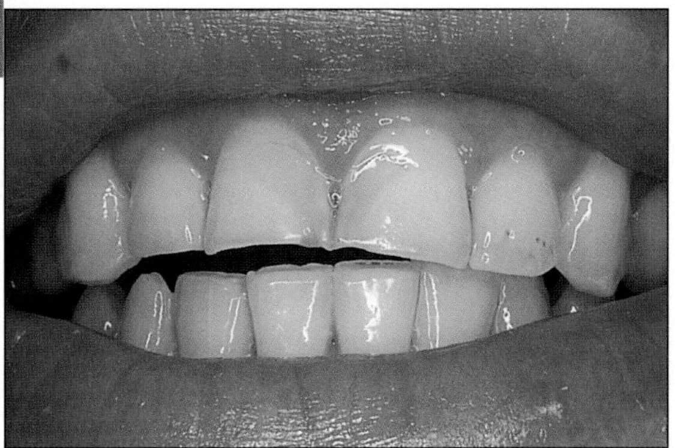

TOOTH WEAR

As an entertainer, this 23-year-old dancer was concerned about her unattractive smile. She had worn her upper teeth so much from grinding, or bruxism, that it appeared her upper jaw was deformed.

After

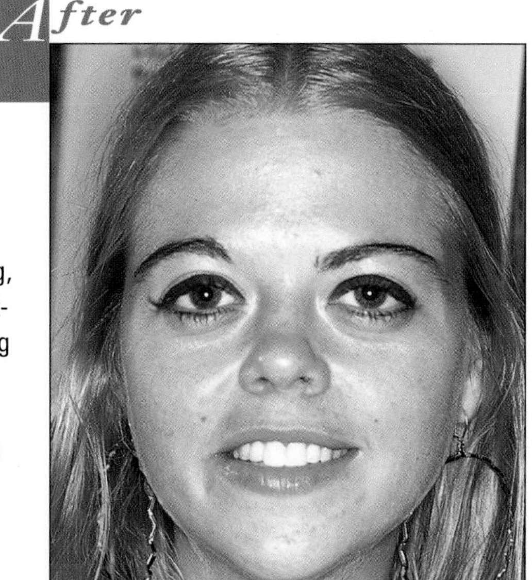

COMPOSITE RESIN BONDING

The most common solutions to this problem are either laminating, crowning or composite resin bonding. Because the patient wanted an economical and immediate result, composite resin bonding was chosen. To achieve the effect of longer-looking front teeth, the biting edges of the lower teeth were cosmetically contoured to compensate for the new length of the upper teeth. There is no harm in adding to the upper teeth and reshaping the lower teeth provided that the bite is compensated for and the patient maintains the same bite relationship. (See p. 186.)

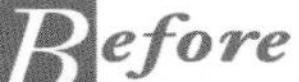

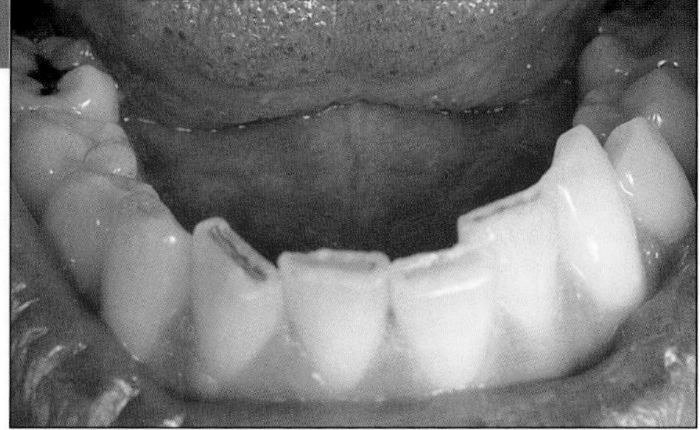

WORN ENAMEL RESULTING IN BROWN STAINS

This 28-year-old computer expert had excessive abrasion caused by bruxism (grinding) of the teeth, and brown stains on the biting edges of the lower teeth due to the erosion of the enamel. Once the enamel wears, the next layer (dentin) becomes exposed, and this layer is more susceptible to stains, such as from smoking. Prevention is the best treatment.

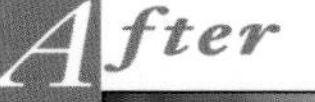

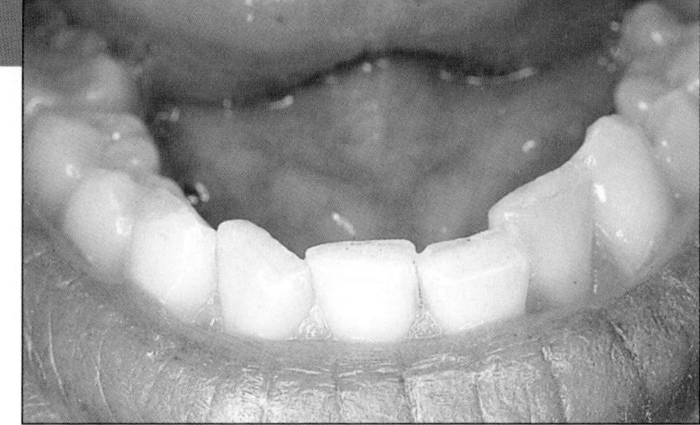

COMPOSITE RESIN BONDING AND COSMETIC CONTOURING

Erosion was inhibited by restoring the area with composite resin bonding. Generally no anesthetic is required, even when the tooth is prepared with a bur (rotating instrument), as there is little sensitivity in this area. In this case, cosmetic contouring to blend the shapes and improve the smileline was performed as well.

Overbite: A Detriment to Facial Esthetics

One of the bite problems that is most detrimental to facial esthetics is the deep overbite, which refers to the almost complete overlapping of the upper front teeth over the lower front teeth. Frequently, the edges of the lower teeth actually bite into the gum tissue of the upper palate. The treatment of choice for deep overbite is orthodontics.

Before

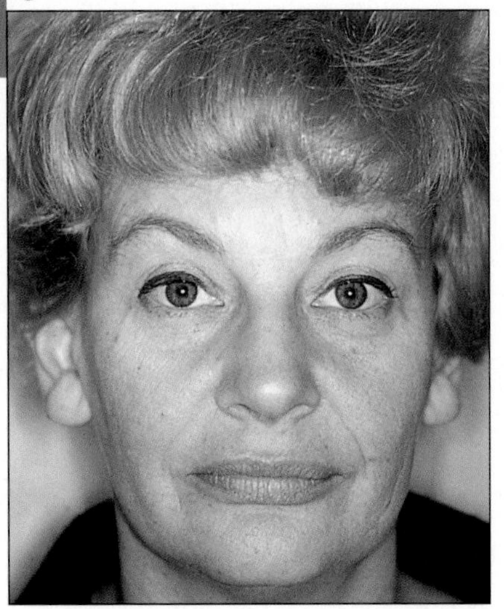

Deep overbite

This 44-year-old woman had a deep overbite, crossbite and several malposed teeth. Her lips appear thicker than they should. Also, the loss of muscle tone caused the muscles in this area to sag, giving an older appearance.

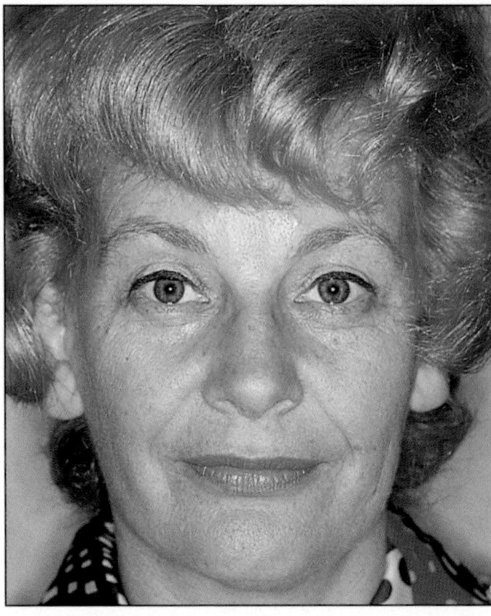

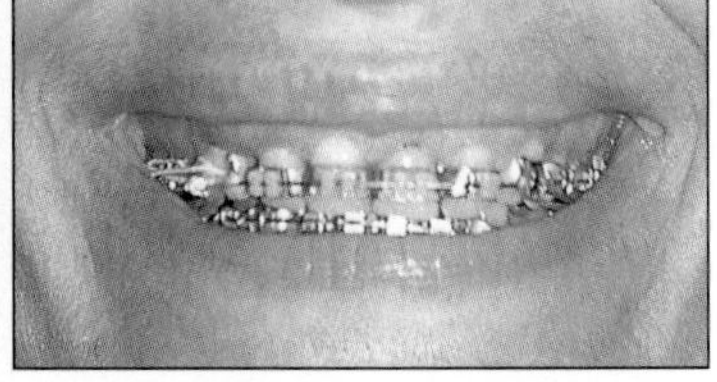

Before crowns could be constructed, orthodontic treatment was necessary to create a more normal bite relationship. Notice the improved appearance even during orthodontic therapy.

After

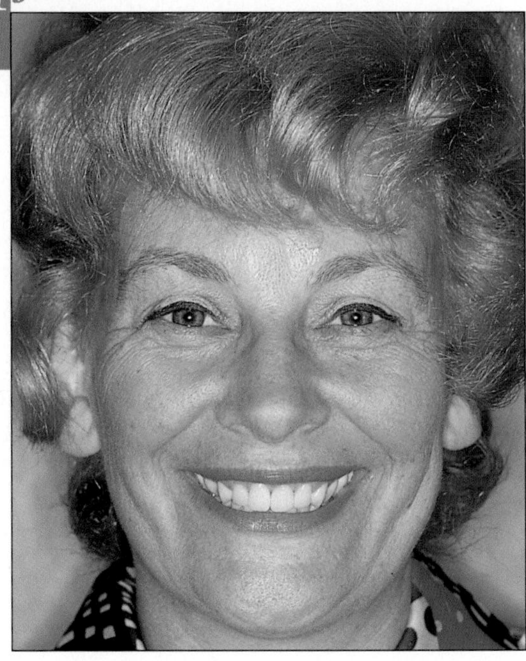

Orthodontics and Full Crowns

A beautiful new smile follows orthodontic therapy and the placement of new crowns. Notice the improved muscle tone permitted by restoring the proper bite, which provided enough room so that properly sized crowns could be placed.

Closed Bite: The Face May Look Collapsed

Some tooth wear is a natural function of aging. As long as it doesn't change your bite, it isn't a functional problem. Occasionally, however, tooth wear causes major bite disorders. For example, extreme erosion in the back of the mouth can result in a "collapsed bite." The inadequate tooth structure causes a partial disintegration of the lower facial tissue, which results in an aged appearance, as if the person had no teeth. This problem can exist even in young people.

If the closed bite is not too severe, the back teeth often can be built up with crowns or onlays, which allows the front teeth to be bonded or crowned. However, opening the bite through orthodontic treatment is typically the best bet. Restorative procedures such as crown and bridge or bonding then can be performed after orthodontic treatment is complete. Orthognathic surgery also may be required if the lower jaw needs to be repositioned.

Crossbite: It Often Causes a Protruding Chin

In a normal bite, the upper teeth slightly overlap the lower teeth. A crossbite results when the opposite occurs, or when the lower teeth overlap the upper teeth. It can occur in both the front and back teeth. When a crossbite develops in the front teeth, the result is an unattractive protruding chin.

If a crossbite is particularly severe, orthognathic surgery may be required

Although full crowns or composite resin bonding often can be used to "build out" the upper arch, this treatment only lends itself to a limited amount of esthetic modification. The best way to correct a crossbite is through orthodontics.

If the crossbite is particularly severe, orthognathic surgery, as well as orthodontics, may be required. This combined approach can result in a dramatic improvement in facial appearance. Best of all, the teeth tend to remain in their new positions once the condition is corrected.

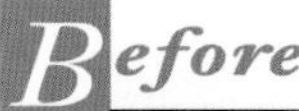

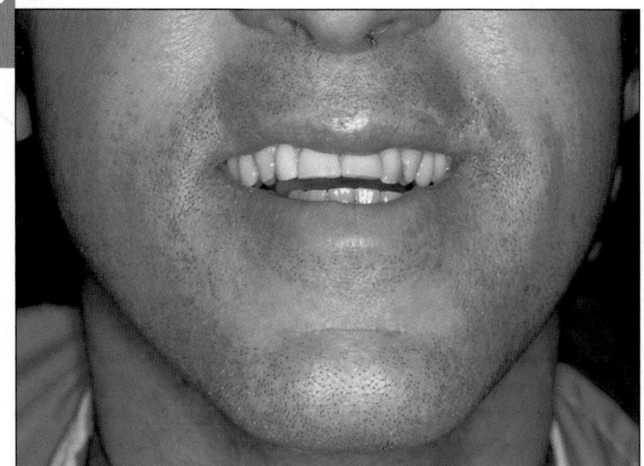

CROSSBITE WITH PROTRUDING CHIN AND JAW

This nationally known sports and television star had a protruding chin complicated by upper teeth that fit behind the lower teeth. The necks of the upper teeth were also severely eroded.

After

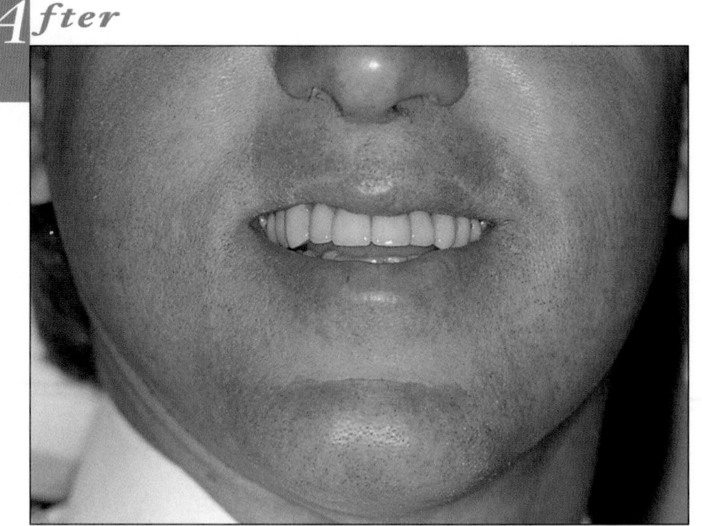

COMPOSITE RESIN BONDING AND FULL CROWNS

The ideal treatment in patients like this would be orthodontics, by itself or combined with surgery, to reposition the jawbone. However, a compromise treatment of recrowning some upper front teeth and bonding others helped improve this man's smile. The lower teeth were cosmetically contoured to look straighter and to permit the additional length of the upper teeth. Building the upper teeth out and down created more emphasis on the upper part of the face, enhancing facial symmetry.

OPEN BITE: IT MAY CAUSE THE UPPER LIP TO PROTRUDE

Occasionally, the upper and lower front teeth cannot come together when the back teeth are touching. This condition creates a space commonly referred to as an open bite. Genetic defects, as well as habits such as tongue thrusting, thumb sucking and pencil biting, can cause open bites.

Although people with open bites aren't always aware of the problem, one telltale symptom is difficulty biting with the front teeth. In addition, open bites cause protrusion of the upper lip, making it difficult for patients with open bites to close their lips over their teeth without straining.

Orthodontics, occasionally combined with orthognathic surgery, is the best treatment for an open bite. It not only corrects tooth deformity, but moves underlying bone inward, enabling the lips to close properly.

Before

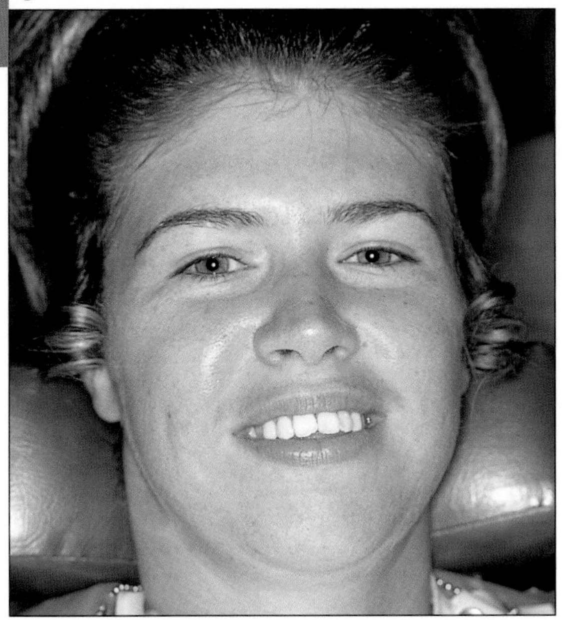

OPEN BITE

This woman was disturbed by the unattractive smile created by her open bite. In fact, it was virtually impossible for her lips to close over the teeth without muscle strain, and it was difficult for her to bite into foods with her front teeth.

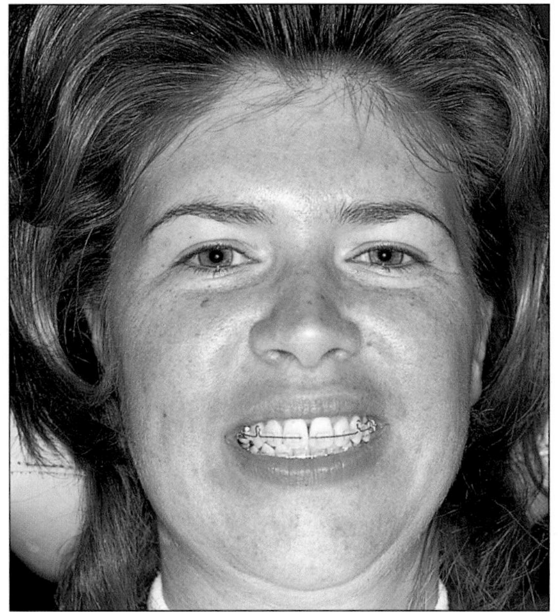

ORTHODONTIC TREATMENT

Orthodontic treatment corrected the open bite, placing the teeth in a more normal relationship. This picture shows the patient near the end of treatment wearing her orthodontic appliances.

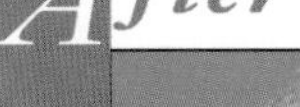

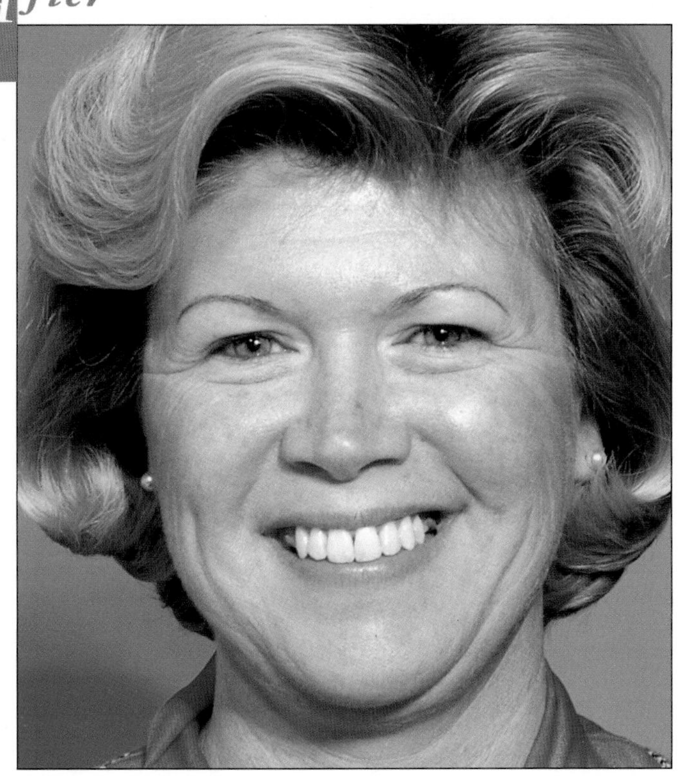

FIFTEEN YEARS LATER

Fifteen years after treatment. A more feminine smile is the result of new tooth position. Lip muscle relaxation is possible when the teeth are properly related. This type of condition is most difficult to correct or to maintain with any treatment other than orthodontics alone, or orthodontics combined with orthognathic (jaw) surgery.

Protrusion: Repositioning Can Change Your Smile

Protruded upper front teeth, often called "buck teeth," can diminish even the best of smiles. In severe cases, protrusion results in facial deformity, and patients cannot close their lips over their teeth.

Orthodontic treatment, combined with orthognathic surgery in severe cases, is the best way to correct protrusion. In some cases, two to four teeth may be extracted to achieve good results. Keep in mind, however, that overcorrection is a major concern when teeth are extracted. Overcorrection occurs when the teeth are moved back too far, resulting in a "dished-in" appearance.

It takes a great deal of planning to decide just how much correction should be undertaken. The upper teeth should be moved into an appropriate position to support the upper lip, but not necessarily into a position where they will touch the lower front teeth. This may well require a functional compromise. Talk to your orthodontist about this problem so that your facial proportions will be balanced.

No matter how severe your protrusion, do not have your upper teeth extracted and replaced with a bridge. This typically won't correct the bone deformity and may seriously impair your chewing ability.

Before

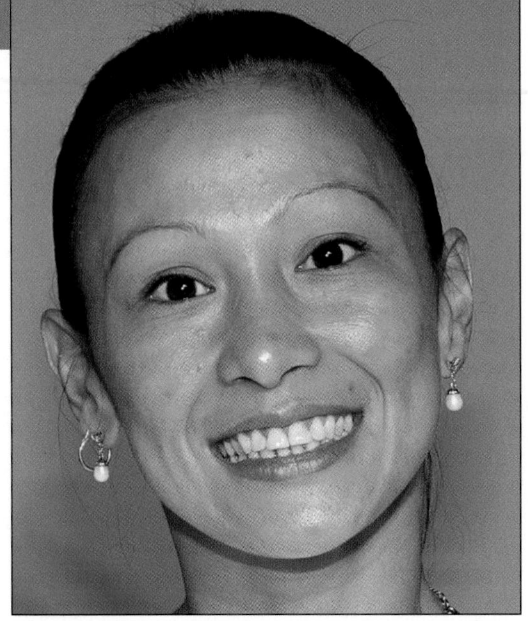

Protruded and Spaced Teeth

This prima ballerina was concerned about her protruding and discolored teeth. Although orthodontic treatment would have been the ideal solution, she opted for immediate results with composite resin bonding.

After

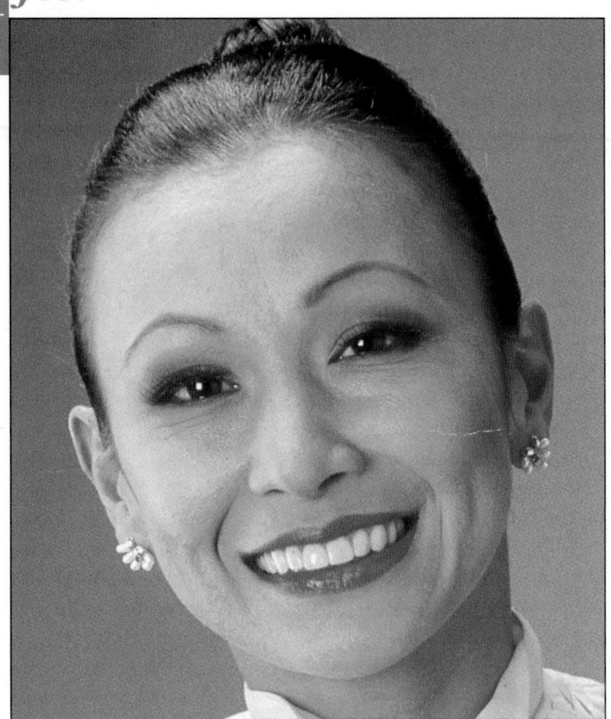

Composite Resin Bonding

Two appointments was all it took to achieve this attractive result. Although the protrusion still exists, the teeth look better. This smile now becomes an important part of this beautiful face.

Before

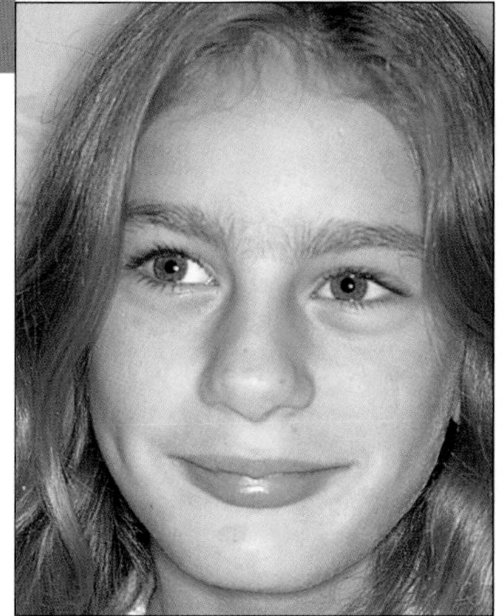

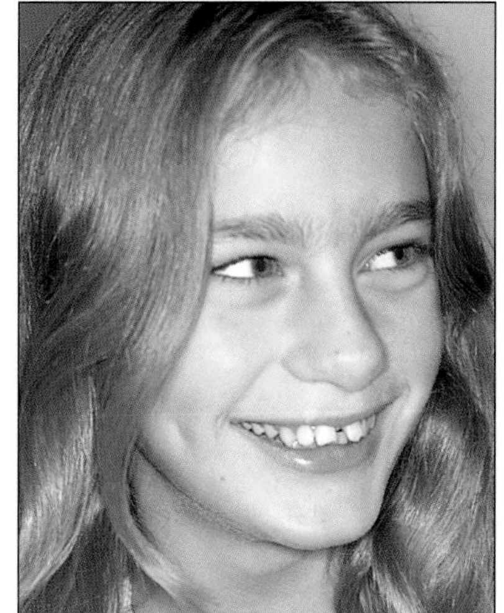

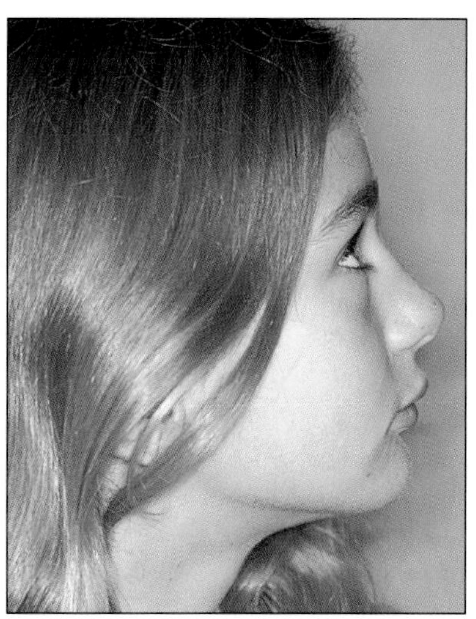

PROTRUDED TEETH

This 13-year-old girl found it difficult to close her mouth because of her protruding teeth.

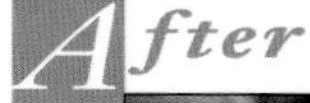

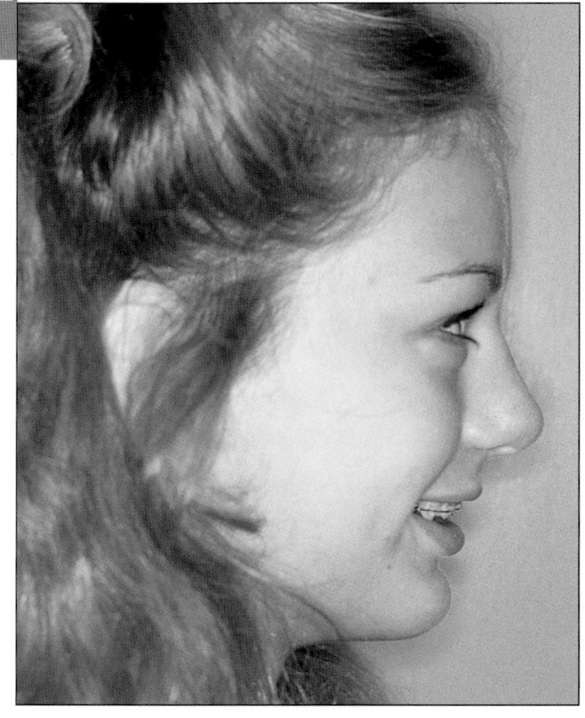

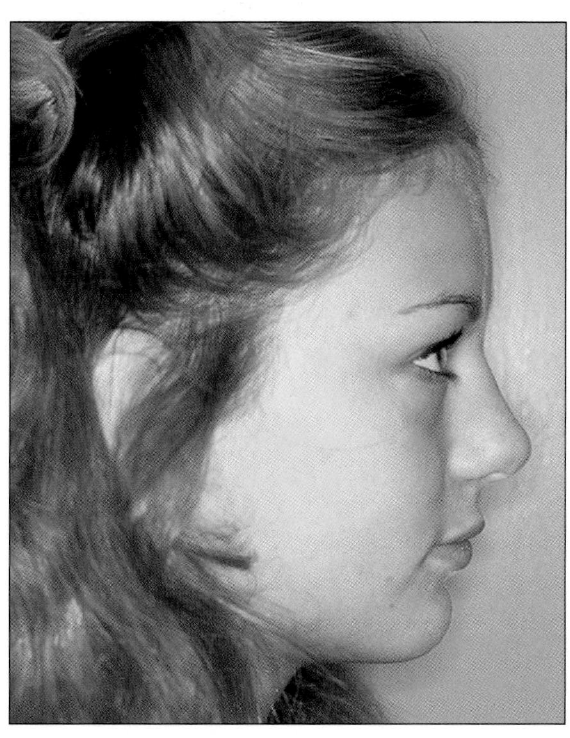

ORTHODONTIC TREATMENT

Two years of orthodontic treatment resulted not only in straighter teeth but a much improved facial profile.

MAKING YOUR TEETH APPEAR LONGER

These diagrams illustrate how the upper teeth can be lengthened to provide a new and prettier smileline. In the case shown on p. 179, the patient's midline was also improved.

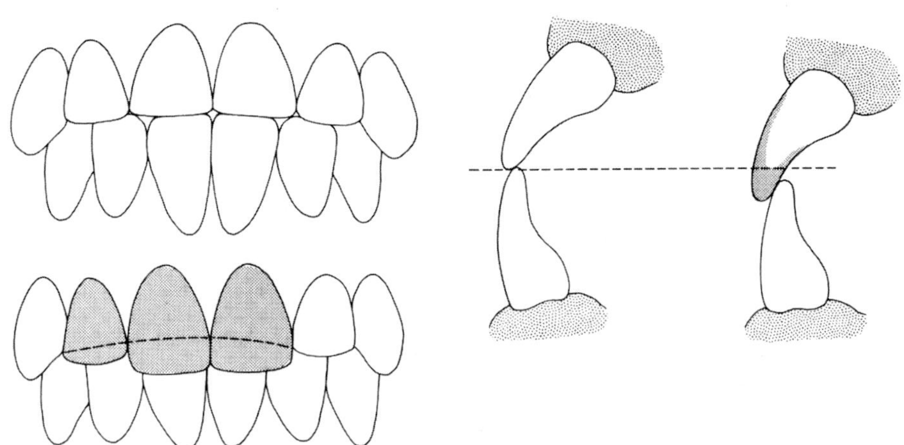

Cosmetic contouring

Cosmetic contouring, or reshaping the natural teeth so that they mesh better, is sometimes the easiest way to correct problems associated with poor bites. Although it isn't always possible, cosmetic contouring can be particularly effective in cases of minor crowding, and it may also provide the finishing touch after orthodontic treatment.

Before

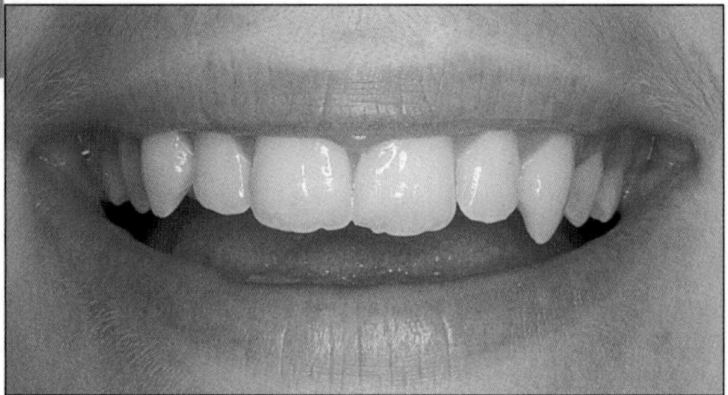

CUSPIDS THAT ARE TOO LONG

This 16-year-old student's smile had a "Dracula" look due to the long, protruding cuspids and chipped front teeth.

After

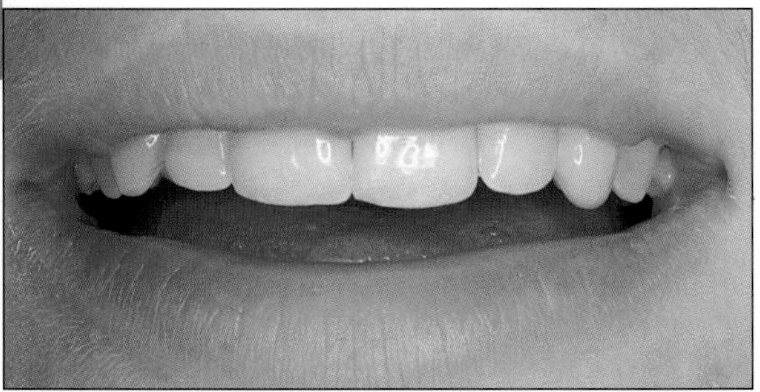

COSMETIC CONTOURING

After cosmetic contouring, in which the cuspids as well as the two front teeth were reshaped, the teeth look more proportionate to one another. If the patient's bite permits reshaping the teeth (something the dentist will determine), cosmetic contouring is a painless and economical treatment.

TREATMENT SUMMARY

COSMETIC CONTOURING

Treatment Time One hour.

Patient Maintenance Normal brushing and flossing.

Results of Treatment Can eliminate minor bite problems within a matter of minutes and may prevent headaches or other associated problems of bad bites.

Average Range of Treatment Life Expectancy Indefinite. (See footnote on p. 50.)

Cost $100 to $950. (See footnote on p. 50.)

Mouth appliances

If you experience bruxism or temporomandibular joint problems, your dentist may suggest that you wear a customized plastic mouth appliance that interrupts grinding. Although the appliance may not break you of the habit, it will prevent further wearing of your teeth and allow your muscles to rest.

After a period of time, your dentist actually can improve and "rebalance" your bite through adjusting the mouthpiece. It also may be necessary to rebuild your teeth so that they fit this new position and so that the muscles operate correctly and comfortably. Chances are your bite will also need readjusting.

As your facial appearance improves, you may find some of your wrinkles disappearing, as well. That "collapsed" look will diminish, and you'll start looking younger almost immediately.

TREATMENT SUMMARY

MOUTH APPLIANCES

Treatment Time Three months to one year for most patients. Some take considerably longer, even indefinitely for certain problems.

Patient Maintenance Appliance must be worn either nightly or full time for a specified time.

Results of Treatment Prevents wearing and tooth loss as well and can alleviate such symptoms as head, neck, ear or back pain.

Average Range of Treatment Life Expectancy Indefinite. (See footnote on p. 50.)

Cost $750 to $4000, depending on amount and frequency of treatment. (See footnote on p. 50.)

Orthodontics

Orthodontics, or repositioning the teeth so that they come together properly, is by far the best treatment for most bite problems. In some cases, orthognathic surgery is combined with orthodontics to achieve faster and better-looking results.

Before

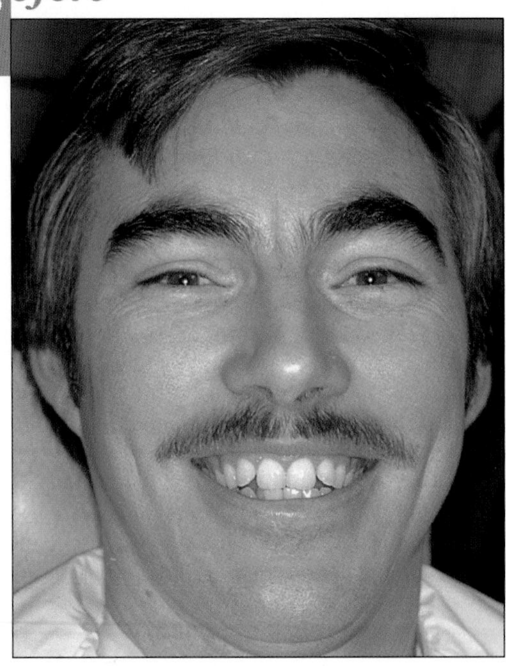

NARROW ARCH

This television personality wanted to enhance his smile.

After

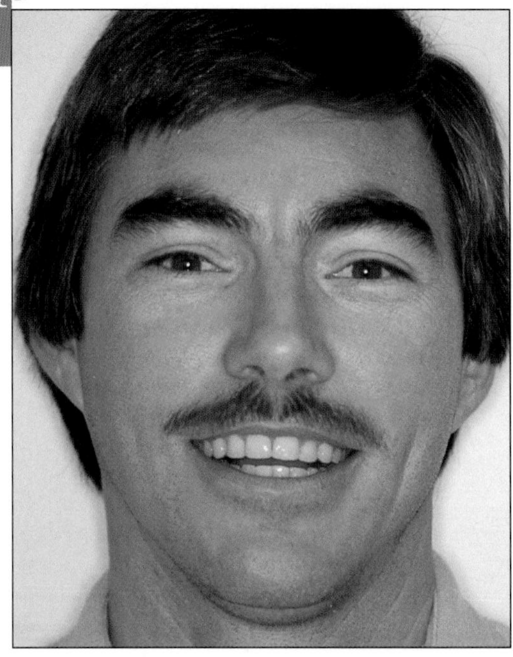

ORTHODONTIC TREATMENT

With the expansion of his arch and the repositioning of his teeth, a good-looking smile that harmonized with the rest of his face was achieved.

TREATMENT SUMMARY

ORTHODONTICS

Treatment Time Six to twenty-four months in most cases.

Patient Maintenance Special care to daily cleaning, checkups every three months after movement is completed. Retainers need to be worn for an indefinite time to make sure the teeth stay in their new positions.

Results of Treatment Bite problems can be solved by realigning the teeth so they meet properly.

Average Range of Treatment Life Expectancy For many, this is a relatively permanent treatment for correcting bites. Life expectancy depends on your cooperation in wearing retainers. (See footnote on p. 50.)

Cost $1500 to $7500. (See footnote on p. 50.)

Bonding

Bonding can be used for certain types of crossbites to build out the upper teeth so that they are in proper relationship with the lower teeth. Or, in selected cases, bonding can be used to build out lower front teeth so that the illusion of protruding upper teeth is diminished.

However, bonding is generally a weak compromise treatment for most bite problems. It is more effective as a way to make discolored, chipped, crowded, worn or irregularly spaced teeth look better in the existing bite relationship.

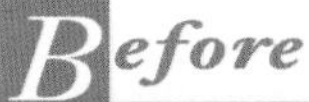

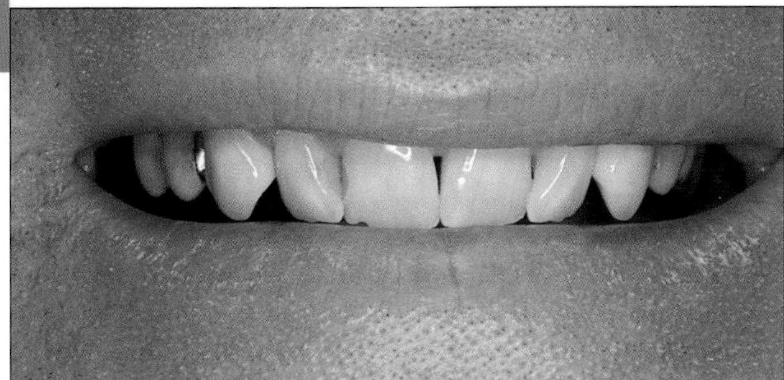

DISHED-IN FRONT TEETH

A dished-in look spoiled the smile of this otherwise handsome 45-year-old businessman. He also objected to the shiny silver filling on the right side. The inward angle of the teeth makes them look shorter than they really are because of downward rather than horizontal light reflection.

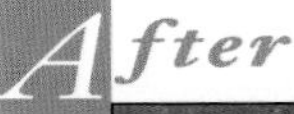

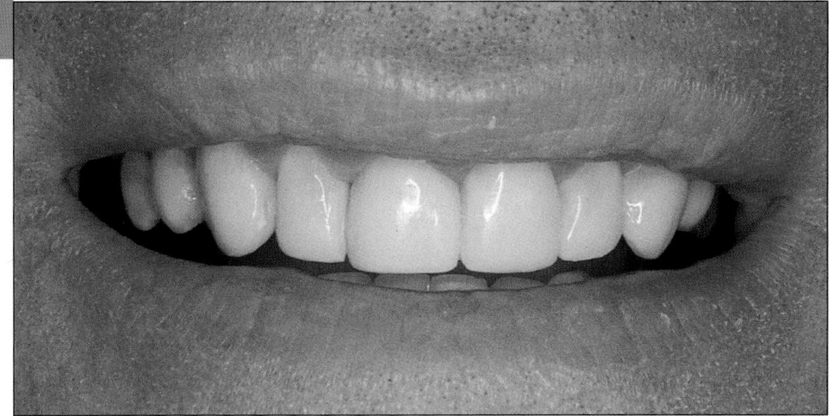

COMPOSITE RESIN BONDING

Composite resin bonding on the ten upper teeth produced a new smile immediately. One appointment was all it took to build out and fill in the front teeth and replace the silver filling with a tooth-colored posterior composite material. However, this material has a shorter life (about three to five years) than other materials. This patient was also advised to avoid smoking, coffee and tea to help reduce staining.

Before

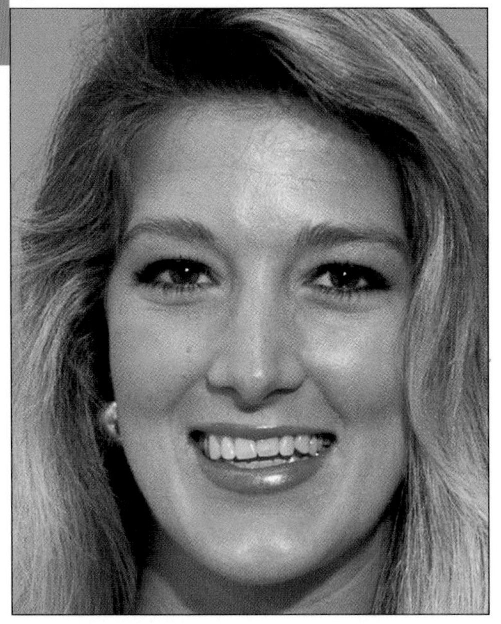

Arch asymmetry

A bad bite can account for an asymmetrical smileline. This beauty contestant wanted to improve her smile for an upcoming pageant.

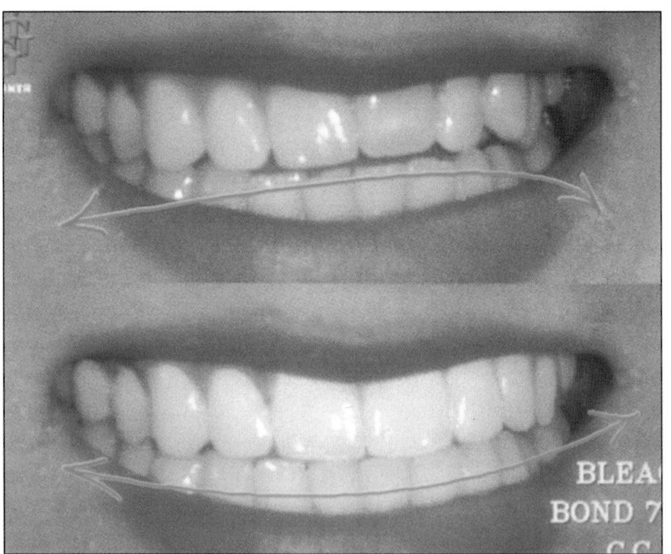

Computer imaging

Computer imaging analysis showed that a good result could be achieved with a combination of composite resin bonding and cosmetic contouring.

After

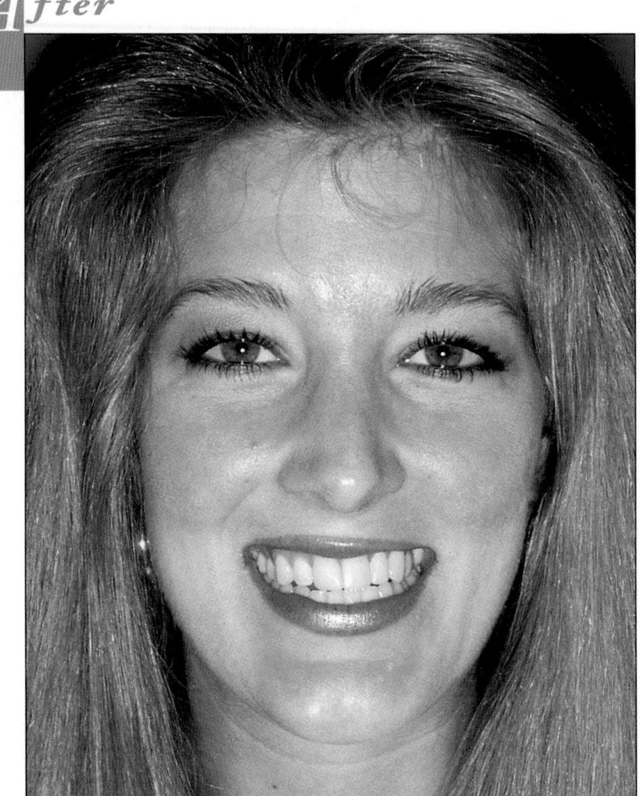

Composite resin bonding and cosmetic contouring

The final result shows just how much a new smile can contribute to total facial harmony and success in life (she won the pageant a few days later).

Before

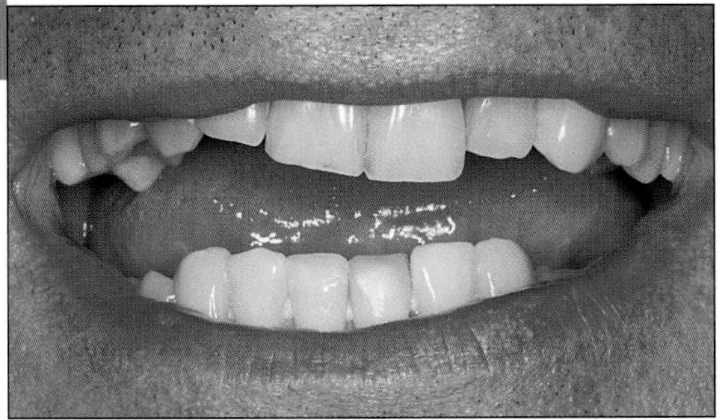

ASYMMETRICAL ARCH CAUSED BY CROWDED AND WORN TEETH

This minister wanted to improve his speaking appearance, which was marred by a crooked smile.

After

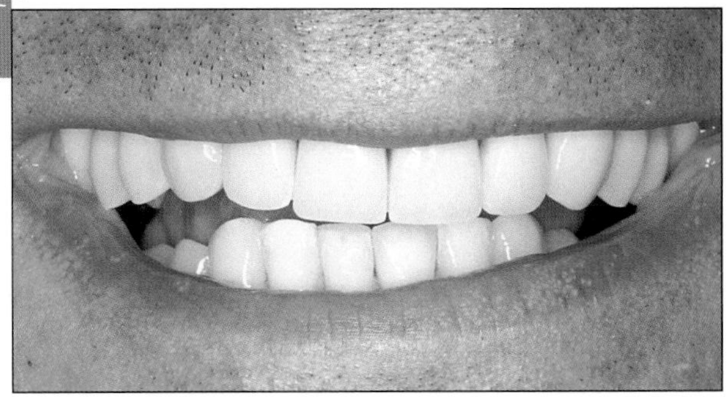

PORCELAIN LAMINATE VENEERS AND COSMETIC CONTOURING

The smileline was greatly improved by first reshaping the existing teeth and then placing ten porcelain laminate veneers. The new smile resulted in an overall more-handsome look, which greatly helped his speaking appearance.

Before

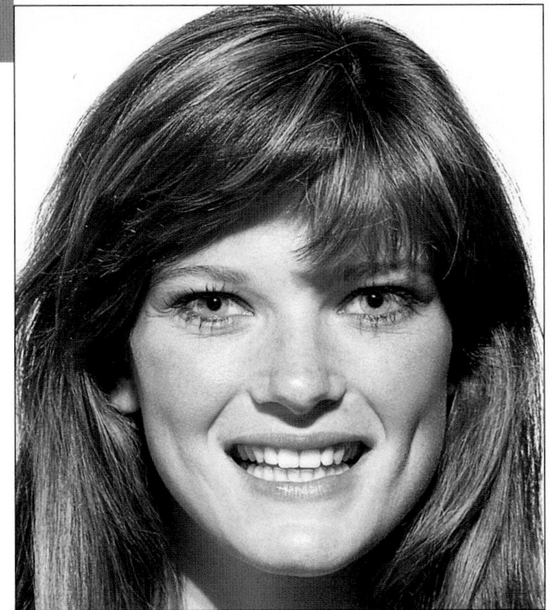

CONSTRICTED ARCH

This model had front teeth that were slanted inward, causing dark spaces at the sides of her smile.

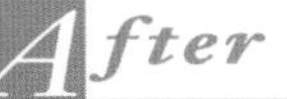

After

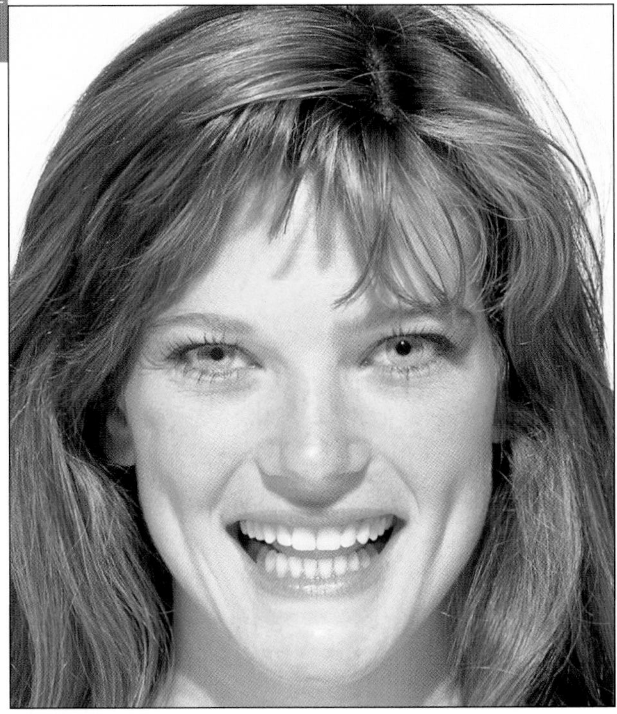

COMPOSITE RESIN BONDING

Immediate building out of the back teeth with composite resin gave this model a wider and brighter smile.

Before

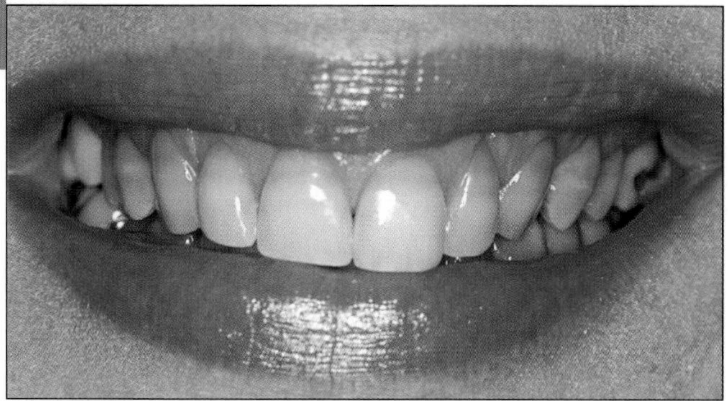

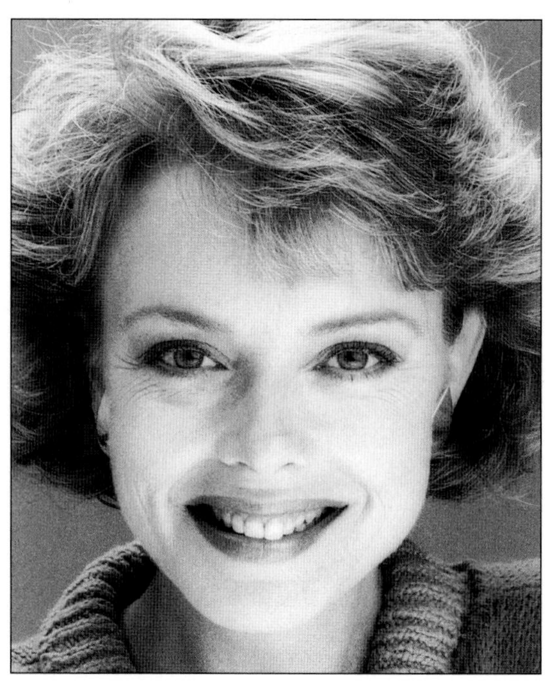

NARROW ARCH

This actress and model was displeased with the dark spaces (she called them "caves") that she saw on each side of her mouth when she smiled.

After

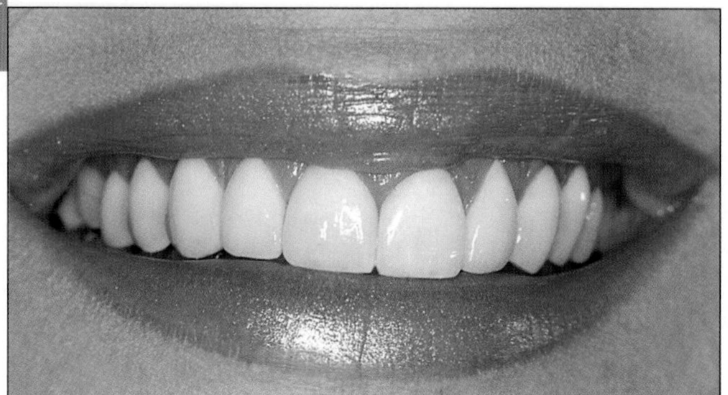

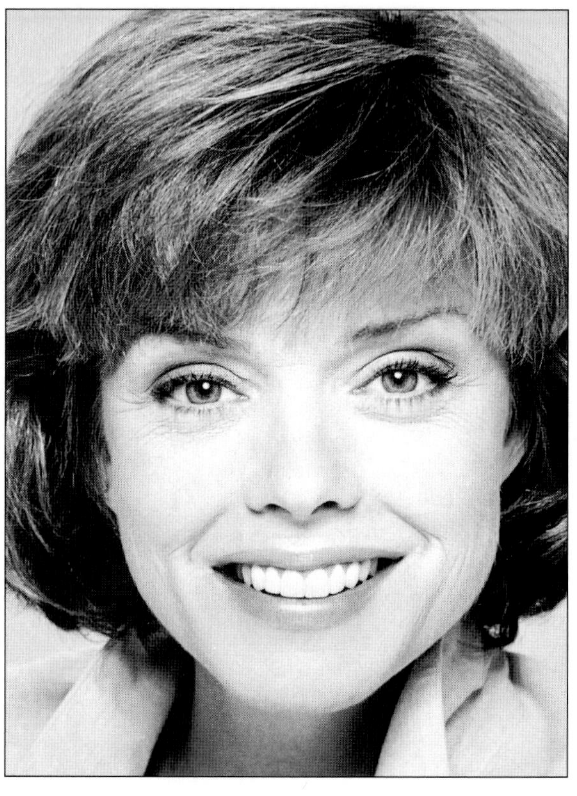

PORCELAIN LAMINATE VENEERS

The solution to this cosmetic problem involved building out the back teeth with lighter-colored porcelain laminate veneers. Lighter colored teeth tend to stand out, whereas darkly stained teeth appear recessive.

Crowning

In cases of extreme wear due to age or bruxism, crowns rather than orthodontics may be the treatment of choice. Crowns can also be used in conjunction with orthodontics to move the lower teeth back or to improve the look of protruding upper teeth.

Before

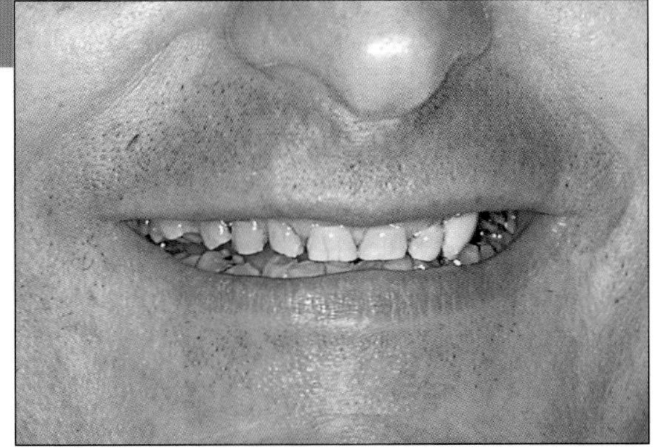

SEVERE WEAR ON LOWER TEETH

This sixty-eight-year-old insurance executive's back and front teeth had been worn almost flat and needed rebuilding. The advanced wear made his teeth appear too small for his face.

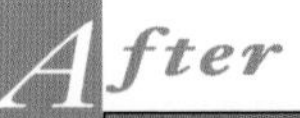

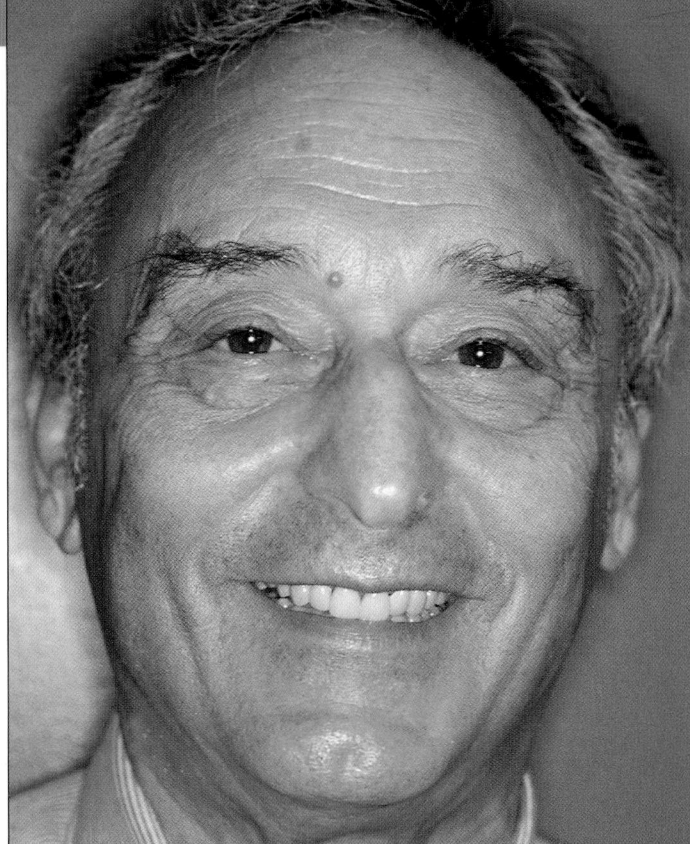

FULL CROWNS

All the upper and lower teeth were crowned to build back the lost tooth structure and help create a younger-looking and more handsome smile.

Treatment Summary

Crowning

Treatment Time Usually two appointments of approximately one to four hours on up to four teeth. Expect to spend more time as additional teeth or more extensive treatment are included.

Patient Maintenance Take care not to bite down on hard foods; the crowns containing porcelain can fracture. Fluoride treatments should be given once a year. Brushing and flossing every day are essential.

Results of Treatment Crowning can sometimes correct within a matter of weeks misaligned teeth that are causing a bad bite.

Average Range of Treatment Life Expectancy Five to fifteen years. Life expectancy is directly proportional to problems with tissue, fractures and danger of decay. Also depends on patient home care. (See footnote on p. 50.)

Cost $550 to $3000 per tooth. (See footnote on p. 50.)

Bridges

When a tooth is missing due to loss or extraction, other teeth usually shift in only a few years. This change in tooth position can cause a variety of bite and gum problems that can be expensive and time-consuming to correct. It is wise, therefore, to replace missing teeth as quickly as possible. One way to do so is with fixed or removable bridges.

Fixed bridges are generally preferable because they cause less trauma to existing teeth than removable bridges. Fixed bridges can also be used as compromise solutions in certain bite problems such as severe protrusion. If the offending teeth are extracted, a fixed bridge can be used to replace the missing teeth in an improved position.

A Word of Caution

Occasionally, even properly constructed restorations can contribute to bite problems. This typically occurs when a disharmony that is barely tolerated already exists in the mouth. In such cases, any irritation or change—even as minor as that which may be caused by crowns or orthodontics—can initiate a muscle spasm and TMJ disturbance.

Such problems may be unforeseen by dentists. When noted, however, they should be corrected quickly. If allowed to persist, they can be extremely difficult to repair.

Comparative Treatments of Open Bite

Advantages	Disadvantages
Orthodontics	
Will improve ability to bite Can improve lip position Can be combined with orthognathic surgery to reduce treatment time and even improve facial results	Time of treatment Retention may be a problem depending on severity of bite and habits Requires retainer for some time
Orthognathic surgery	
Can improve facial esthetics May be only method available to correct deformity Results are usually permanent	General anesthesia required Jaws may require fixation following surgery; limited jaw opening for the first several weeks Requires orthodontic treatment as well
Bonding	
Can lengthen the teeth in mild conditions Can improve color and shape of teeth	Limited amount of benefit Does not improve lip position Usually needs replacement every three to eight years Can chip or stain
Crowning	
Can lengthen the teeth in mild conditions Can improve color and shape of teeth	Limited amount of benefit Teeth require reduction May need replacement in five to fifteen years
Extraction and replacement with bridge	
Could be indicated in patients with advanced periodontal disease or bone loss	Loss of teeth lessens chewing efficiency Can make replacement teeth too long Does not adequately correct lip position May be larger expense to replace teeth

Comparative Treatments of Closed Bite or Deep Overbite

Advantages	Disadvantages
Orthodontics (deep overbite)	
Most preferable Longest lasting Can help cure or prevent TMJ pain Can prevent excessive wear if treated early enough	Takes six months to two years Usually requires wearing retainer for some time
Orthognathic surgery (deep overbite)	
May be necessary in severe cases If too much gum shows, may be indicated May be the only method available	Requires orthodontic treatment as well General anesthesia is usually necessary **Jaws usually require fixation following surgery; limited jaw opening for the first several weeks**
Bonding (both)	
Mainly useful to improve color or shapes of teeth	Does not correct bite problem Can chip or stain Usually needs replacement after three to eight years
Crowning (closed bite)	
In certain cases, can reshape bite and improve facial esthetics by crowning back teeth and creating a space to allow more natural anterior teeth	May be difficult, if not impossible, to open bite Requires tooth reduction May need replacement in five to fifteen years
Extraction and replacement with bridge (both)	
None	Does not correct or improve condition

Comparative Treatments of Protrusion ("Buck Teeth")

Advantages	Disadvantages
Orthodontics	
Most preferable Longest lasting Can be combined with orthognathic surgery to reduce treatment time	Takes six months to two years Retention may be a problem, depending on severity of bites and habits Requires wearing retainer for some time
Orthognathic surgery	
Can shorten treatment time Can improve gross facial deformities May be the only method available to correct deformities	Requires orthodontic treatment as well General anesthesia is usually necessary Jaws usually require fixation following surgery; limited jaw opening for the first several weeks
Bonding	
One-appointment procedure May slightly improve alignment	Can make teeth appear too thick May need replacement after five to eight years Can chip or stain
Crowning	
Can improve the angle of tooth as well as color and shape	Cannot compensate for jawbone differences in relation to the lower jaw May need replacement every five to fifteen years Requires loss of natural tooth structure May involve removal of nerves in teeth to accomplish improved lipline Local anesthesia is required
Extraction and replacement with bridge	
In some cases can improve lipline Can be indicated in patients with advanced bone loss	Can overcorrect by removing too much bone Loss of teeth lessens chewing efficiency May not correct protrusion of bone May not improve facial esthetics Can be most expensive type of correction

Comparative Treatments of Crossbite

Advantages	Disadvantages
Orthodontics	
Most preferable Longest lasting	Takes four to six months if only one or two teeth are involved Requires six to twenty-four months if more than two teeth are involved May need to be combined with orthognathic surgery
Orthognathic surgery	
May shorten treatment time in severe crossbites May be necessary in severe cases Results are usually permanent	Not indicated in one or two teeth crossbites Requires orthodontic treatment as well Jaws usually require fixation following surgery; limited jaw opening for the first several weeks General anesthesia is usually required
Bonding	
Can sometimes build out upper teeth to widen arch One-appointment procedure	Can chip or stain Has limited esthetic life and usually needs to be replaced after three to eight years Does not correct defect Only indicated for mild conditions
Crowning	
Can alter shapes and color of teeth	Local anesthesia is required Requires tooth reduction Does not correct defect Lasts about five to fifteen years
Extraction and replacement with bridge	
None	Does not correct crossbite except in one or two tooth situations Loss of teeth lessens chewing efficiency Expense may be more than better solutions like repositioning

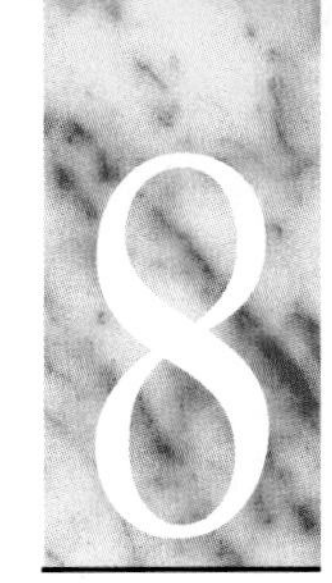

Improving the Jaw and Face Through Surgery

Louis S. Belinfante, DDS

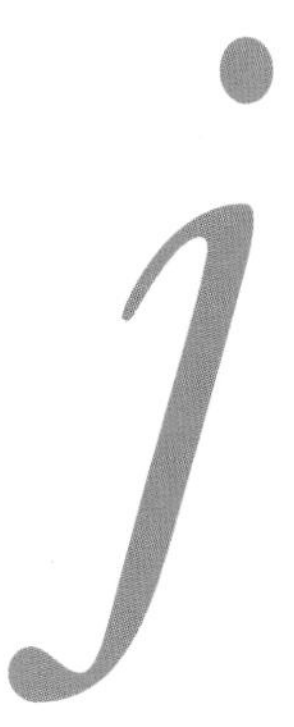

Jaws that don't fit together properly are not only a medical problem, but an esthetic problem. In addition to causing difficulty in biting and chewing, these "bad bites" may make people self-conscious about their smile and their overall appearance. This chapter focuses on the esthetic benefits of correcting such problems.

What Is a Bad Bite?

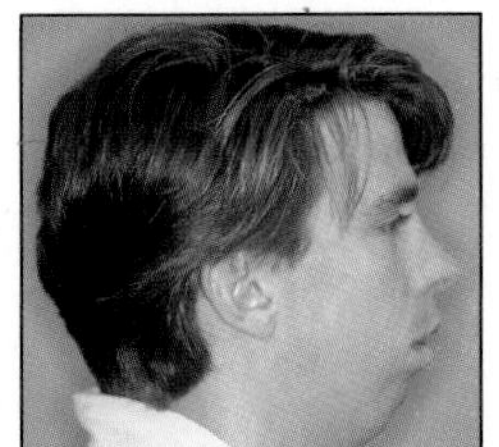

There are many types of bad bites, with some having a greater effect on facial esthetics than others. The good news is that they need not be permanent. While some bite problems can be resolved through orthodontic treatment, more complicated problems require surgery. Improvement, and often correction, can be attained with the proper procedure.

There are many types of bad bites:

- Recessive lower jaw relationship to upper jaw
- Protruding lower jaw relationship to upper jaw
- Open bite relationship, where teeth do not meet
- Asymmetry, where the jaw is "off" to one side or another
- Combinations of the above

Before

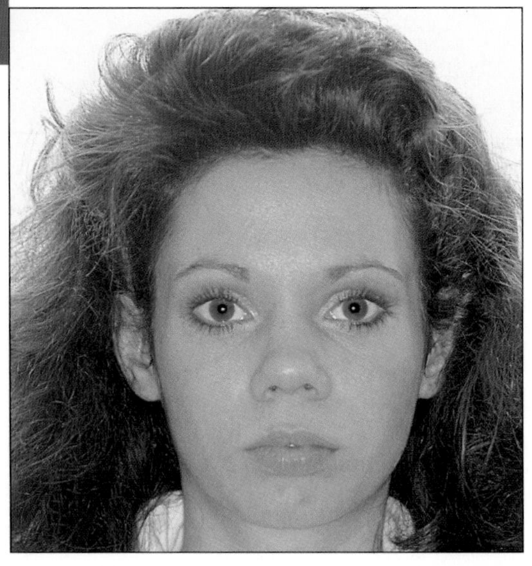

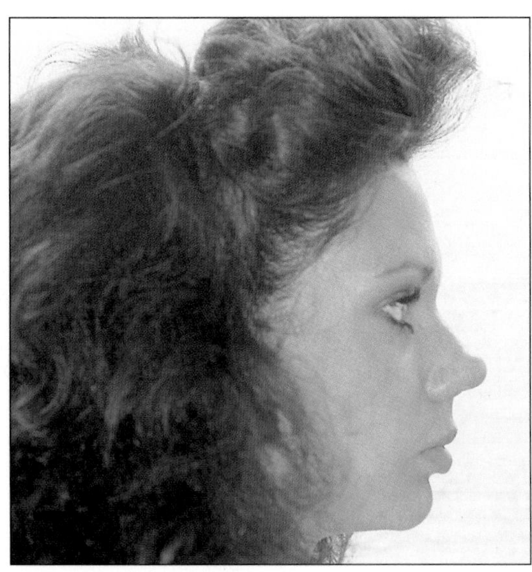

Recessive lower jaw and nasal deformity

This twenty-one-year-old woman sought correction of her recessive lower jaw and deformed nose.

After

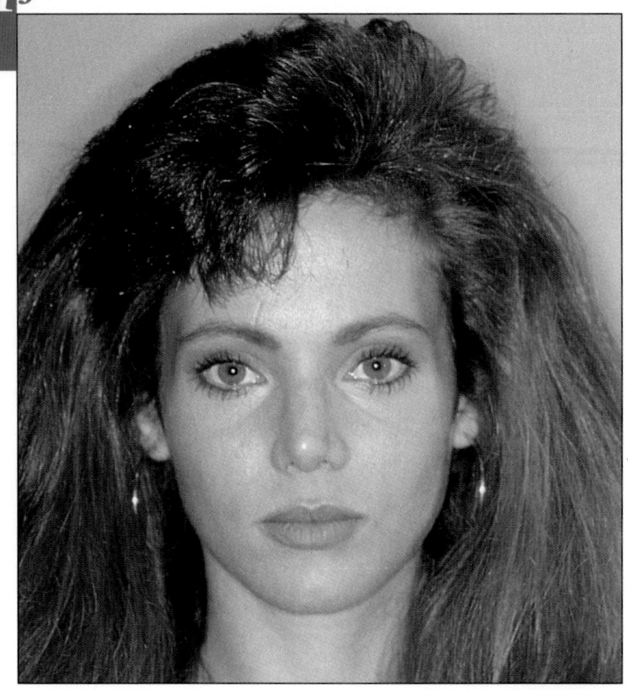

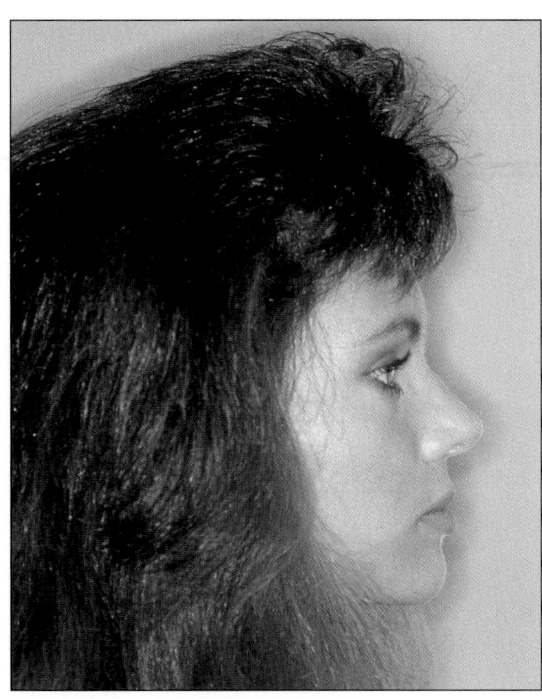

Multiple jaw osteotomies (bone incisions) and rhinoplasty (nose surgery)

After approximately one year of presurgical orthodontics, the patient underwent surgery to have the lower jaw bone brought forward. Her nasal deformity was corrected at the same time. This involved thinning the tip and the entire width of the nose.

Who Can Help?

There are basically six types of specialists whose services include changing facial features. Depending on your problem, you may need only one doctor, or several specialists may work together as a team to provide you with the best results.

Oral and maxillofacial surgeon

The oral and maxillofacial surgeon changes facial features by performing surgery on the underlying bone structure. This may be accomplished by rearranging the jaw bones or adding some form of plastic material or implants to the bones to enhance a particular feature, such as the cheekbones or chin. The oral and maxillofacial surgeon may also perform other types of facial surgery such as rhinoplasty (nasal reshaping), blepharoplasty (removal of fat and tissue from baggy eyelids), rhytidectomy (facelift), liposculpture (selected fat removal), chemical peel, laser resurfacing and scar revision.

Before

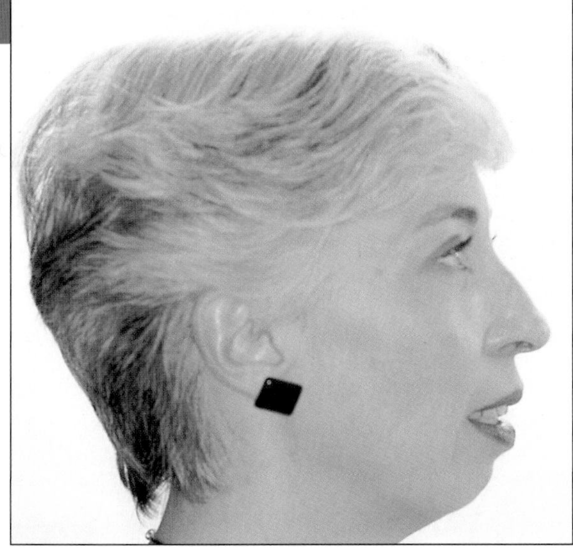

Recessive chin and chronic TMJ dysfunction

This woman had both a recessive chin and chronic temporomandibular joint (TMJ) pain.

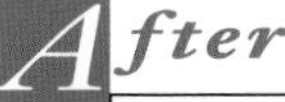

After

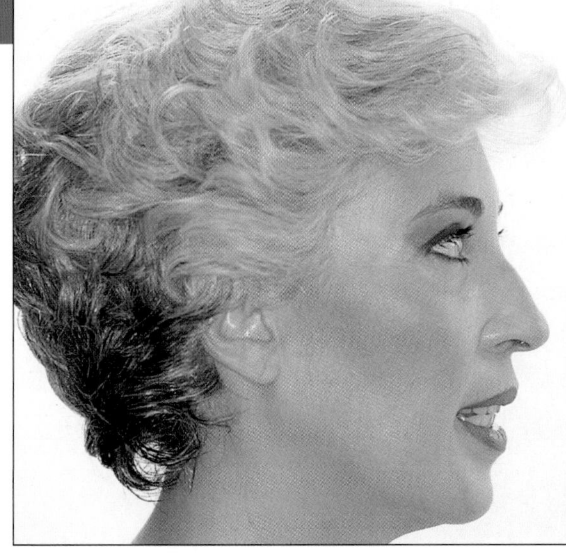

Surgery

Surgery included advancing the chin forward using the patient's own bone and surgically correcting her TMJ problem. All surgery was performed at one time.

Orthodontist

Orthodontists work with individual teeth by applying forces that place them in proper position in the jaw bones. They also align teeth so that they are in a correct relationship with one another. Orthodontists can often alter the facial bones of very young patients.

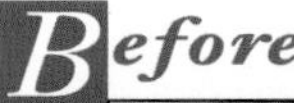

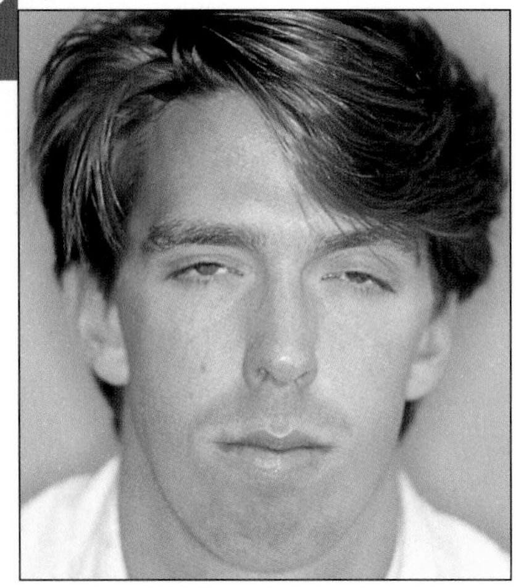

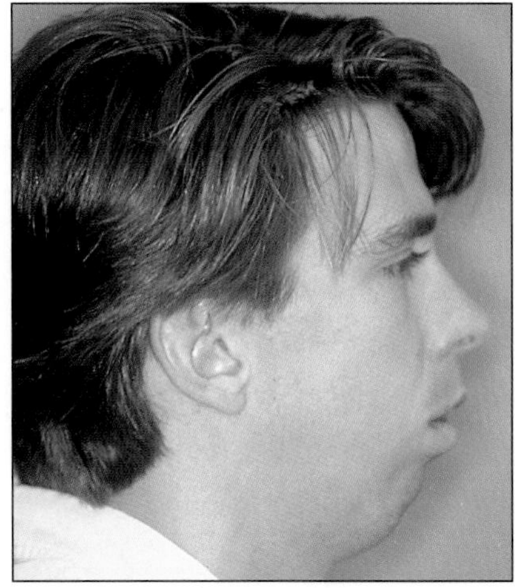

RECESSIVE LOWER JAW, RECESSIVE CHIN, GUMMY SMILE AND OPEN BITE

This twenty-four-year-old man wanted correction of his upper jaw and chin.

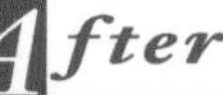

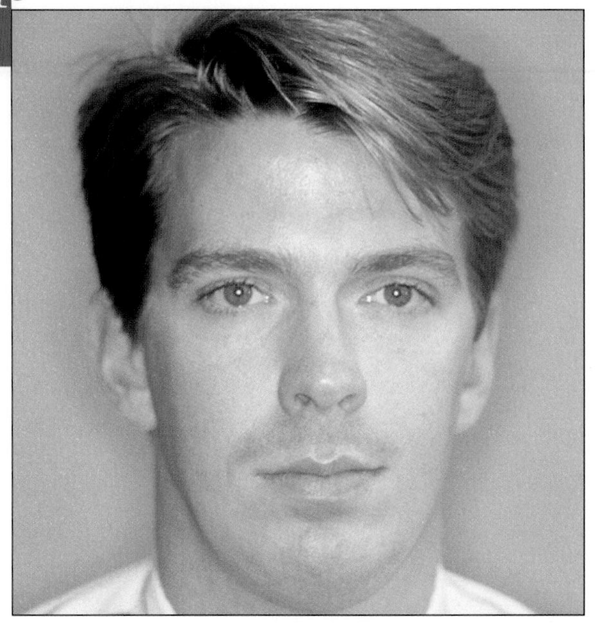

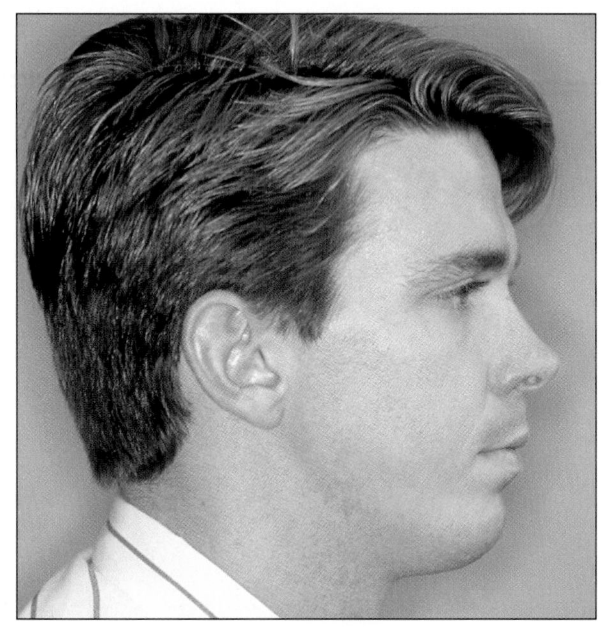

SURGERY AND ORTHODONTICS

He underwent orthodontic therapy for about a year before surgery. At the time of the surgery, a wedge of bone was removed from his upper jaw to reduce his gummy smile and open bite. The lower jaw was placed in a more forward position, and his chin was advanced.

Before

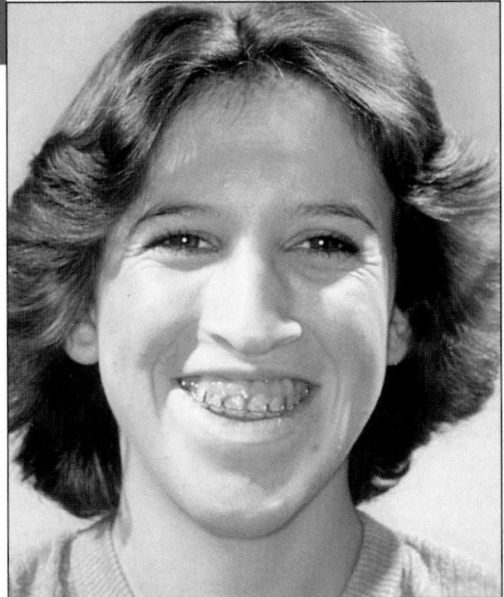

GUMMY SMILE, PROTRUSIVE LOWER JAW AND OPEN BITE

This eighteen-year-old woman sought correction of her high lipline and protrusive chin area.

After

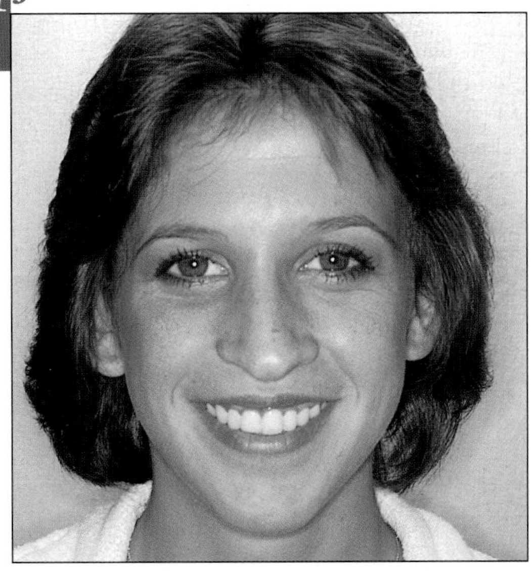

ORTHODONTICS AND SURGERY

The patient underwent about eighteen months of presurgical orthodontics. Surgery involved removal of a wedge of bone from the upper jaw to help reduce her gummy smile, her open bite and the protrusiveness of the lower jaw.

Before

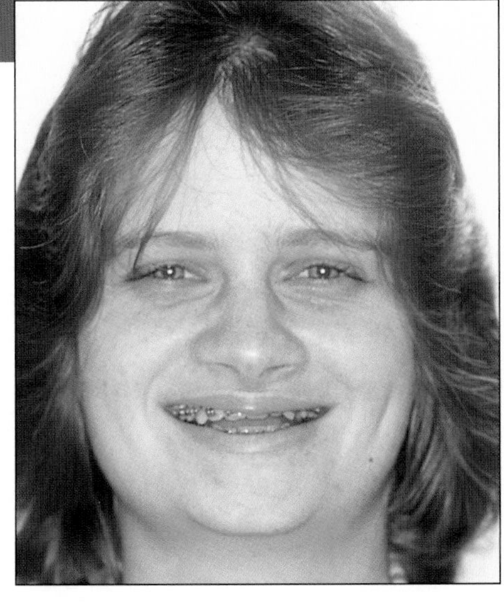

UPPER TEETH NOT VISIBLE

This 25-year-old woman had an upper jaw problem. Her upper teeth were not visible when her upper lip was relaxed.

After

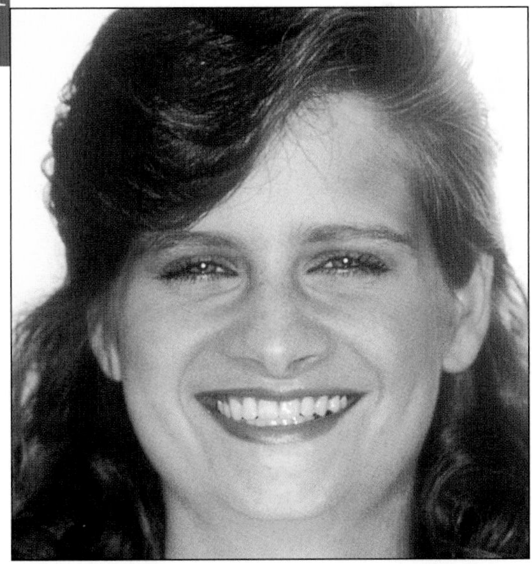

ORTHODONTICS AND SURGERY

After extensive presurgical orthodontic therapy, a bone graft was constructed to lengthen her upper jaw. The patient is shown here about eighteen months after surgery. Her smileline is much closer to normal and enhances her overall appearance.

General dentist or prosthodontist

The general dentist or prosthodontist (specialist) achieves esthetic results by adding or removing teeth or realigning them through cosmetic contouring. They may also bond, laminate or crown the teeth to improve their appearance.

Plastic surgeon

Plastic surgeons typically reconstruct body parts that are defective or in need of repair. For example, they may reduce or enlarge breasts, perform liposuction, revamp scars, perform facial surgery or repair defective tissues.

Otolaryngologist

Otolaryngologists work primarily on functional areas of the head such as the tonsils, inner ears and sinuses. They may also perform cosmetic surgery.

Dermatologist

Dermatologists change facial features by altering skin texture and form. They may do this with chemical peels, dermabrasion, liposuction, laser resurfacing or through medical treatment. Some dermatologists also perform general plastic surgery procedures.

What Is Orthognathic Surgery?

The term *orthognathic* means "straight jaw." Orthognathic surgery is usually performed in a hospital by an oral and maxillofacial surgeon. Typically, the surgeon makes incisions from inside the mouth and cheeks so that there are no scars on the face. In cosmetic oral and maxillofacial surgery, which addresses the soft tissue drape of the face, incisions are sometimes made on the facial skin itself.

Cuts in the bone, or osteotomies, are made with specially designed instruments. The bones are then properly rearranged and wired internally for several weeks so that the parts can "set" in their new positions. In some cases, stainless steel wires are left in position. Occasionally the surgeon will correct bony problems and may even perform surgery on the nasal passages, eyelids, cheeks or chin.

Another approach to orthognathic surgery involves the use of internal rigid fixation, in which screws and plates are used instead of wires, or are used in addition to them. This often allows the patient to regain jaw mobility more quickly. In such cases, small incisions in the skin may be necessary.

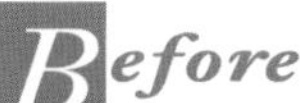

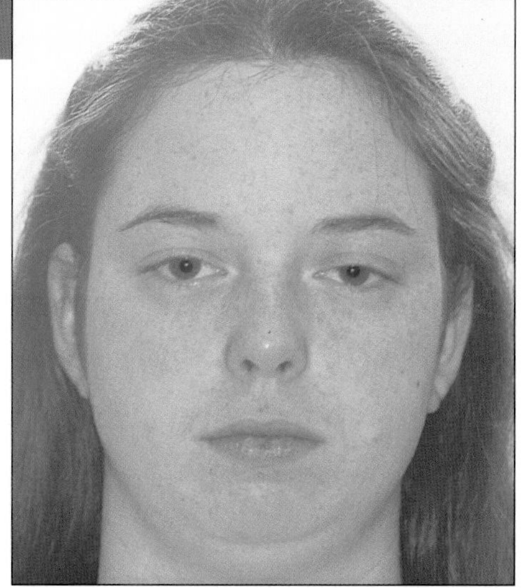

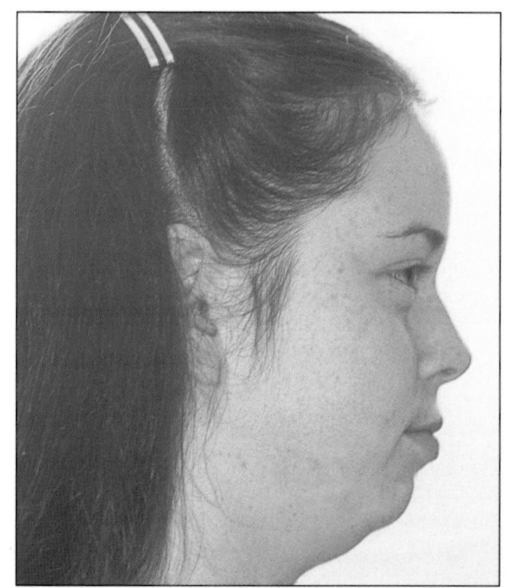

EXCESSIVE FACIAL FATTY TISSUE, GUMMY SMILE AND RECESSIVE LOWER JAW

This young woman had reduced chewing ability as well as excess facial fat tissue.

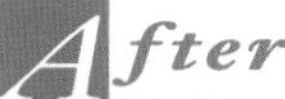

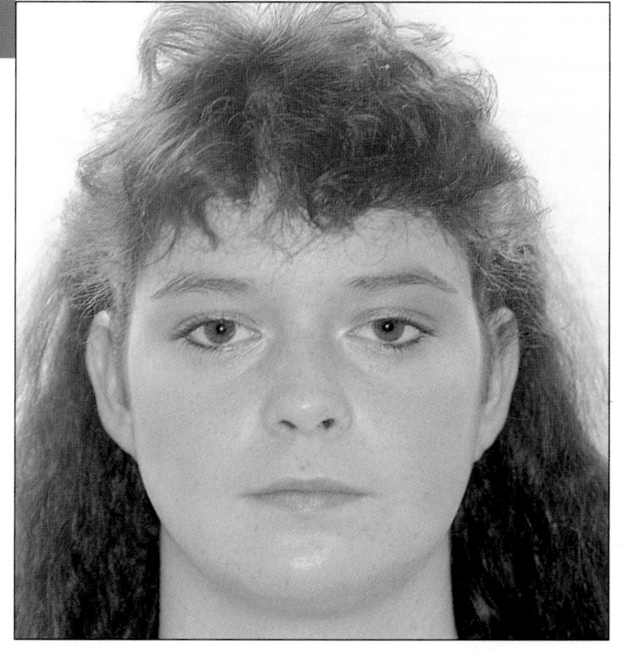

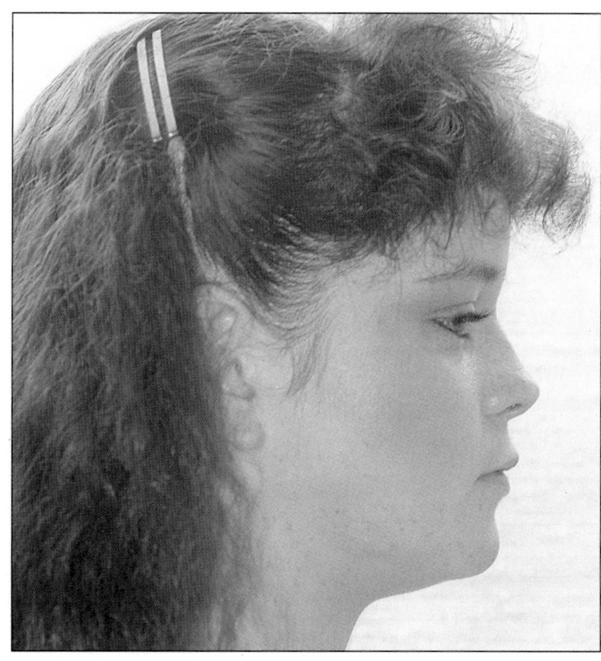

LIPOSUCTION AND SURGERY

Facial liposuction, along with upper and lower jaw surgery, were performed at the same surgical appointment. The relationship of facial tissue to bone is now more harmonious.

Before

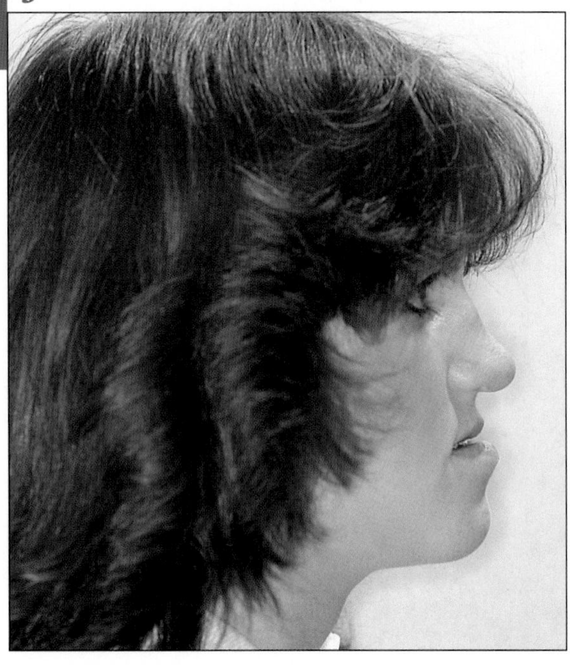

PROTRUDING LOWER JAW

This 16-year-old girl was disturbed by her bad bite—her lower jaw was too far forward and to one side.

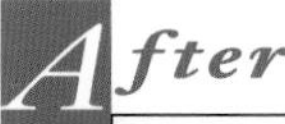

After

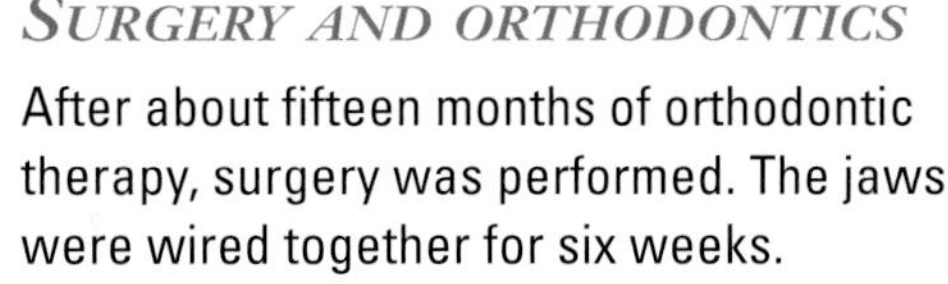

SURGERY AND ORTHODONTICS

After about fifteen months of orthodontic therapy, surgery was performed. The jaws were wired together for six weeks.

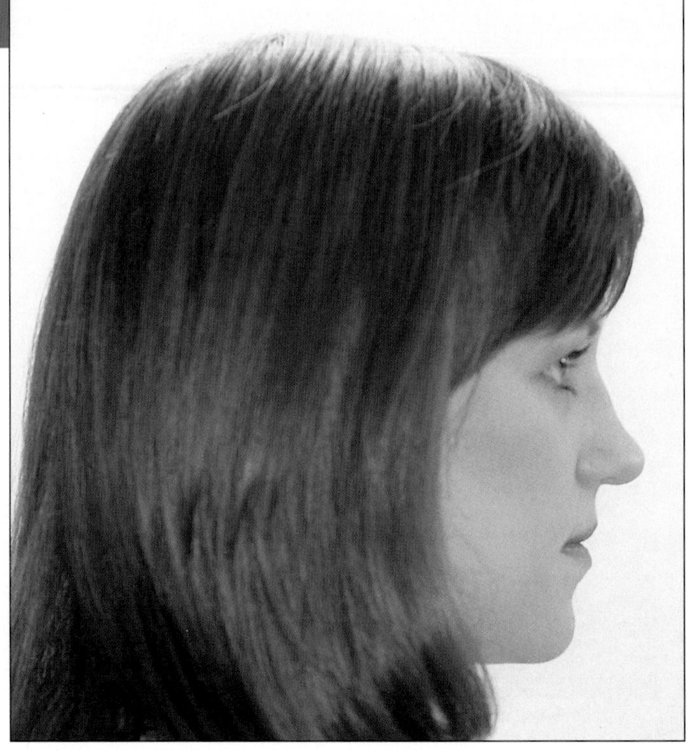

Before

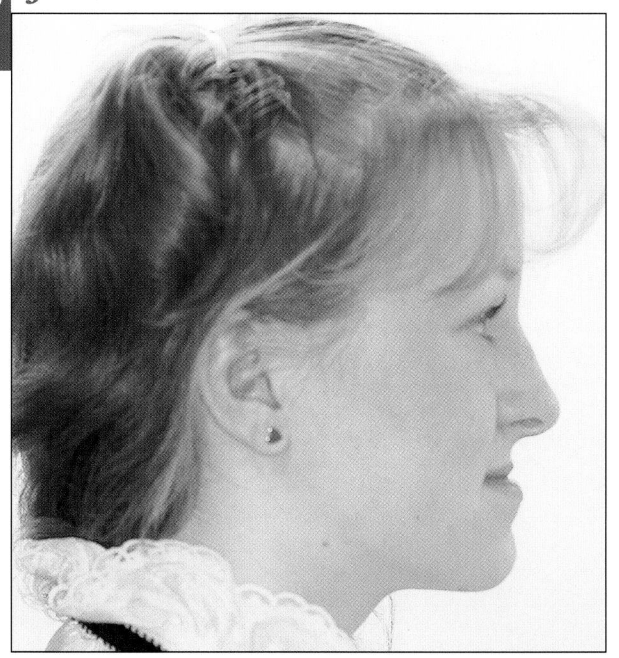

PROTRUDING LOWER JAW

This young woman's complaint was twofold. She had difficulty chewing her food properly, and she felt that the length of her lower jaw was unattractive.

After

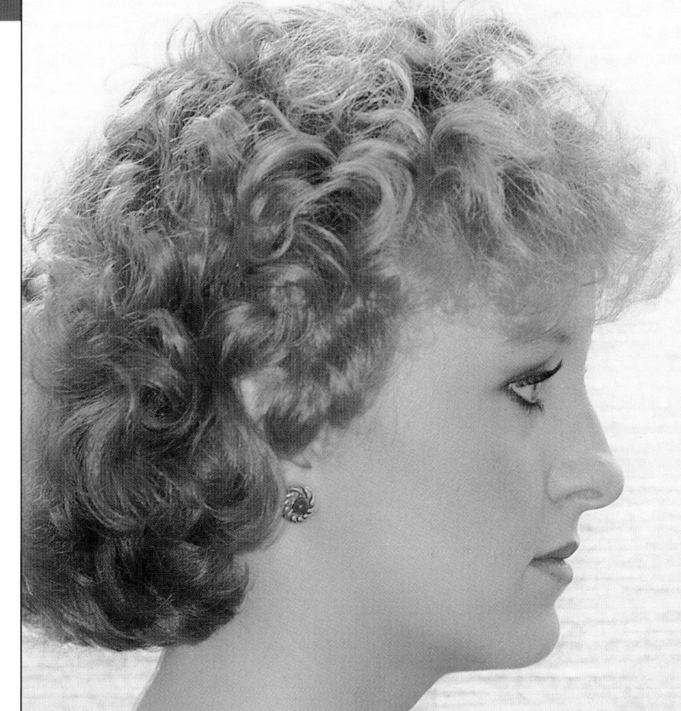

SURGERY AND ORTHODONTICS

Orthodontic therapy prepared the patient to have the proper type of corrective surgery. The surgery allowed the lower jaw to be placed in a more backward position.

Communication Is Critical to Success

It is important that you tell your doctor exactly what you want to correct. He or she may zero in on a particular problem, but what if that problem is not your primary concern? And while the surgeon's treatment may be exquisite by professional standards, you'll be disappointed if the final result isn't what you expected.

Your surgeon will need special records in order to evaluate your problem. These records typically include models of your teeth, photographs, video images and special X-rays. These records may point to additional problems that you and your doctor should also discuss. For example, you may have seen an oral and maxillofacial surgeon because you have a protruding jaw. Your records, however, may indicate that additional problems exist. Using your records, your surgeon will design a highly specialized treatment plan for you.

SOME SURGEONS USE VIDEOIMAGING TO GIVE YOU A GOOD IDEA OF WHAT YOU'LL LOOK LIKE AFTER SURGERY

Because it is so important that you get an idea of the final result, some surgeons use videoimaging to give you a good idea what you'll look like after surgery. Other doctors trace your profile based on your X-rays.

It is also important that you understand each step of the surgical procedure that you are to undergo. Your doctor may show you a model of a skull to illustrate the actual operation. The main risks and possible outcomes of the procedure should be explained thoroughly. It is then up to you to decide which procedures you wish performed.

Fees and Insurance Coverage

Costs for the initial phase of orthognathic treatment may range anywhere from several hundred to several thousand dollars. You should discuss fees before surgery takes place. Insurance may often cover hospitalization or clinic charges, as well as most of the surgeon's fees, if the procedures are performed for functional reasons.

Ask your doctor or the office's insurance coordinator to write a letter to your insurance company stating the nature of your problem, the planned correction and the fee. The letter should also ask the insurance company to specify how much of the procedure it will cover.

Many patients with jaw deformities also need orthodontic treatment to rearrange the teeth before or after surgery or both. In fact, it is almost impossible to obtain ideal results unless presurgical and postsurgical orthodontics is performed.

Before

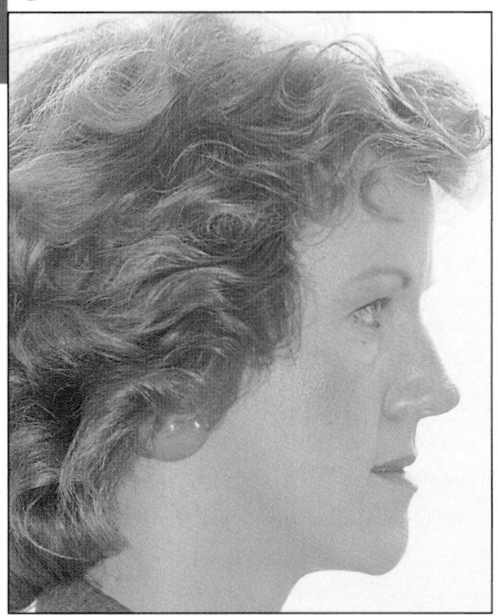

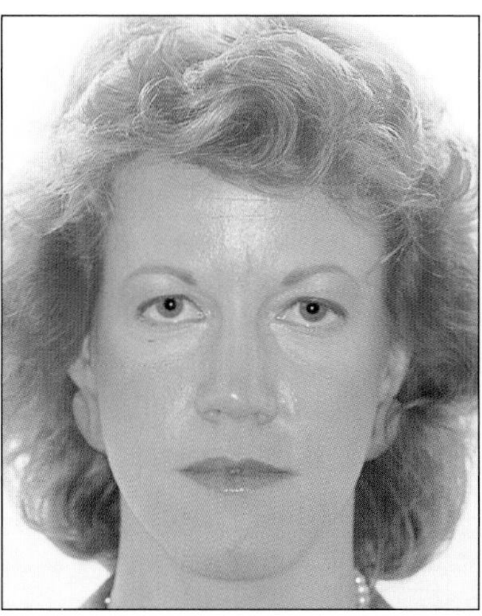

Baggy eyelids, flat cheek bones and protruding lower jaw

This twenty-eight-year-old woman was concerned about her baggy eyelids; even when well rested, she looked tired. In addition, she had a protruding lower jaw, which was emphasized by her flat cheeks.

After

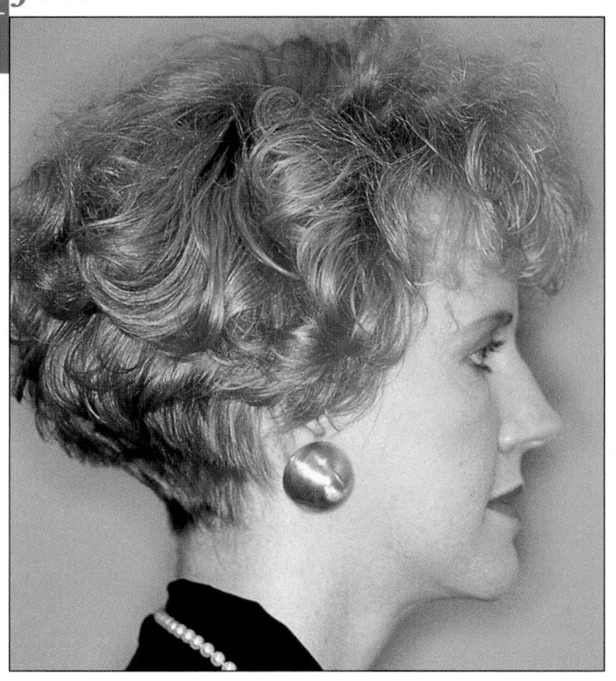

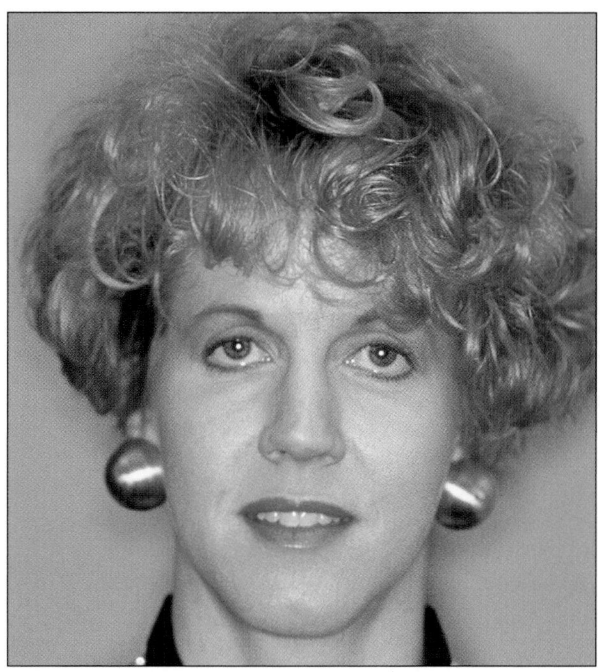

Blepharoplasty (eyelid recontouring), build up of cheek bones and repositioning of lower jaw

Excess fat, skin and muscle were removed from the eyelid tissue. Cheek bone implants were placed to enhance the middle of her face. Lastly, the lower jaw bone was positioned backward via a series of cuts (osteotomies) in the bone.

Surgery

Some orthognathic surgical procedures can be accomplished on an outpatient basis, which means you don't have to spend a night in the hospital or surgical facility. Although some complex procedures require remaining in the hospital for two or three days, the typical hospital stay is one to two days.

Regardless of where you have your surgery, routine laboratory tests will be performed before the procedure. The actual operation may take from one hour to several hours, depending upon its complexity as well as the severity of your condition. Immediately after the surgery, you will go to the recovery room where you will stay until your doctor feels you are ready to go back to your own room or be discharged.

If you require a hospital stay, you will probably be fed intravenously at first. However, as soon as you indicate that you can drink the liquids prescribed, the intravenous fluids will be discontinued.

Because the bones are rearranged during surgery, the jaw is typically wired in place for six to eight weeks. This allows the jaws to heal in proper position, much like a cast helps a fractured arm heal correctly. However, internal pins or screws can, in most instances, eliminate the need for the jaws to be wired together.

SOME ORTHOGNATHIC SURGICAL PROCEDURES CAN BE ACCOMPLISHED ON AN OUTPATIENT BASIS

Although you can expect some swelling and soreness, they are well controlled with medication. Because there are so many nerves in the mouth and facial area, there may also be some numbness after the operation. In most instances, normal feeling returns within a few weeks.

You will probably experience some weight loss at first. However, a specific number of calories will be planned for you on a daily basis, and your diet will be supplemented with vitamins and minerals. As you regulate the calories you take in, your weight loss will level off.

If wiring is used to keep the jaw in place, it will be removed in three to eight weeks. If plates or screws are used, that time span is much less. Because the jaws will have been closed for a long time, you may experience some stiffness at first. After several weeks, however, you should be able to chew comfortably. Your surgeon will then direct you back to your general dentist and orthodontist for the completion of treatment.

Before

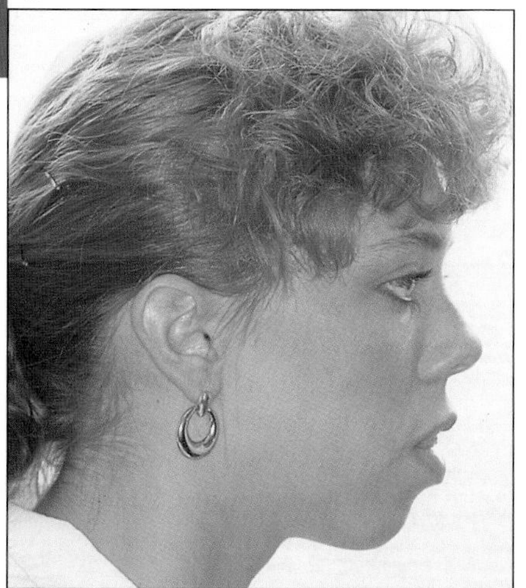

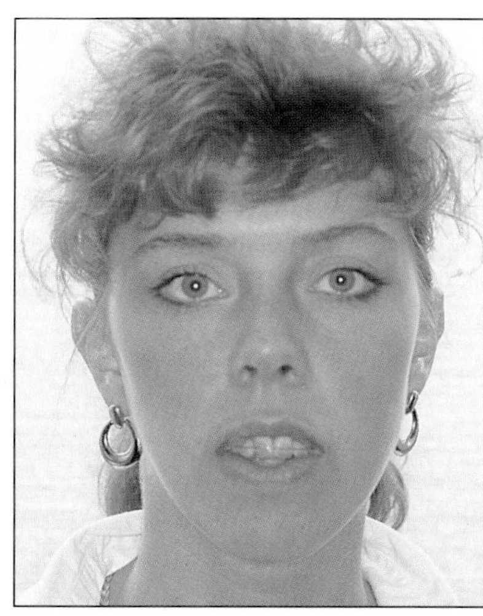

Gummy smile, open bite and recessive lower jaw and chin

This twenty-four-year-old woman sought to enhance her facial features and correct her functional deformities.

After

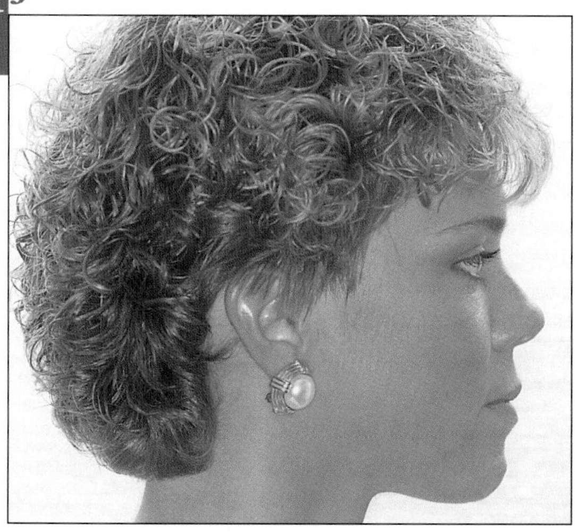

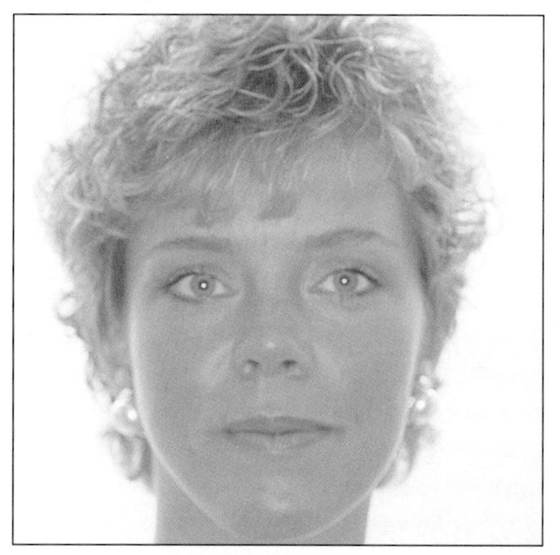

Surgery

Orthodontics and surgery

The patient underwent presurgical orthodontic therapy for one year before surgery. Surgical reduction of her upper jaw was done to reduce her gummy smile and open bite. Surgical alignment was performed on her lower jaw and chin. The patient also opted for a new hair style and make-up.

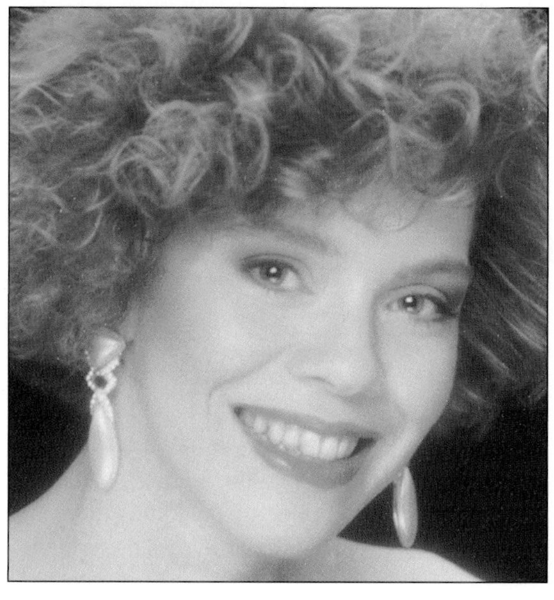

Before

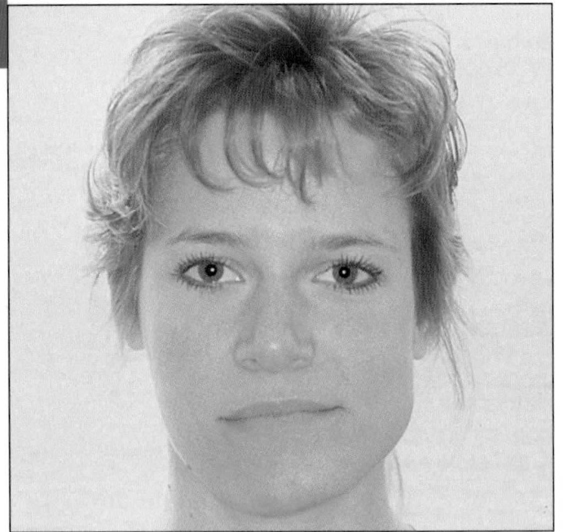

ASYMMETRY OF THE FACE

This twenty-four-year-old woman had major facial asymmetry, mostly due to a bony protrusion on the right lower half of her face. This deformity also involved her upper jaw, lower jaw, chin and bite plane.

After

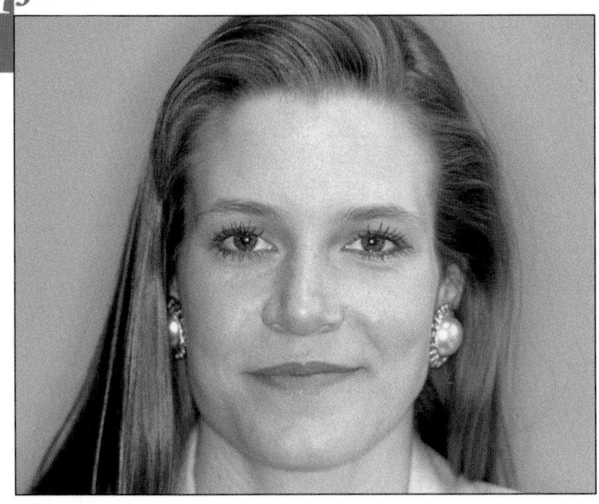

SURGERY TO UPPER JAW, LOWER JAW AND CHIN

Surgery was performed to correct the unevenness of the upper jaw. The lower jaw was surgically treated to match the new bite. The overgrown portion of the lower jaw was removed and reused as a graft for the upper jaw.

Before

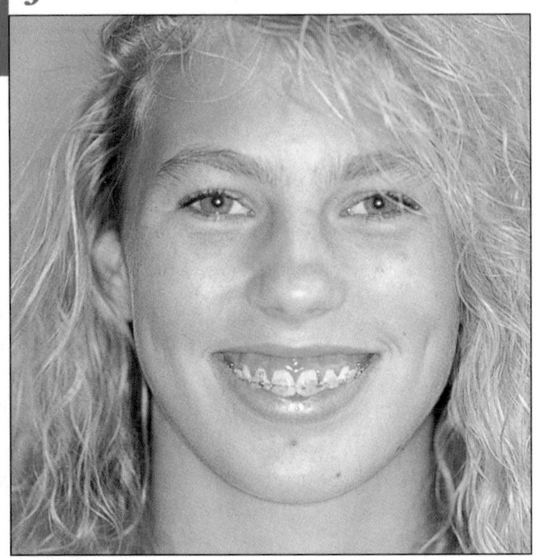

RETRUSIVE LOWER JAW, RETRUSIVE CHIN, WIDE NOSE AND GUMMY SMILE

This thirteen-year-old girl had a lack of growth of her lower jaw. A physical examination, X-rays, videoimaging and dental mold analysis revealed the problems described.

After

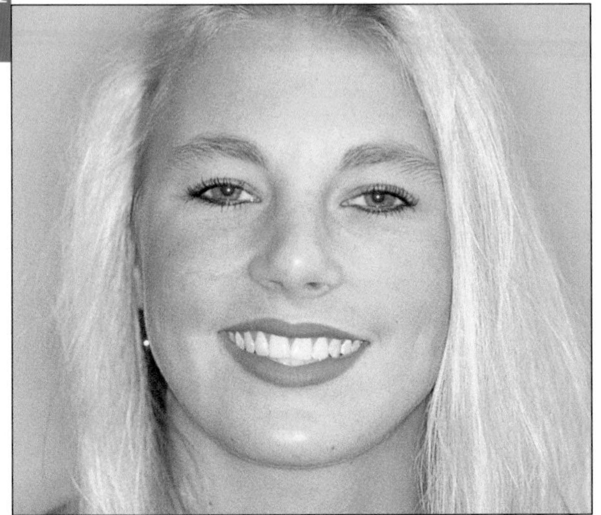

ORTHODONTIC THERAPY, NASAL SURGERY AND SURGERY TO BOTH JAWS AND THE CHIN

Surgery was performed to lengthen the lower jaw and chin. During the one hospital procedure, nasal surgery was also performed to reduce the width of the nasal tip along with upper jaw surgery to reduce the gummy smile.

Before

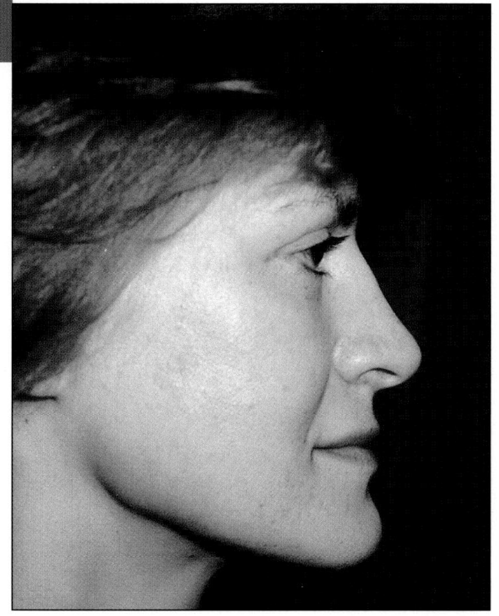

FACIAL REJUVENATION DESIRED

This young woman was dissatisfied with her facial appearance.

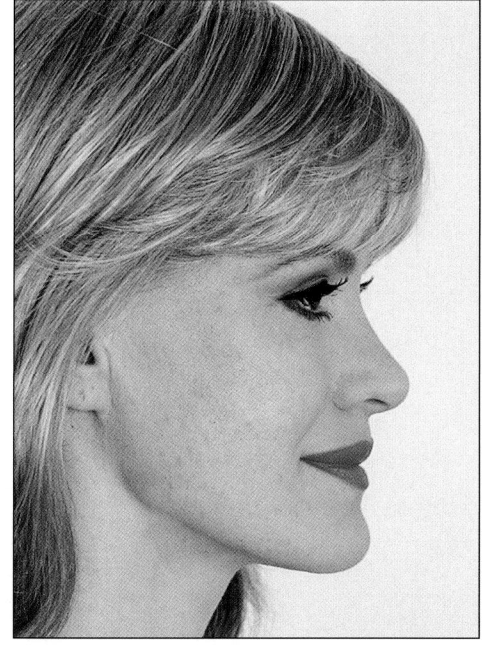

FACE-LIFT AND EYELID, NOSE AND SKIN IMPROVEMENTS

Multiple procedures were performed by plastic surgeons, including a face-lift, eyelid, nose and skin alterations. However, the woman felt that her chin was still too prominent.

After

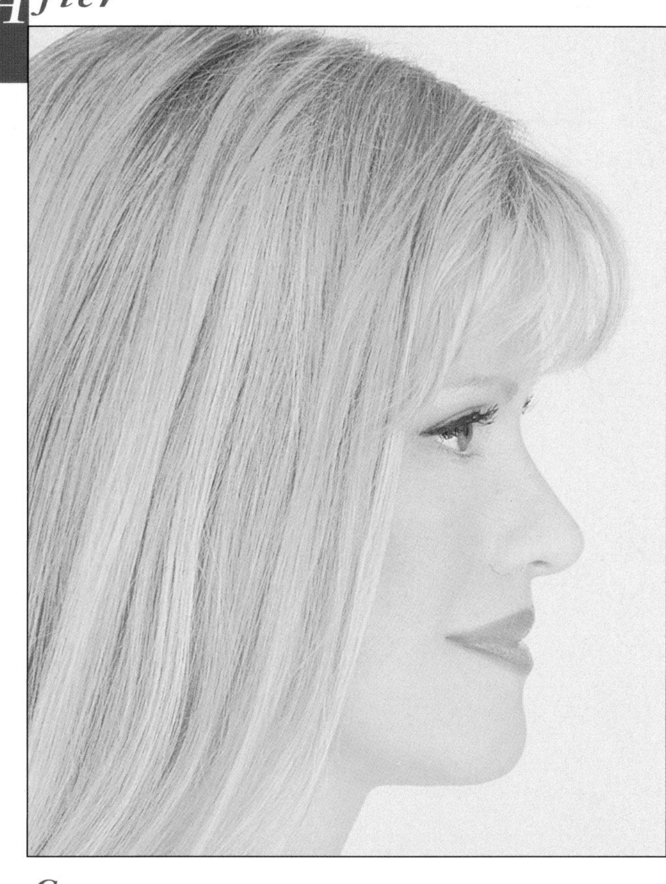

CHIN REDUCTION

A chin reduction was later performed by the chapter author to improve facial harmony.

Surgery

TREATMENT SUMMARY

ORTHOGNATHIC SURGERY

Treatment Time One to three months.

Patient Maintenance Meticulous daily care of the mouth and teeth while the jaws are wired together.

Results of Treatment Usually jaw problems and facial esthetics are improved by rearranging the jaw bones and possibly adding implants, removal of fatty tissue, etc.

Average Range of Treatment Life Expectancy For the most part, the treatment is permanent. (See footnote on p. 50.)

Cost Several hundred to several thousand dollars, depending upon the treatment. (See footnote on p. 50.)

ADVANTAGES

1. Some jaw problems can be treated only by surgery
2. The procedures are usually accomplished in one or two visits at either a hospital or office surgical suite
3. Although surgery can be costly, it may be covered by insurance
4. In most cases, self image is greatly improved, which may help relationships, career advancement and quality of life

DISADVANTAGES

1. Surgery is required
2. Jaws may be wired together for six to eight weeks
3. Surgery may be costly, especially if not covered by insurance
4. Facial swelling and discomfort, with associated inconveniences, may last several weeks
5. May cause a negative personality change in unstable individuals
6. If plastic implants are used, they may become infected or shift
7. Facial numbness may result temporarily or permanently

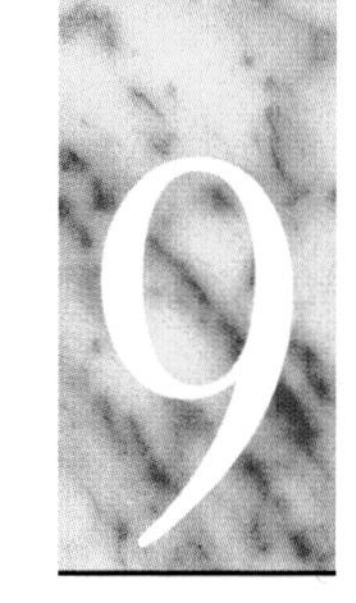

How Your Gums Affect Your Smile

If the teeth can be described as the canvas of a painting, then the gum tissue is the frame around the canvas. In other words, the gum tissue can make or break a smile. Before learning more about healthy and diseased gums, it helps to understand the integral relationship between the jaw bone, the teeth and the gums.

Teeth are supported in the upper and lower jaw bones by fibers that run between the tooth and the bone. The teeth are surrounded by tissues that provide additional support. Gum tissue, also known as gingiva, covers a portion of the jaw bone, forming a collar around the neck of each tooth.

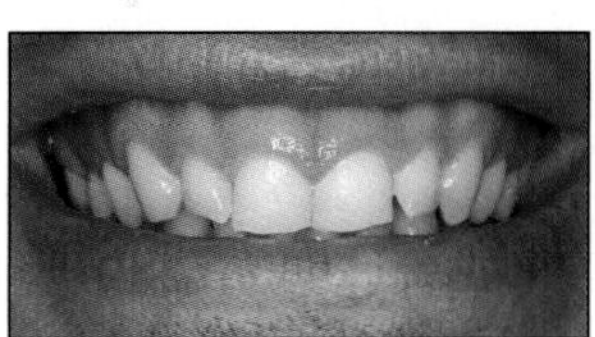

What Is Gum Disease?

Healthy gingival tissue appears pink, knife-edged and stippled like an orange peel. Various shades of pink may be characteristic of healthy tissue depending on a person's ethnic background and skin tone. Stippling may also vary according to age and gender.

Gum disease, commonly referred to as periodontal disease, is a condition that affects the tissues surrounding the teeth. It is caused by excessive bacteria building up in the mouth. The collection of bacteria and their by-products is

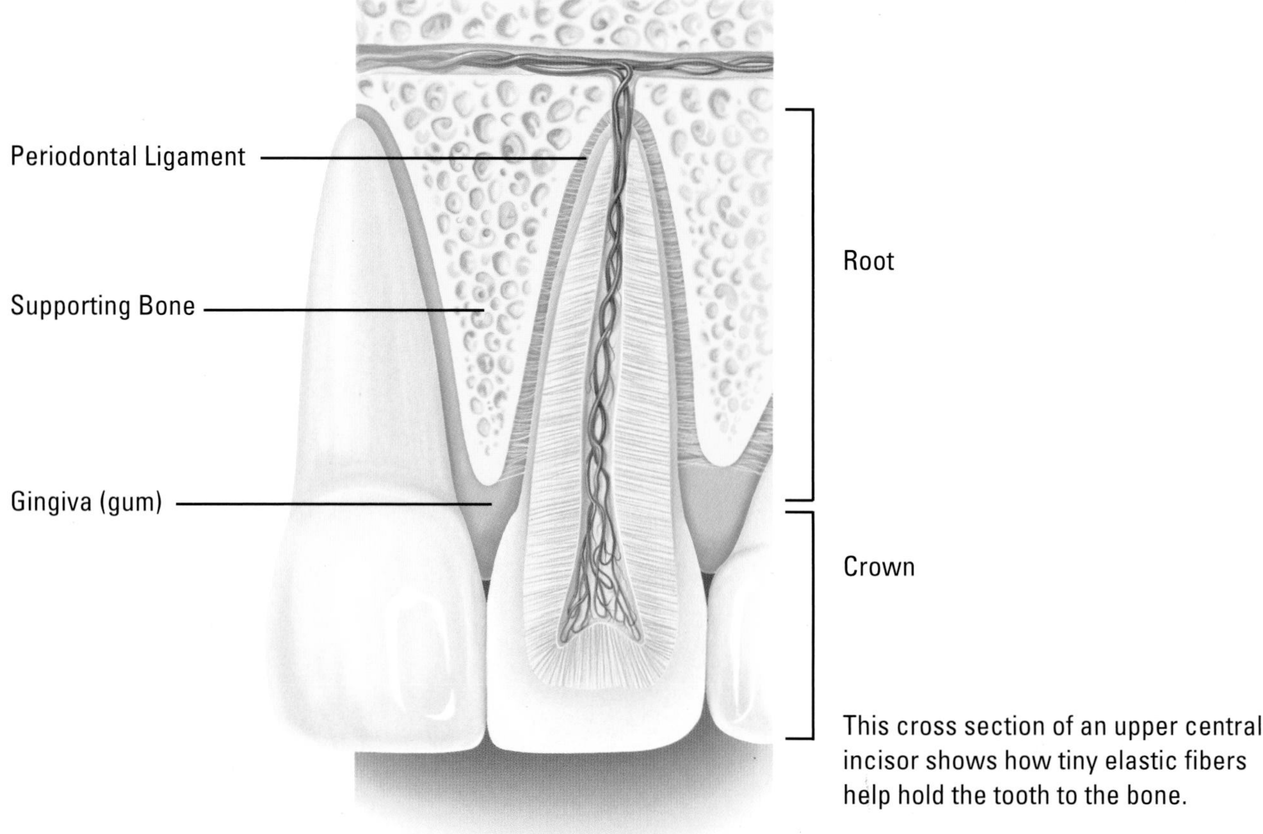

This cross section of an upper central incisor shows how tiny elastic fibers help hold the tooth to the bone.

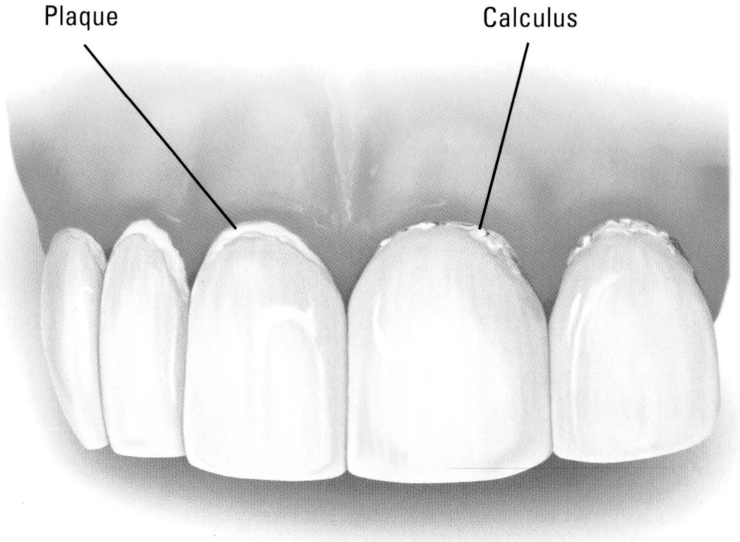

The bacterial plaque shown could have been removed by brushing and flossing. When the plaque is allowed to remain, the minerals from saliva cause the plaque to harden and cause calculus (tartar). This must be removed by the hygienist or dentist to prevent further disease.

commonly referred to as plaque. If plaque is allowed to remain in the mouth for too long, the minerals from the saliva cause it to harden, forming what is known as calculus or tartar.

The presence of either plaque or tartar can lead to periodontal disease. In the early stages, gums may bleed easily and appear red, tender, spongy and slightly swollen. One or all of these symptoms may be present at the same time.

If the bacterial build-up under the gumline is allowed to increase, pockets will form under the gum. Eventually, the disease may lead to a recession of the gingival tissue, destruction of the underlying bone, loosening of the teeth and ultimately tooth loss. *Periodontal disease is the primary cause of tooth loss in the adult population.*

Certain systemic changes can also increase your chances of getting periodontal disease. These include pregnancy, hormonal changes, psychological stress and certain medications.

Be aware that gums occasionally bleed for reasons other than periodontal disease. For example, during pregnancy, hormonal changes can cause the gums to bleed. Although the cause of the bleeding should be determined by a dentist, there is usually no cause for alarm in these cases. An anxiety-related condition called trench mouth, or Vincent's infection, also mimics periodontal disease. It causes bleeding, pain, severe odor and can result in esthetic deformities. Unlike other gum diseases, however, it is usually treated effectively with a combination of antibiotics and periodontal therapy.

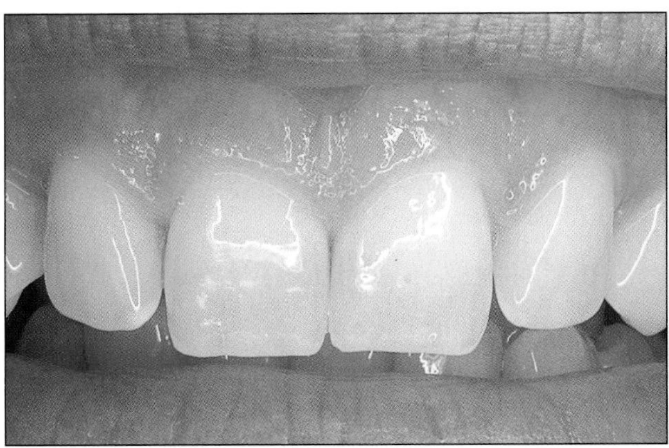

Healthy gum tissue is usually pink, knife-edged and stippled like an orange peel. Notice how it curves around the neck of the tooth and frames it.

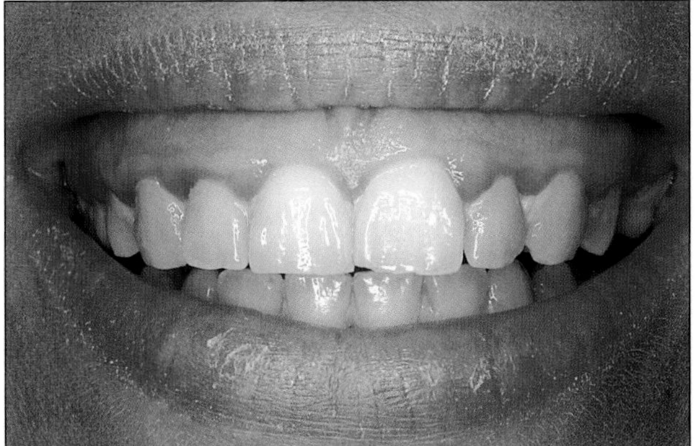

An attractive smile can be ruined by unsightly gums that are red, swollen or puffy. Treatment for this patient would consist of several professional cleaning appointments with the hygienist, followed by scaling with her general dentist or periodontist. Finally, good home-care practice consisting of proper brushing and flossing can result in a healthy smile.

Treatment of Periodontal Disease

Treatment of periodontal disease is directed at halting the disease at the point at which it is diagnosed. Because it is difficult to cure advanced forms of the disease, the sooner it is detected, the better. Therefore, if you have any of the symptoms mentioned, seek the help of either your family dentist or a periodontist, a practitioner who specializes in the treatment of gum disease. If allowed to progress, periodontal disease can cause the loss of every tooth you have.

The most significant step in therapy is plaque removal. You should see a dentist or hygienist regularly for professional cleanings. This, combined with diligent home care that includes brushing, flossing and other therapies prescribed by your dentist, often prevents periodontal disease or stops it in its early stages.

If periodontal disease is more advanced, it may be necessary for a professional to perform root planing, also called root scaling. Scaling removes plaque and calculus from the crowns of the teeth and the surfaces of the roots; curettage removes the diseased tissue that lies next to the tooth. Scaling and curettage combined with meticulous home care may be sufficient to control the disease, depending on its severity.

In later stages of the disease, scaling and curettage may not produce adequate results. In these cases, surgery is often required. During surgery, the dentist surgically lifts sections of gum so that a direct view of the diseased root and bone is permitted. Plaque and calculus are removed from the area, and bone defects are corrected. The tissue is then positioned in a way that allows more efficient cleaning after healing. Often, the procedure requires only a local anesthetic.

When the exposed area reveals extreme bone loss, however, bone grafting or guided bone regeneration (GBR) is sometimes required. Bone grafting involves building up the bone with bone marrow from another part of the mouth or an artificial bone implant material. This procedure is typically performed over the course of several appointments, but in some cases it may be done all at once in a hospital or an outpatient facility with the aid of general anesthesia.

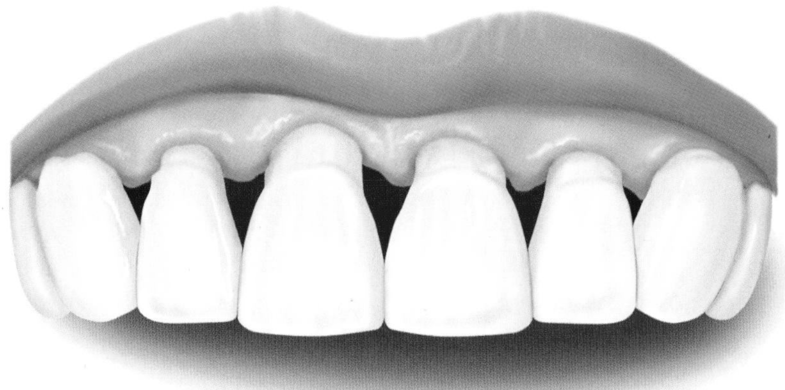

When periodontal disease causes the gums to shrink away from the teeth, the teeth appear longer and unattractive spaces between them can show. The gums of some older people recede without periodontal disease.

Prevention Is Best

The best way to head off periodontal disease is through careful home care. This includes regular brushing, flossing, vigorous rinsing and massaging the gums. In other words, keep your mouth as clean as possible so that bacteria can't accumulate.

Treatment for Loose Teeth

Loose teeth don't always mean gum disease, but if when you press on your teeth they fall back into your gums, gum disease is probably the culprit. If the disease has not progressed so far that the teeth are severely loose, then the treatment of the inflamed and infectious gums will usually correct the problem.

If the shifting of teeth persists, your dentist may suggest splinting. Splinting involves holding the teeth together with plastic or a similar material so they can withstand the pressure of chewing while the gum and bone are healing. Later a long-term solution will be suggested, such as interconnected crowning.

Sometimes there is simply too much bone loss, however, and regeneration isn't possible. In such cases, the teeth may be splinted together with a bonding material for increased stability. This is often an effective temporary solution that gives the teeth time to stabilize. If this is successful, crowns linked together may be placed on the loose teeth as well as those that adjoin them. This solution provides support while also allowing retention of most of the natural tooth.

Treatment for Gum Loss

Gum tissue can be lost due to a variety of causes including periodontal disease, severe infection, or trauma or tooth extraction. In many cases, the gum tissue recedes, creating esthetic problems. In such cases, grafting of soft-tissue gum can be performed either to correct the esthetic deformity or to prevent the recession from getting worse.

If gum loss is severe, a removable artificial interdental tissue appliance may be used. Made of gum-colored flexible plastic, the appliance is contoured to the shape of the teeth, fitting over the teeth and covering the spaces. It must be cleaned frequently.

Full crowning, or sometimes laminating, can also be used to mask a loss of interdental tissue, but it is not generally recommended unless the teeth themselves need to be restored. Whenever possible, composite resin bonding is used to build up the teeth and fill in the spaces. It is usually preferable to crowning because it is less costly and requires little tooth reduction. However, like all acid-etch procedures, this process must be repeated after several years and is susceptible to staining.

Before

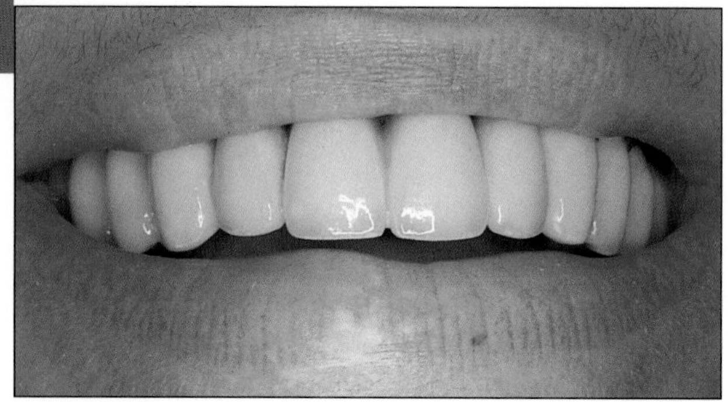

SMILELINE THAT REVEALS UNATTRACTIVE SPACES

An automobile accident caused this 24-year-old student to lose her four upper front teeth as well as supporting bone. Although the teeth were replaced with a fixed bridge, because of her high lipline unattractive spaces between the teeth showed when she smiled.

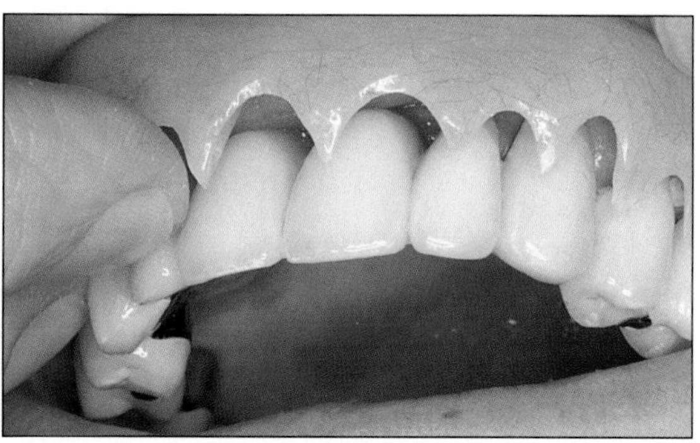

A removable artificial tissue appliance was made for this woman. The pink acrylic, which closely matches the patient's own gum tissue, can be easily inserted or taken out at will. The patient wears it by locking it into the spaces between her teeth. The appliance can be worn as long or often as desired.

After

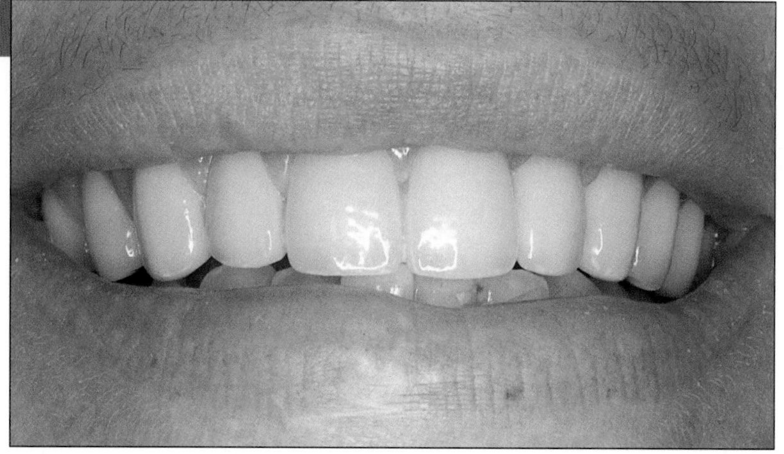

ARTIFICIAL GUM APPLIANCE

Notice the improvement in the smile with the appliance in place. The appliance allows the wearer to eat and speak normally. The result is a pretty smile that looks young and natural.

Before

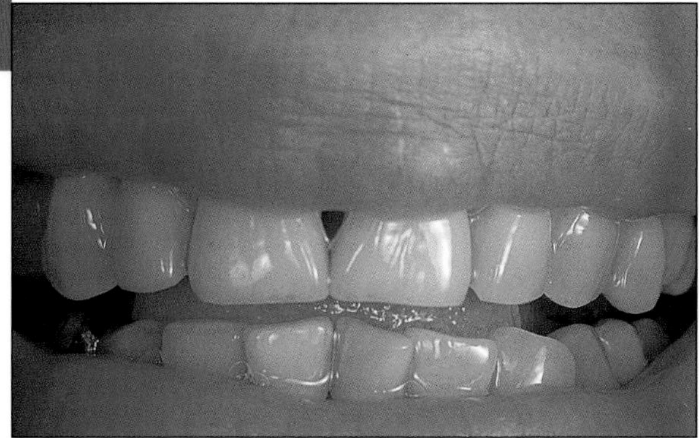

LOSS OF GUM TISSUE BETWEEN TEETH

This 55-year-old woman had periodontal disease and underwent surgery to save her teeth. However, she was concerned about the resulting unattractive spaces between her teeth.

After

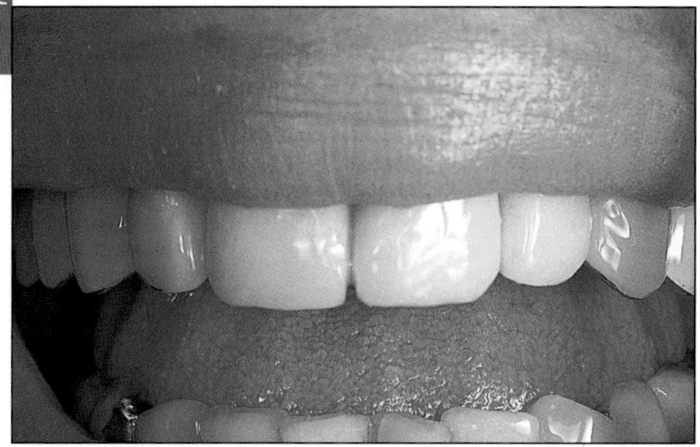

FULL CROWNS

Since the teeth were loose, full crowns were made to splint the teeth together. At the same time, the porcelain was built to hide the spaces. The final result with connecting porcelain crowns shows a new smile without spaces and with more attractively colored teeth.

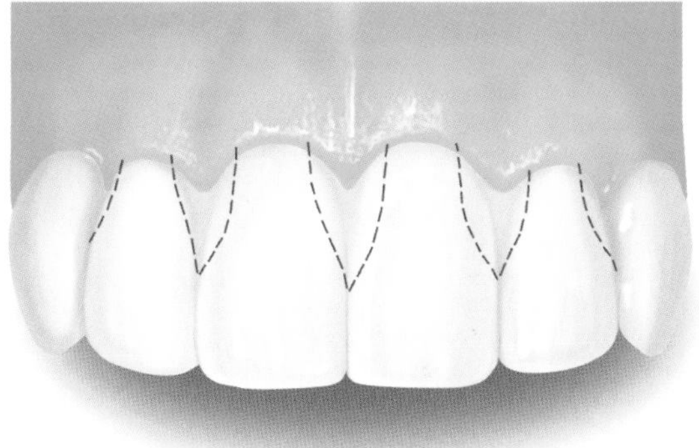

This drawing illustrates how either porcelain or composite resin is built out to help mask the spaces between the teeth.

Before

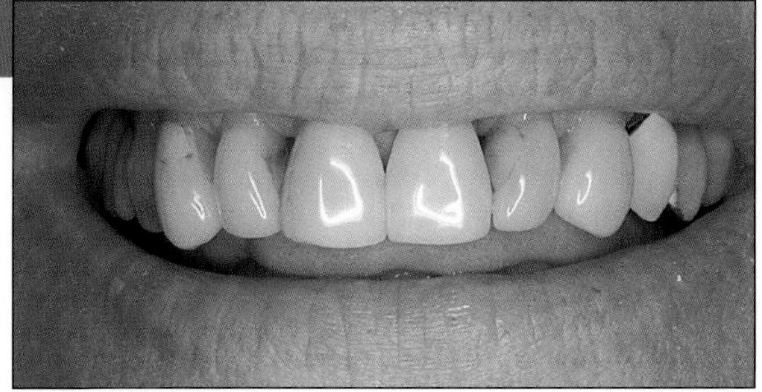

LOST GUM TISSUE CAUSING UNSIGHTLY SPACES

This 45-year-old television performer disliked her smile after gum surgery, but she did not want to have her teeth crowned. She wanted to hide the unsightly spaces between her teeth where gum tissue had been removed during the surgery.

After

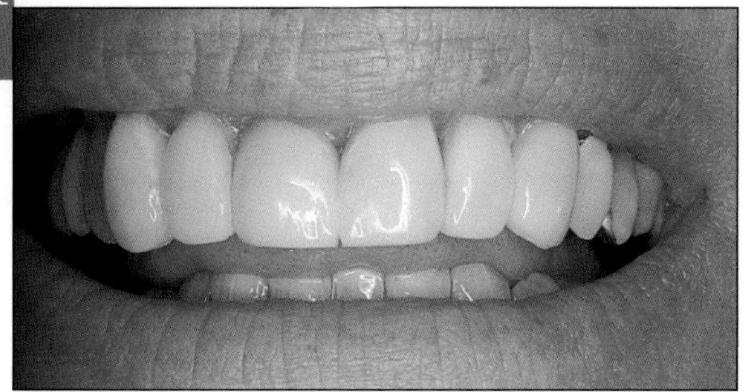

COMPOSITE RESIN BONDING

Since enough enamel remained on her teeth, the older fillings were removed and composite resin bonding was placed around the necks of the front six teeth. In addition to concealing the spaces, the bonding material lightened her teeth.

Treatment for Receding Gums

Receding gums are a common periodontal problem. They also can be an esthetic problem if you have a high lipline, especially if you have crowns. If tissue recedes, the previously hidden junction where tooth and crown meet may become visible. The root of your tooth, which is typically darker than the crown, may be unsightly. Or you may find that a metal or porcelain margin shows (see p. 73). Whatever the cause, even the most natural-looking crowns can't stand up to exposure like that.

Unfortunately, gum tissue usually doesn't grow back. Therefore, your dentist may suggest cosmetic gum surgery. Although procedures designed to replace tissue *between* the teeth are not very predictable, your dentist may be able to mask the area.

Masking typically involves removing part of the crown and root and bonding over the area with composite resin to hide the metal margin or exposed root. However, because it's difficult to obtain a good esthetic match this way, a better alternative is to dull the metal slightly or hide it with a darker colored composite resin. If the junction is porcelain and the root is dark, a better color match, although not a perfect one, will probably be obtained. The ideal solution is to replace the crown.

The best way to avoid tissue recession is to practice good oral hygiene at home and to have professional tooth cleanings three or four times each year. Also, begin proper cleaning immediately after a crown is placed even if the tissue is sore. If bacteria accumulate around the gumline, the tissue will only become more sensitive and recession may occur.

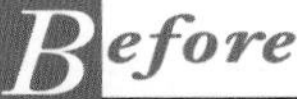

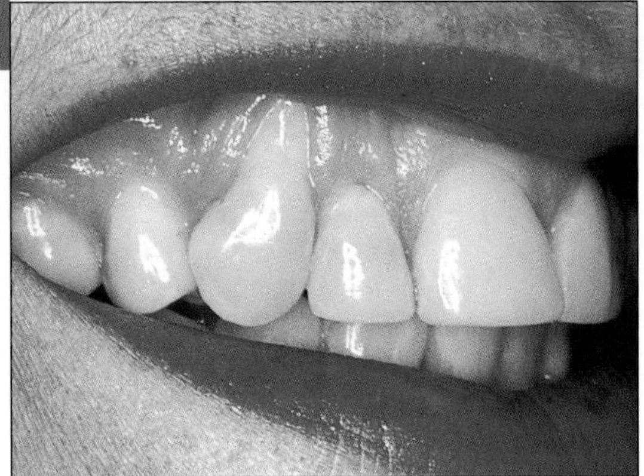

Severe tissue loss

This woman had a high lipline that revealed the severe clefting of gum tissue on her right canine.

After

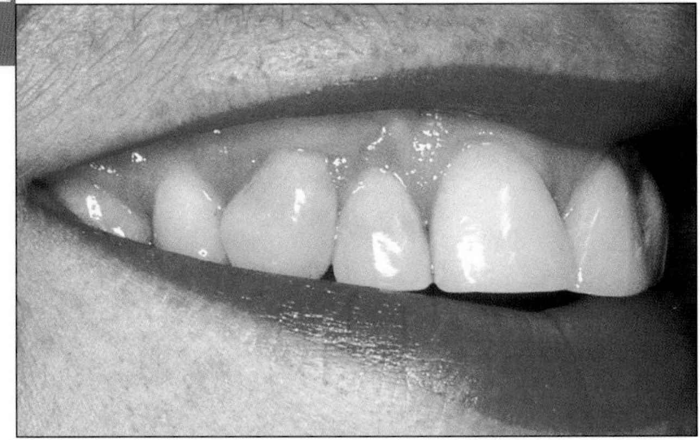

Cosmetic gum surgery

Cosmetic gum surgery, consisting of a graft, was used to enhance both function and esthetics.

Before

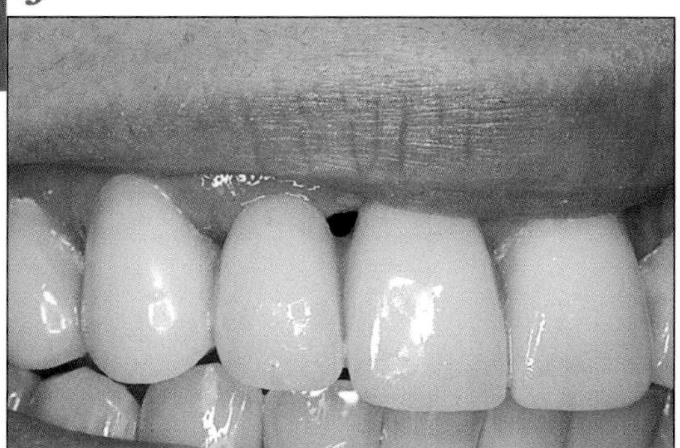

Loss of gum tissue between teeth

This radiant young woman's smile was marred due to a horseback-riding accident that left her with unattractive spaces between her teeth.

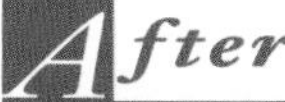

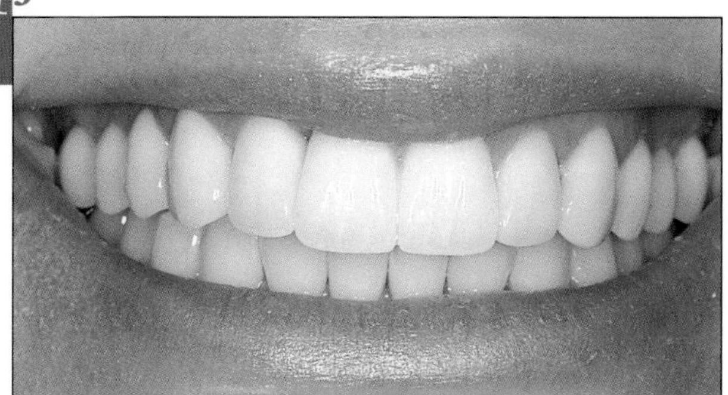

Cosmetic gum surgery, bleaching and a new bridge

Cosmetic tissue surgery built down the missing gum tissue. The lower teeth were then bleached, and a new upper fixed bridge with improved tooth contour was placed.

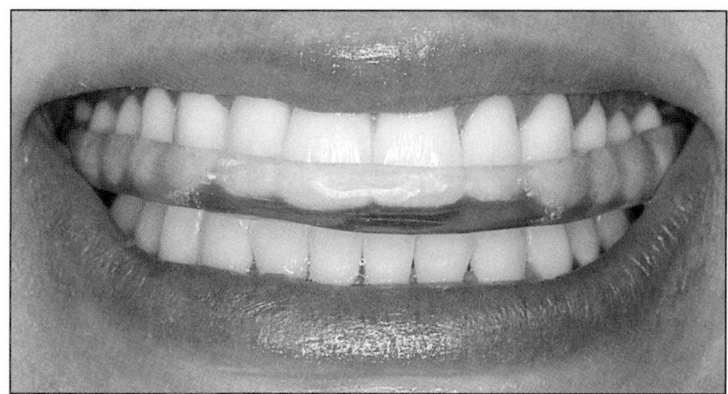

A custom-fitted bite appliance was fabricated for wear during sleep to keep the porcelain from fracturing due to possible bruxism or tooth clenching.

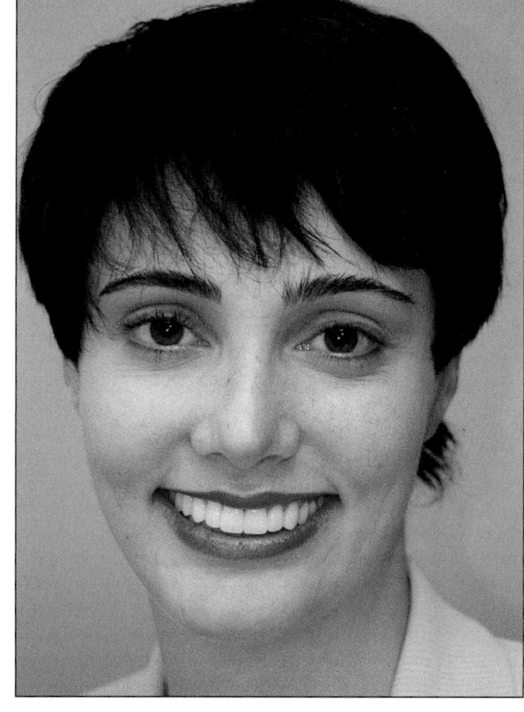

The final result shows how both the shape and color of teeth complement this woman's facial proportions.

Before

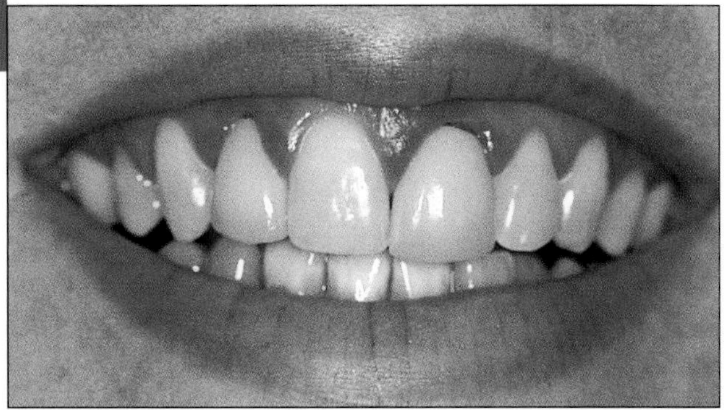

GUM DISEASE DUE TO POORLY FITTING CROWNS

This young woman had crowns that did not fit properly, causing the gum disease shown here.

After

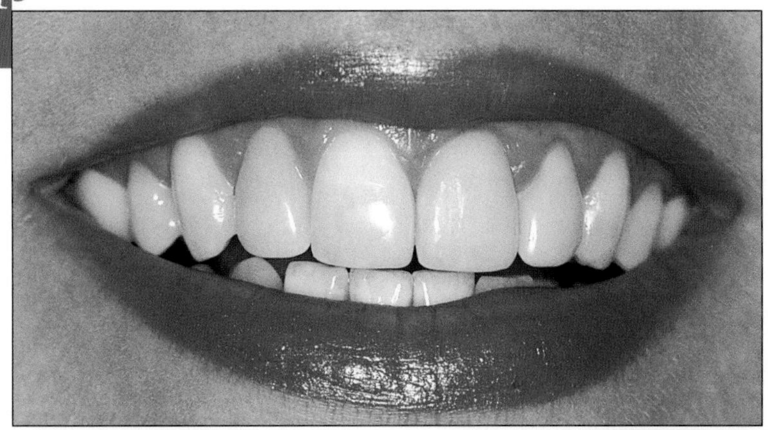

NEW, PROPERLY FITTING CROWNS

Two new, perfectly fitting crowns were all that was necessary to clear up this woman's gum disease.

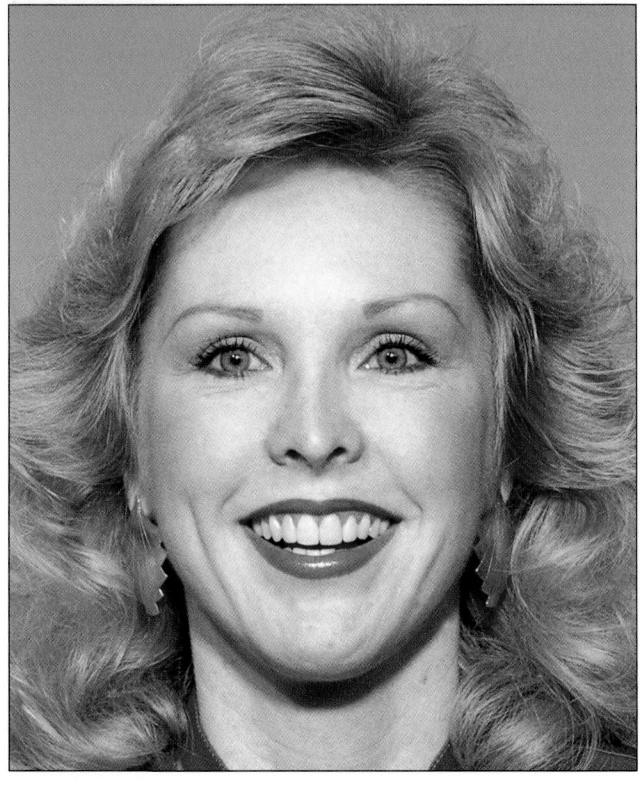

*B*efore

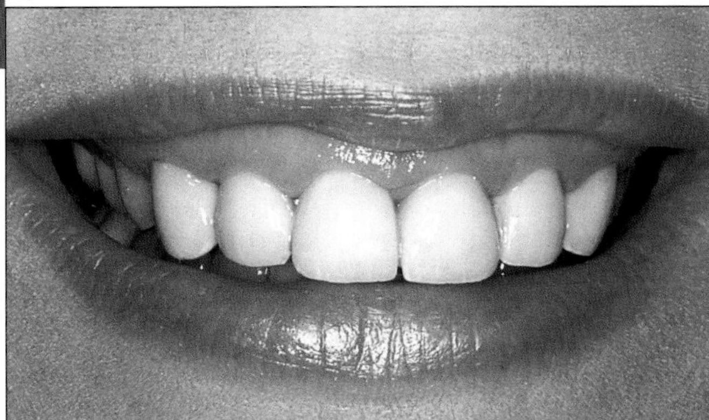

NARROW ARCH, HIGH LIPLINE WITH GUMMY SMILE, DISCOLORED AND POORLY PROPORTIONED CROWNS

This woman was concerned about showing too much gum when she smiled. Her back teeth are not visible behind the poorly constructed front teeth.

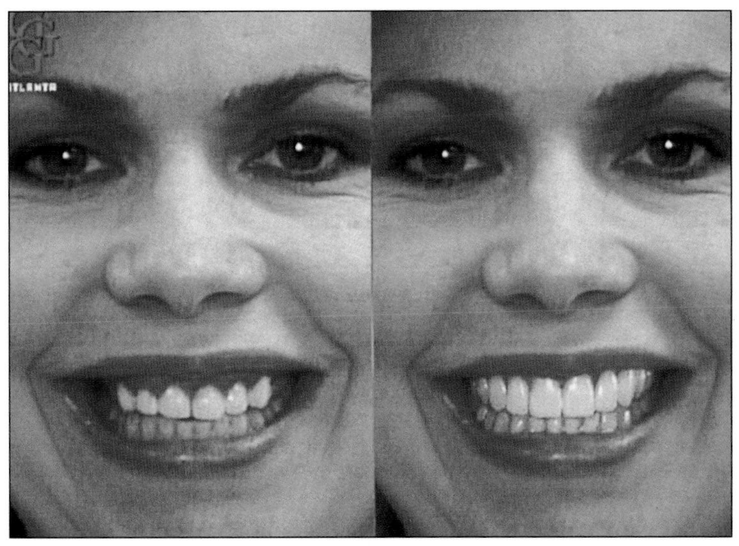

COMPUTER IMAGING

The treatment plan included surgical removal of some gum tissue, combined with new crowns correctly proportioned and built out laterally to fill up the smile.

*A*fter

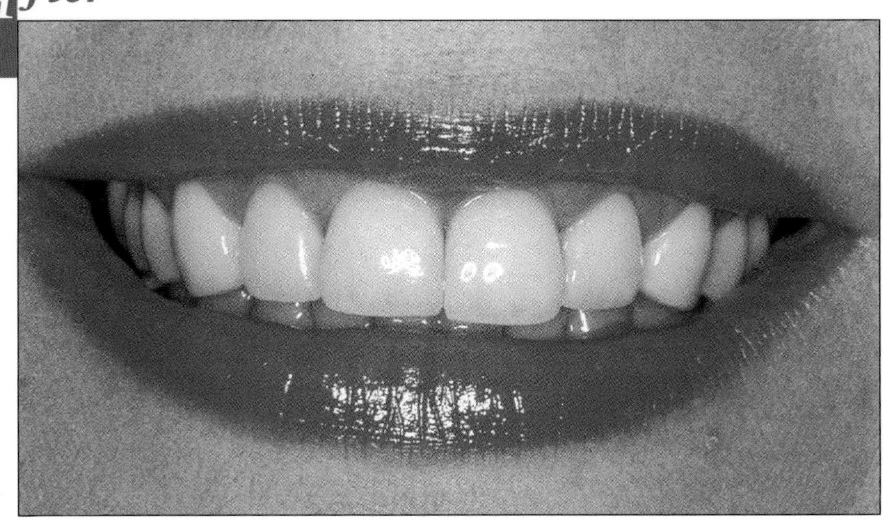

COSMETIC GUM SURGERY AND NEW CROWNS

This view shows a much improved smile two years after the surgical procedure and placement of the new crowns. Always invest in the finest ceramics to help achieve your most natural smile.

Treatment for Ridge Resorption

After tooth extraction, the affected tissue heals to a slightly lower height than the tissue adjacent to it. When a tooth is lost due to an accident or advanced bone loss, this tissue loss or ridge resorption can be even more pronounced. In fact, a bone defect often results, making replacement with a fixed bridge difficult, if not impossible. Unless something is done to mask the defect, the teeth will look much too long. In these cases, three techniques can be used to mask the defect.

Fixed porcelain interdental addition

A fixed porcelain interdental addition involves adding gum-colored porcelain to the bridge to mask the space between the restoration and the gum. The main challenge is obtaining a good color match. Expect to pay about 25 percent more for your bridge when this procedure is required.

Removable artificial tissue appliance

This appliance may be the easiest and least expensive way to mask missing tissue. Because it's made of flexible plastic, however, it is fragile. It also requires maintenance. Cost of the appliance typically ranges from $350 to $1500.

Ridge augmentation

Several new techniques have recently been developed for replacing missing ridge tissue. They involve the addition of either transplanted tissue or implant material. This surgical procedure ensures the creation of a more esthetically pleasing and better-fitting fixed bridge, where the replacement teeth emerge from the transplanted tissue as do normal teeth. Cost for the procedure can range from $985 to $4000, depending on the severity of the defect.

Before

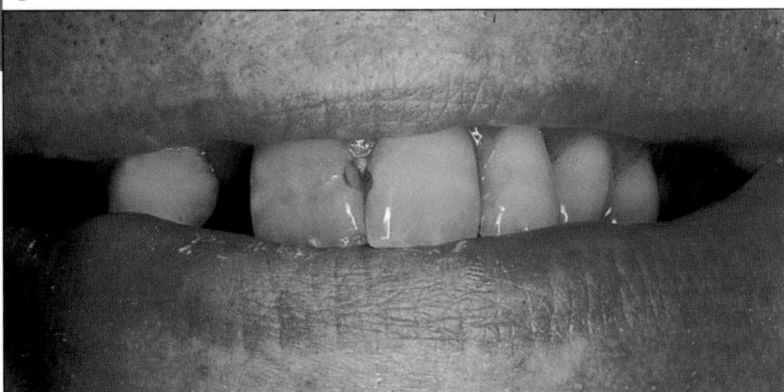

Missing tooth and receding gum tissue

This 45-year-old man had a missing right lateral incisor, which made him smile self-consciously. When he smiled, he kept his upper lips as far down as possible.

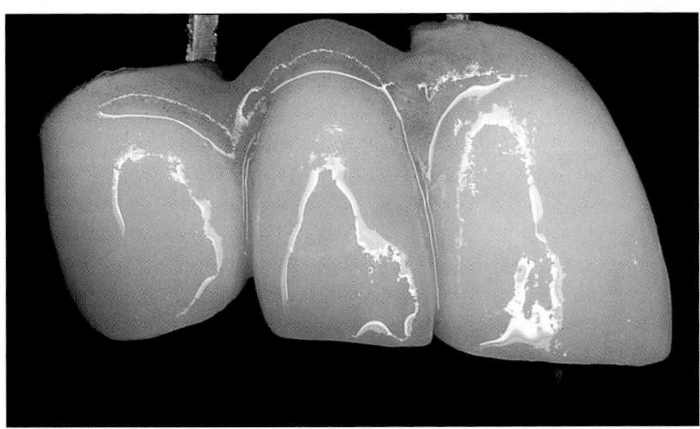

A three-unit conventional bridge was made with a fixed porcelain interdental addition to simulate the missing gum tissue.

After

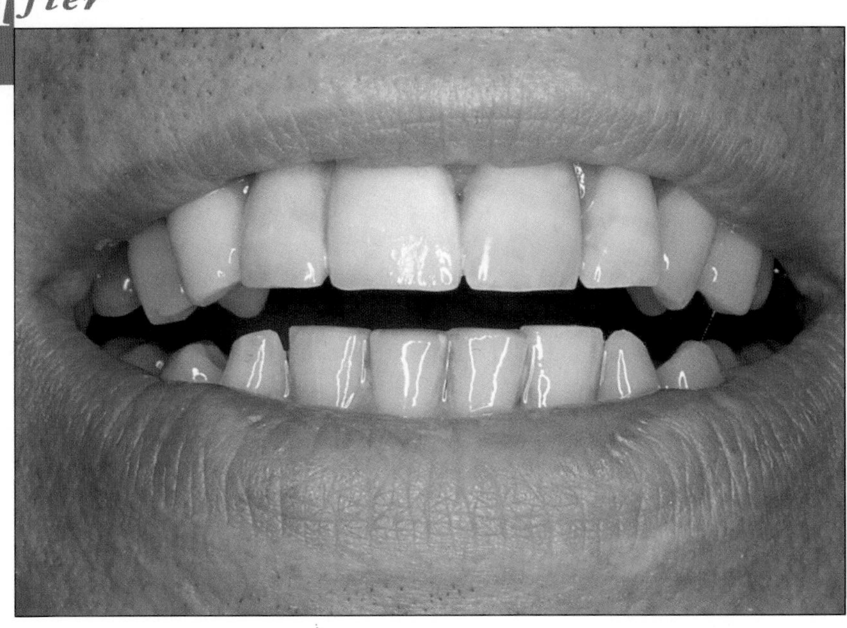

Fixed porcelain addition

The new porcelain-bonded-to-metal bridge enabled the patient to have a relaxed lipline and, as a result, his smile improved considerably.

Before

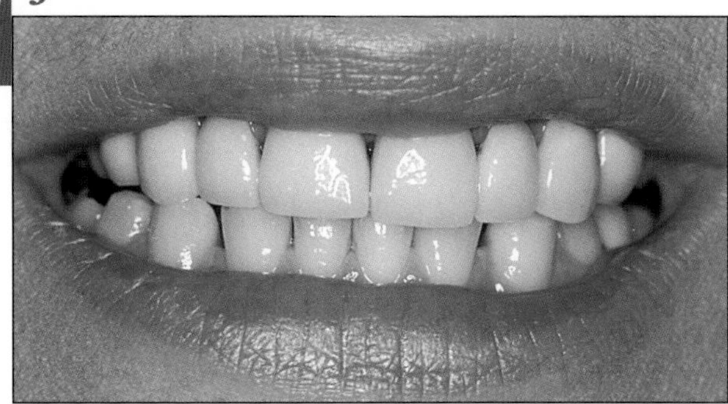

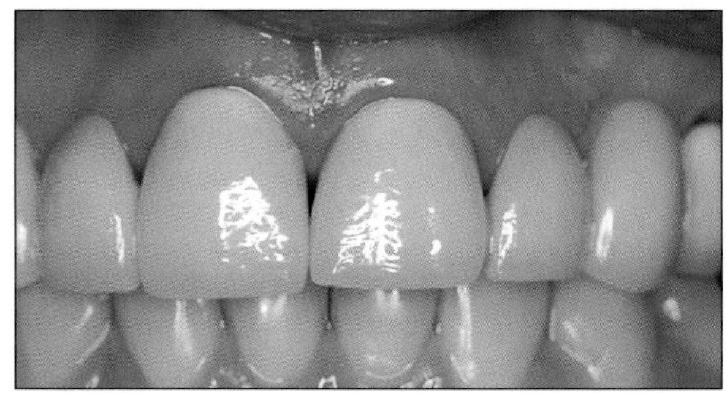

UNATTRACTIVE BRIDGE AND LOSS OF INTERDENTAL TISSUE

This woman disliked the unattractive spaces that showed when she allowed herself to smile fully. The spaces were due to earlier tooth loss of the right and left lateral incisors and cuspids, resulting in bone and gum tissue loss around and in between the missing teeth.

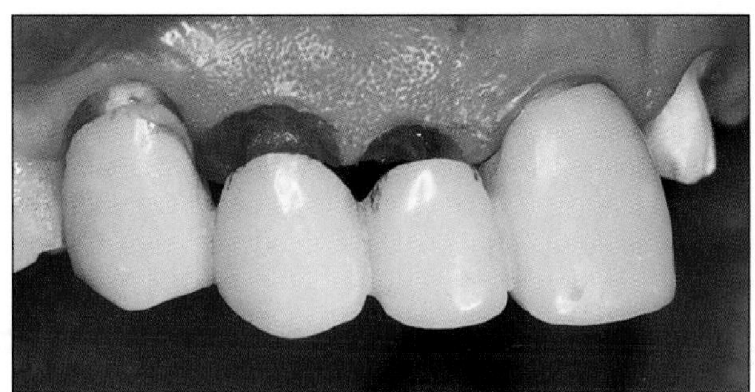

TRY-IN OF TEMPORARY BRIDGE

As the temporary bridge is being fitted, the missing lateral and cuspid are better visualized.

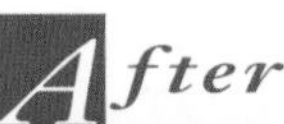

After

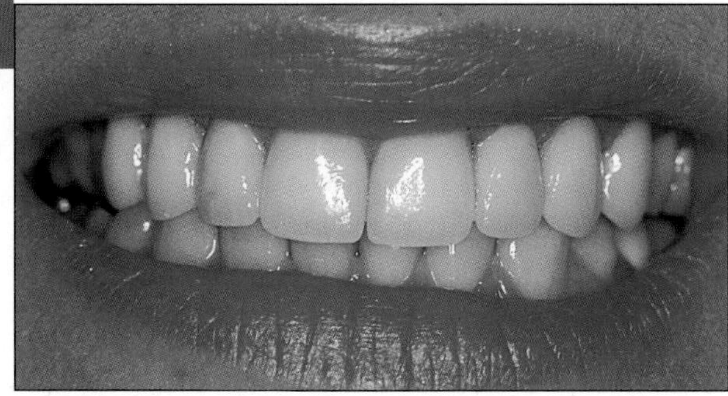

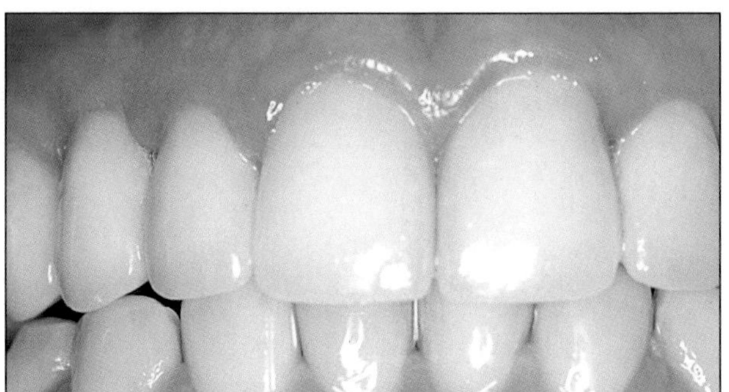

RIDGE AUGMENTATION AND NEW CERAMO-METAL BRIDGES

Cosmetic dental surgery consisting of ridge augmentation allowed for a more natural-appearing fixed bridge. This permitted the woman to smile again with renewed confidence.

If you show unattractive spaces at the gum line, consider having a ridge augmentation procedure before being fitted for a new bridge.

TREATMENT SUMMARY

RIDGE AUGMENTATION

Treatment Time One to four appointments of one hour or more.

Patient Maintenance Routine daily brushing and flossing and professional cleanings.

Results of Treatment Creates the illusion of normal gums, which allows the replacement tooth to appear as though it is naturally emerging from the gum tissue.

Average Range of Treatment Life Expectancy Indefinite/long lasting. (See footnote on p. 50.)

Cost Depends on number of teeth; usually $985 to $4000. (See footnote on p. 50.)

ADVANTAGES

1. Can achieve a more esthetic, natural-looking result
2. Can make gum tissue easier to clean under bridge
3. May improve speech
4. Can help prevent food traps

DISADVANTAGES

1. Takes extra time to construct a bridge
2. Extra cost

TREATMENT FOR EXCESSIVE GUM TISSUE

Too much gum tissue can be the result of disease, or, for some people who have high liplines, it can be normal. If the problem is due to periodontal disease, the overgrowth is usually thick and swollen, and it may bleed. This kind of inflammation is usually treated with scaling and curettage by your dentist or periodontist.

After the tissue responds to treatment, it will be reevaluated to determine if additional treatment is needed. If it is, your dentist is likely to suggest one of the following surgical procedures.

Gingivectomy

A gingivectomy involves surgically removing some of the gum tissue. It is performed only if an adequate amount of attached gum tissue will remain.

Gingivoplasty

A gingivoplasty is a reshaping of the gum tissue. It can improve the contour of the gums around the teeth.

Flap surgery

Flap surgery involves surgically lifting sections of the gum tissue so that the underlying bone and surrounding tissue can be treated. The flap is then re-attached at a higher point so that less gum tissue shows when you smile.

Orthognathic surgery

Orthognathic surgery involves removing a section of bone above the roots of the teeth and closing up the entire arch so that the gum tissue is not visible when you smile. Although this is the most extreme and costly surgical alternative, if other procedures fail to provide the result you want, orthognathic surgery may be an option (see p. 214).

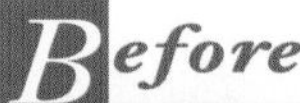

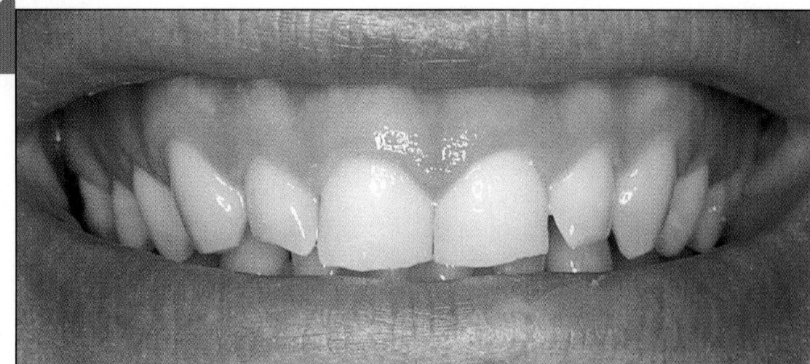

HIGH LIPLINE WITH SMALL AND DISCOLORED TEETH

Big, beautiful, white teeth is what this man wanted most; instead, he had short, stubby, discolored teeth covered by a great deal of gum tissue.

After

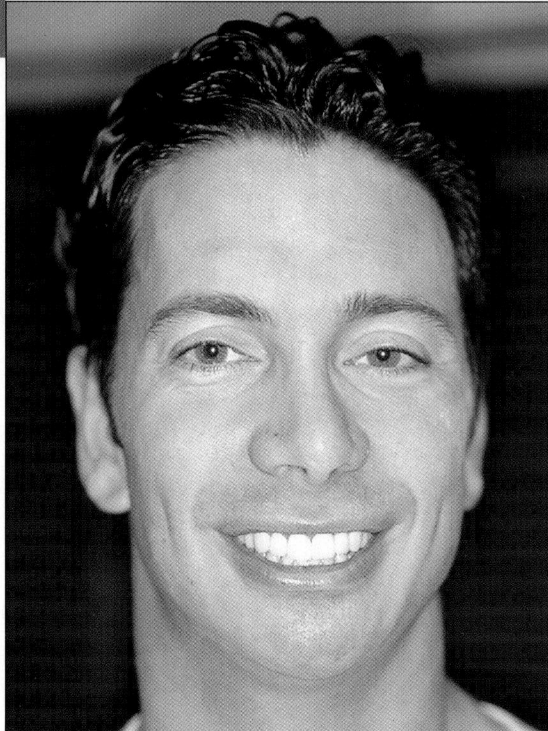

COSMETIC GUM SURGERY AND PORCELAIN LAMINATE VENEERS

Cosmetic gum surgery was performed. The teeth were then fitted for twelve porcelain laminate veneers. Several days later, the patient's preselected shade was bonded to his teeth, giving him the bright, white smile he'd always wanted.

Before

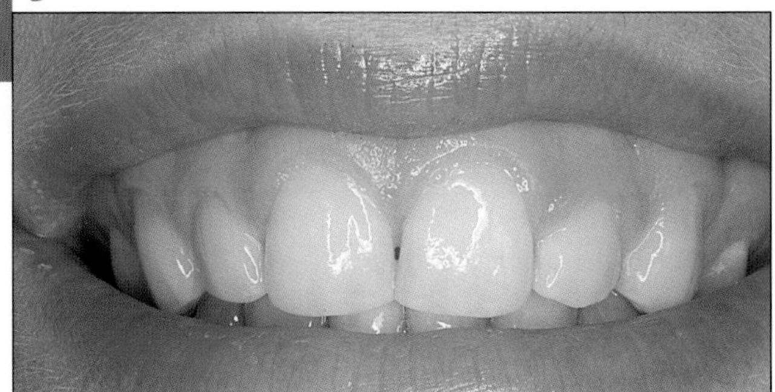

Gummy smile or high lipline

This 20-year-old Miss America beauty contestant was disturbed about the amount of gum tissue that showed when she smiled. She wanted longer teeth, but lengthening the teeth from the biting edge would not eliminate the show of gum tissue. Instead, cosmetic gum surgery was decided upon to lengthen the teeth from the necks upward.

After

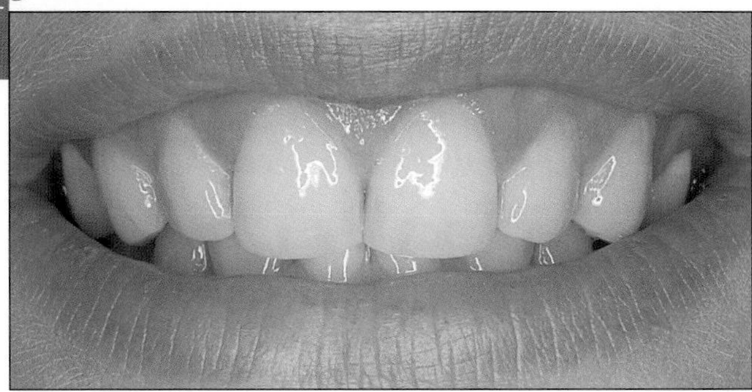

Cosmetic gum surgery

After cosmetic gum surgery, her teeth appear longer with much less gum tissue showing when she smiles, giving her more self-confidence.

Unattractive fixed bridge

This 23-year-old model was extremely unhappy with her unattractive fixed bridge, which replaced the right front central incisor. The incorrect shapes of the two front teeth called attention to the bridge. The upper front teeth were discolored, and the cuspids stuck out, producing a bulldog look. Furthermore, the plastic on the false tooth was beginning to wear and show gold.

Before

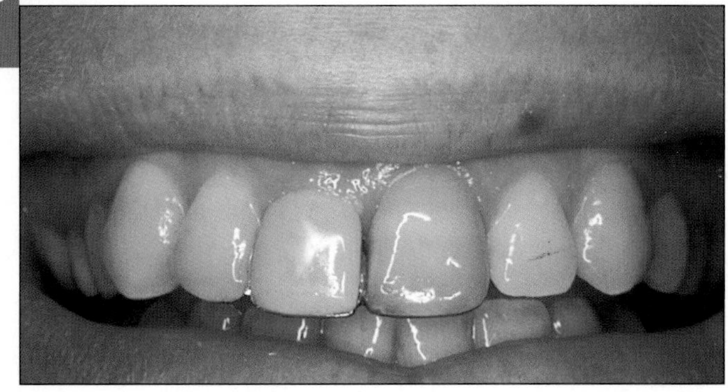

Cosmetic gum surgery, a new fixed bridge and cosmetic contouring

The old bridge was removed and cosmetic gum surgery was done on the ridge where the missing tooth was to permit a more natural-looking bridge to be placed. A new three-unit porcelain bridge was inserted, which provided a more attractive smile. Notice how removing bulk from the cuspids through cosmetic contouring also helped her overall smile. **Often it takes a combination of treatments to achieve the best results.**

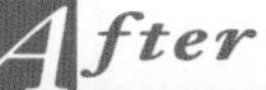

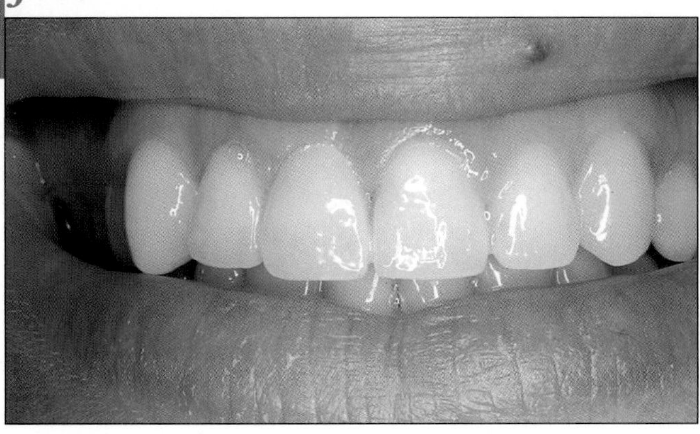

Before

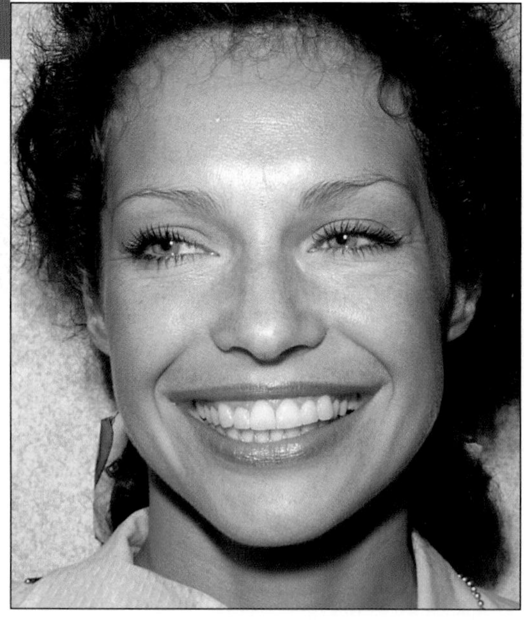

UNEVEN GUMS AND TOO-EVEN TEETH

This dentist had worn her teeth down, producing a "sawed off" look. In addition, her gum tissue covered too much of her front teeth, making the lateral incisors appear shorter than they were.

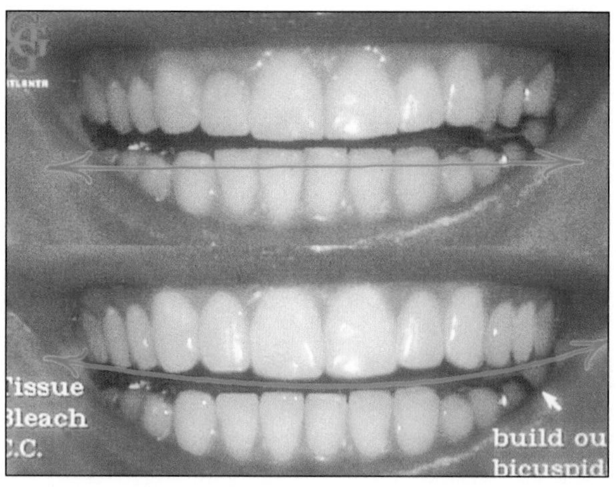

COMPUTER IMAGING

This computer imaging photograph illustrates the difference in the smileline created by tissue surgery, cosmetic contouring, bleaching, new crowns and bonding.

After

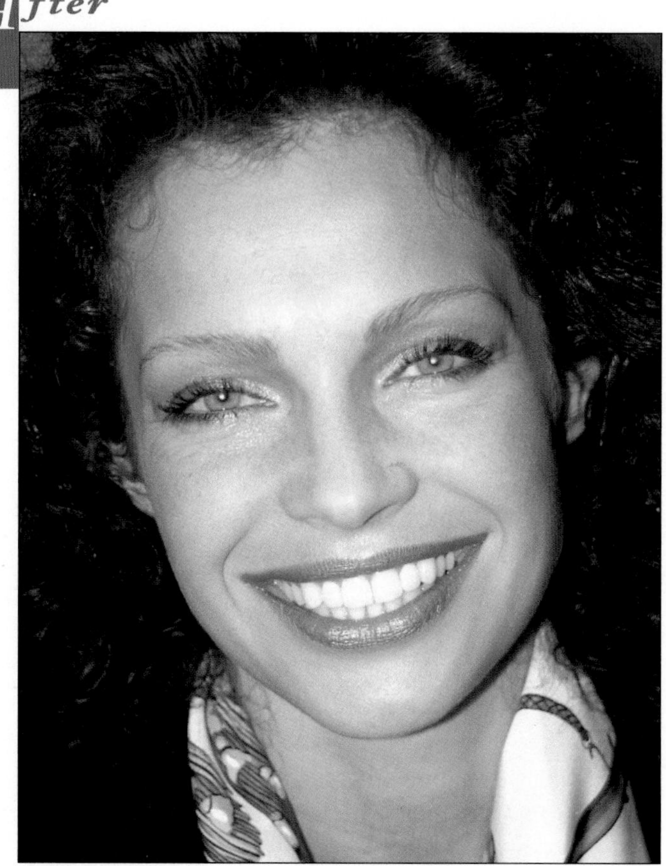

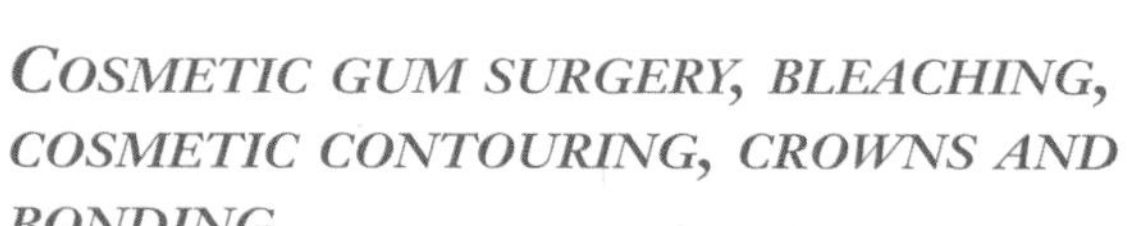

COSMETIC GUM SURGERY, BLEACHING, COSMETIC CONTOURING, CROWNS AND BONDING

Cosmetic gum surgery was first done to raise the tissue around the front teeth, making them appear more proportionate. Bleaching then lightened the teeth. Cosmetic contouring helped shape the teeth before the two lateral incisors were recrowned. Finally the bicuspids were built out to balance the smile. The final result shows how effective integrated dental therapy can be to achieve a dazzling new smile.

Before

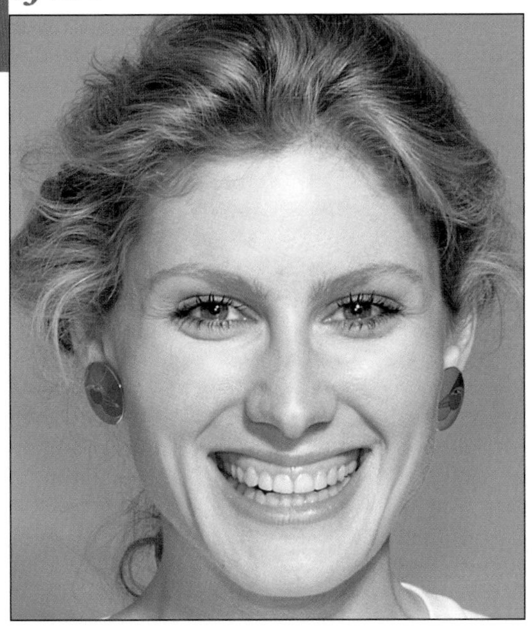

HIGH LIPLINE AND STAINED TEETH

This actress was displeased with her yellow stained teeth and gummy smile.

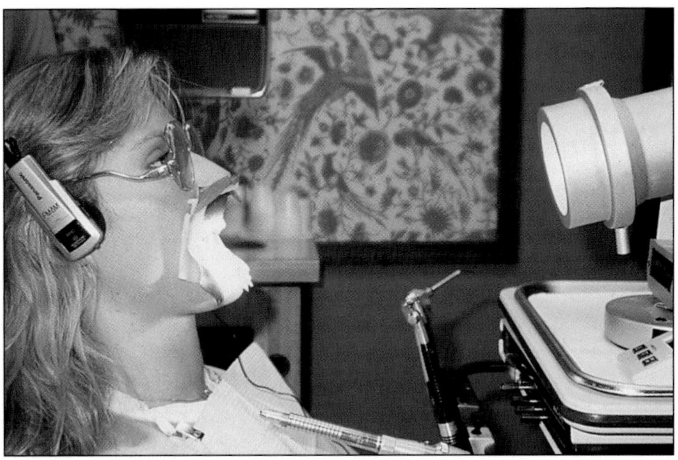

IN-OFFICE BLEACHING

The upper teeth are being bleached with concentrated hydrogen peroxide and a special bleaching lamp. Plain gauze has been applied to the lower lip to protect against accidental solution leakage.

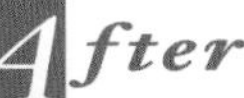

After

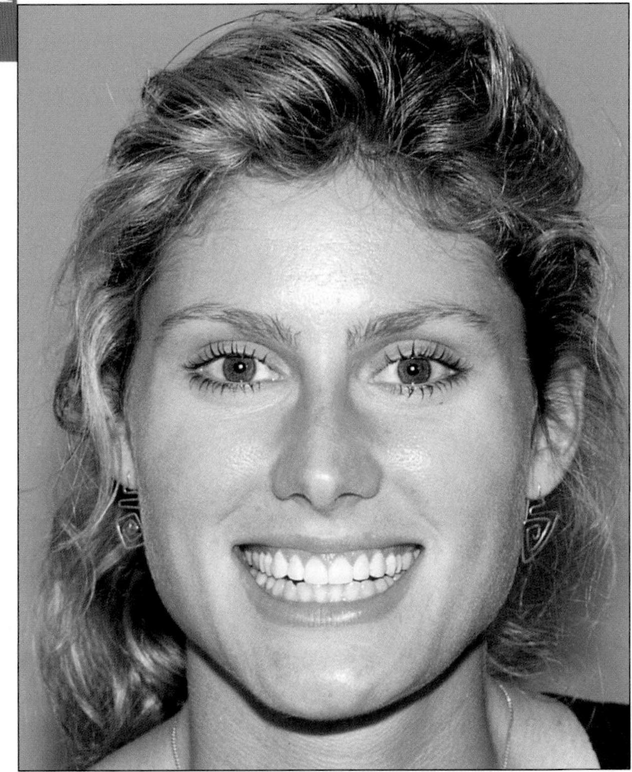

COSMETIC GUM RAISING AND BLEACHING

The smileline was improved by surgically raising the gum tissue and then bleaching the teeth, creating a brighter smile.

Before

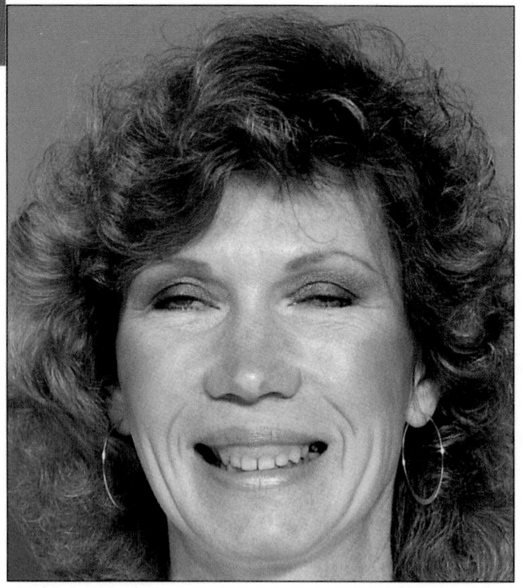

HIGH LIPLINE AND DISCOLORED TEETH

This patient wanted lighter teeth. However, merely making the teeth lighter would not give her as attractive a smile as possible because her teeth appeared too short for her face. Therefore, a cosmetic gum-raising procedure was first planned.

After

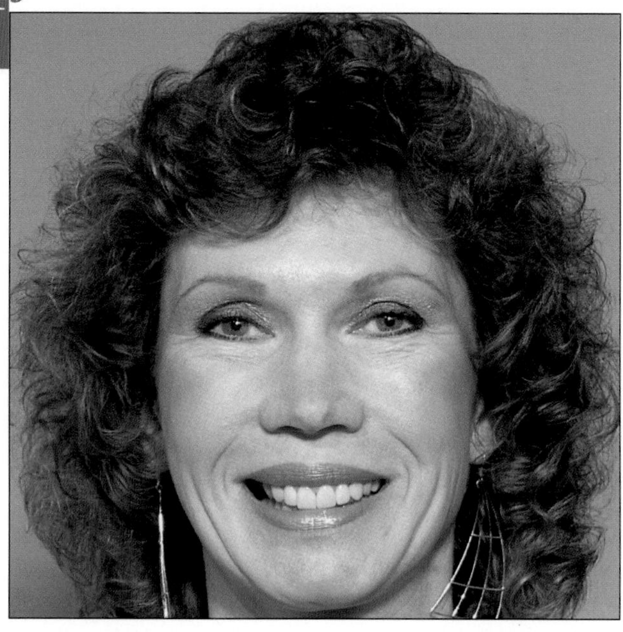

COSMETIC GUM RAISING AND TEN PORCELAIN LAMINATES

By first undergoing a gum-raising procedure, followed by the placement of ten porcelain laminates, this woman's smile is made much more attractive. Well-proportioned porcelain laminates help to make the entire face look much brighter. Consider having your gums positioned in the most attractive relationship to the teeth and lipline before having your teeth restored.

Before

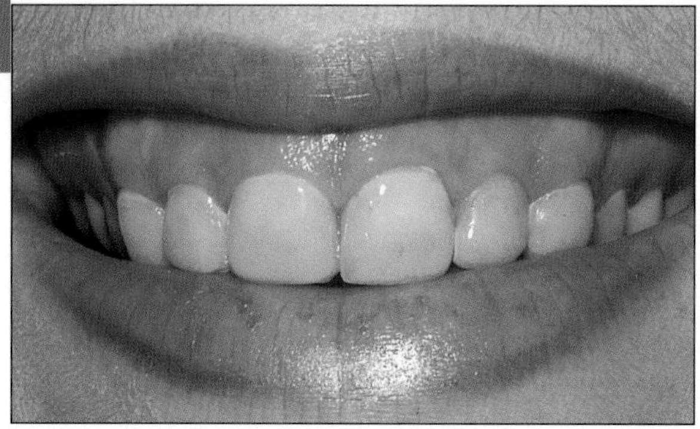

HIGH LIPLINE AND STAINED PLASTIC VENEERS

This 19-year-old student was dissatisfied with her plastic laminates. In addition, she didn't like "all the pink gums showing" when she smiled.

After

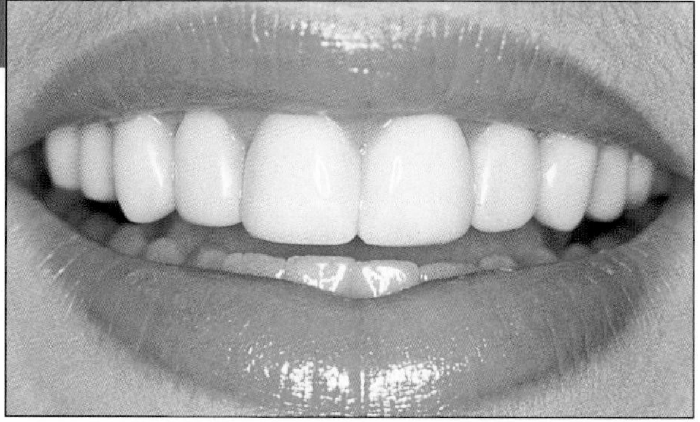

COSMETIC GUM RAISING AND COMPOSITE RESIN BONDING

The contour of the gum tissue was changed to be in harmony with her upper lipline. Next, ten teeth were bonded with a lighter shade of composite resin in a single appointment. A more proportionate smile is the result.

Before

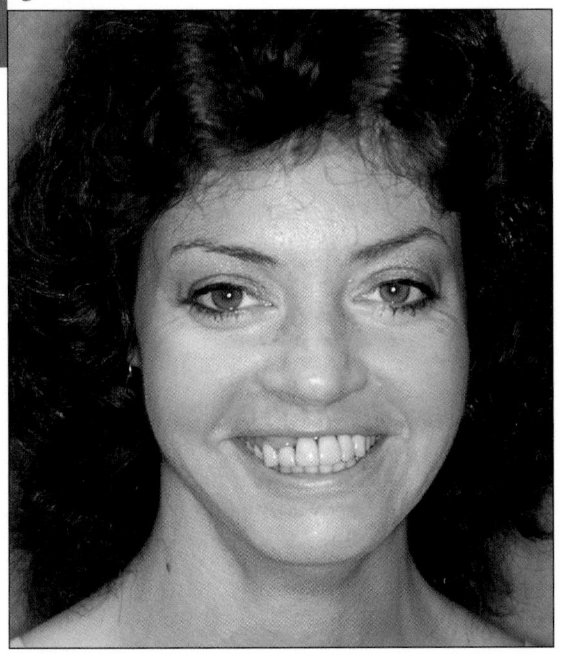

Uneven-Appearing Gums and Too-Large Teeth

This nurse had been in an accident that caused loss of tooth and bone. She felt the replacement disfigured her smile and was esthetically unacceptable.

After

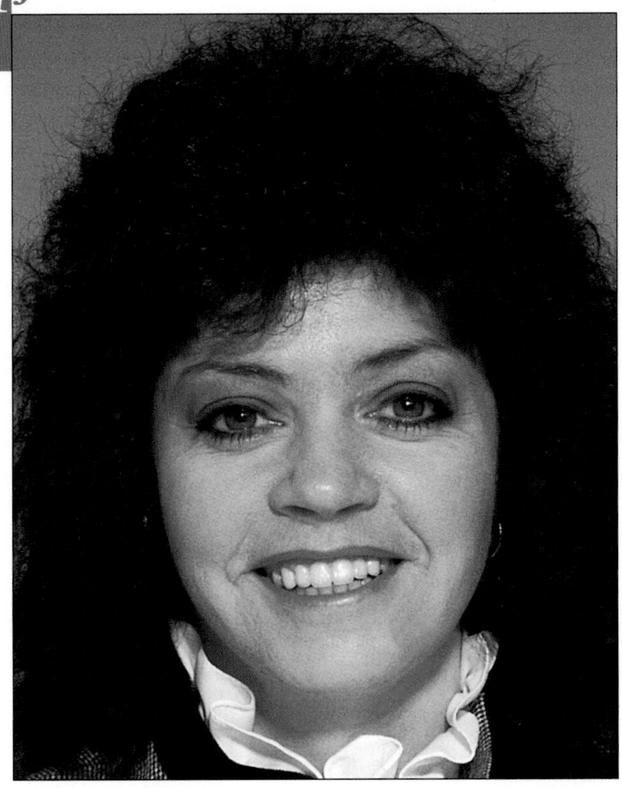

Surgery to Replace Missing Bone and Gum Tissue and a New Fixed Bridge

The patient underwent surgery to regain lost bone and gum. Finally, a new bridge with better tooth proportion and shading was placed to achieve a more attractive smile

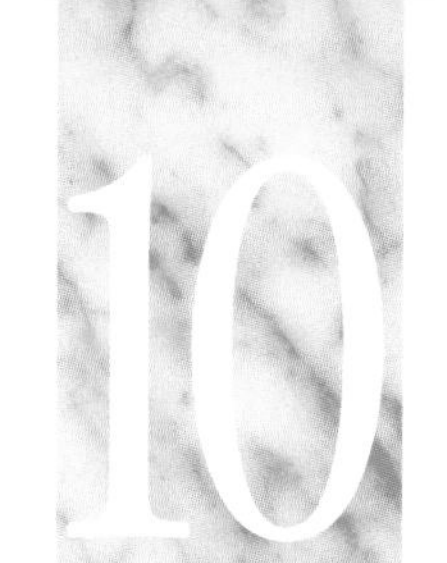

Looking Years Younger with Cosmetic Dentistry

Today, people over 65 make up more than 13 percent of the population. By the year 2030, one in every six Americans will be 65 years or older, yet the emphasis on youth is still embedded in our culture.

Consumers spend billions of dollars each year on services and products designed to make them more attractive. Countless women—and increasing numbers of men—have face-lifts and other plastic surgery procedures in an effort to enhance their appearance and remain competitive in job markets where looking youthful is an asset.

While many patients benefit from plastic surgery, others could be helped with cosmetic dentistry alone. After all, your smile is one of the most important parts of your face. It's what people usually notice first about you. If your smile is attractive and healthy looking, it will take years off your appearance. If, on the other hand, your smile reveals worn, discolored, chipped or missing teeth, you'll look older than you should, and no amount of plastic surgery can change that.

Dentistry's role in improving appearance is often misunderstood and underrated. For example, many people believe that only dentures can alter the appearance of their smile, yet nothing could be further from the truth. Such cost-effective techniques as cosmetic contouring, bleaching or bonding often work wonders—typically in a single office visit!

If you'd like to take years off your smile—and your overall looks—ask your dentist about cosmetic procedures that can help. Chronological age should never stand between you and a more pleasing appearance.

Youth doesn't have to be wasted on the young!

How to Change an Aging Smile

As we age, the edges of the front teeth wear until these teeth are about the same length as the others. At the same time, the upper and lower lips lose muscle tone. The upper lip may sag, covering more of the upper teeth. The lower lip may also drop, allowing more of the lower teeth to show. These conditions create an older smileline.

In many cases, treatment consists of making the upper teeth longer. Your dentist may shorten the lower teeth with cosmetic contouring while lengthening the upper teeth through bonding, laminating or crowning. If the back teeth are worn and need crowning, your dentist can make the new crowns slightly longer provided there is sufficient space in front to lengthen the upper teeth.

If worn and discolored fillings are aging your smile but your teeth don't need crowning, consider replacing your old fillings with tooth-colored composite fillings or with porcelain inlays or onlays (see pp. 77 to 88). The easiest and best way to see how cosmetic dentistry can make your smile and face appear more youthful is through computer imaging.

How to Avoid an Aging Smile

1. Watch for unnatural wear. It ages the smile.
2. Avoid bone and gum loss. Spaces between the teeth can give an older look to the smile. Take proper oral hygiene seriously and request frequent periodontal evaluation from your dentist.
3. Replace fillings when necessary.
4. Don't let your crowns or bridges age you. If they are worn down, replace them.
5. Have any discolored teeth corrected. Staining makes you look older.
6. Replace any missing teeth as soon as possible. Missing teeth can cause your bite to collapse and tissues to sag.
7. Correct your bad bite. As you age, the bad bite tends to become more pronounced. It's never too late to have it corrected!

Bad Bites and Bruxism Can Grind Away Your Smile

Often teeth wear more quickly than they should due to factors other than aging. Some people have incorrect bites that contribute to a wearing down of the enamel. Others have a habit called *bruxism*, or excessive grinding of the teeth, that causes tooth erosion.

If your teeth are worn down, there are several ways to correct the problem. You can lengthen the upper incisors with bonding or laminating and shorten the lower incisors. Alternatively, the upper teeth can be contoured to give an illusion that the front two are longer than they actually are. You can also be fitted with a bite appliance if you grind your teeth at night.

Before

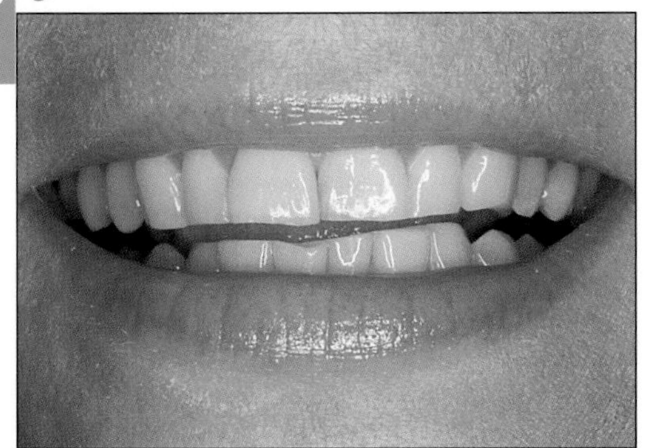

Tooth Grinding (Bruxism) Causing Tooth Wear and an Older Smileline

Bruxism, or grinding the teeth at night, was the chief cause of wear for this 31-year-old executive whose teeth ended up with a sawed-off look. Note how she unconsciously put her tongue behind her front teeth to hide the space that shows a jagged outline. In addition to poor dental esthetics, the patient suffered constant headaches, and neck and back discomfort due to further complication of muscle spasms. The diagnosis was temporomandibular joint dysfunction (TMJ).

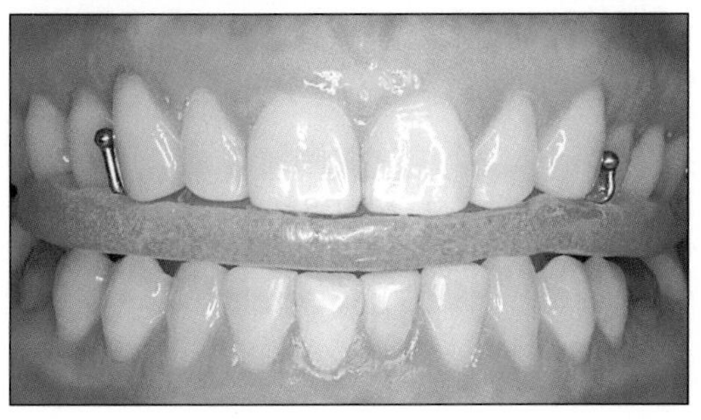

Bite Appliance and Cosmetic Contouring

A removable appliance was made to correct the TMJ dysfunction and prevent the teeth from further wear. Following three months of TMJ treatment to cure the symptoms and relax the muscles, the patient wore the appliance only at night. The square, masculine-looking upper and lower teeth were cosmetically contoured to produce a prettier smile.

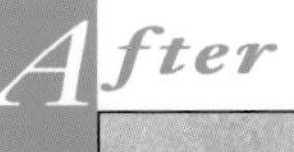

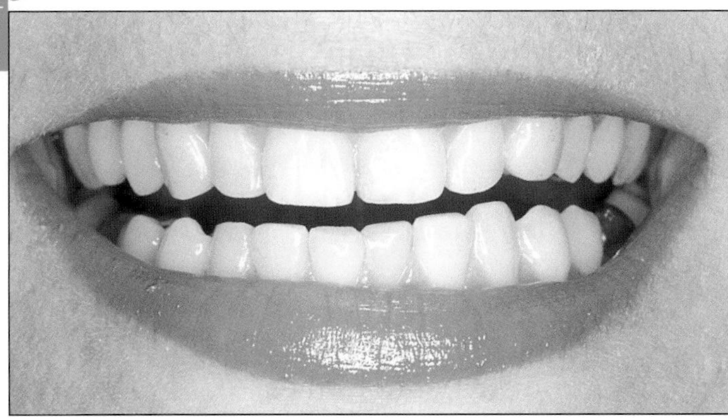

Cosmetic Contouring: An Economical Approach

The most economical way to correct teeth that are simply worn down from wear is with cosmetic contouring. The upper teeth are reshaped to give the appearance that they are longer than they really are. Cosmetic contouring typically takes about one hour and anesthesia is rarely required. Costs may range from $350 to $950.

Bonding: A Younger Smile in Hours

In other cases of tooth wear, the dentist will fuse composite resin or laminate veneers to the front surfaces of the teeth to give the smile a more youthful and healthy appearance. Either procedure can be performed in a matter of hours. Although bonding eventually must be redone, the procedures are relatively inexpensive, particularly when compared to laminating or crowning. Costs per tooth range from $185 to $950 for bonding and $450 to $2500 for laminating.

Before

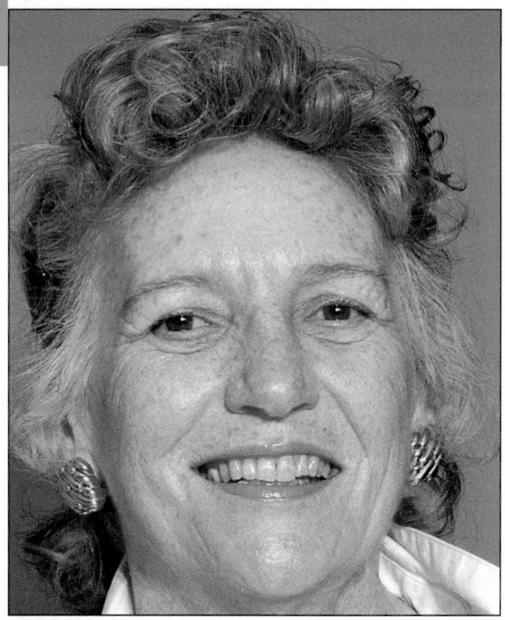

Discolored teeth

This lady realized her stained and discolored teeth were aging her smile.

After

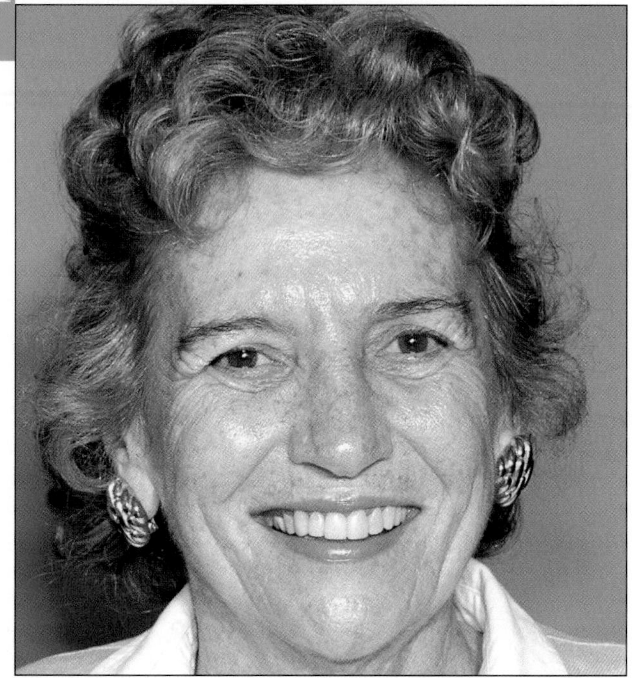

Composite resin bonding and cosmetic contouring

Following composite resin bonding and cosmetic contouring of the upper and lower teeth, her teeth look lighter and more even and her smile more youthful.

Before

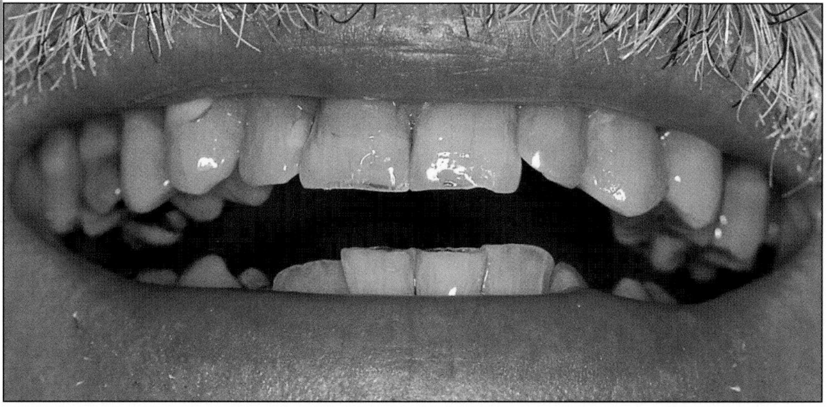

CROWDED, DISCOLORED AND WORN TEETH

This 72-year-old man was unhappy with what he felt was an unattractive smile.

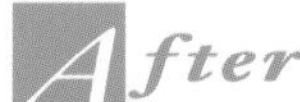

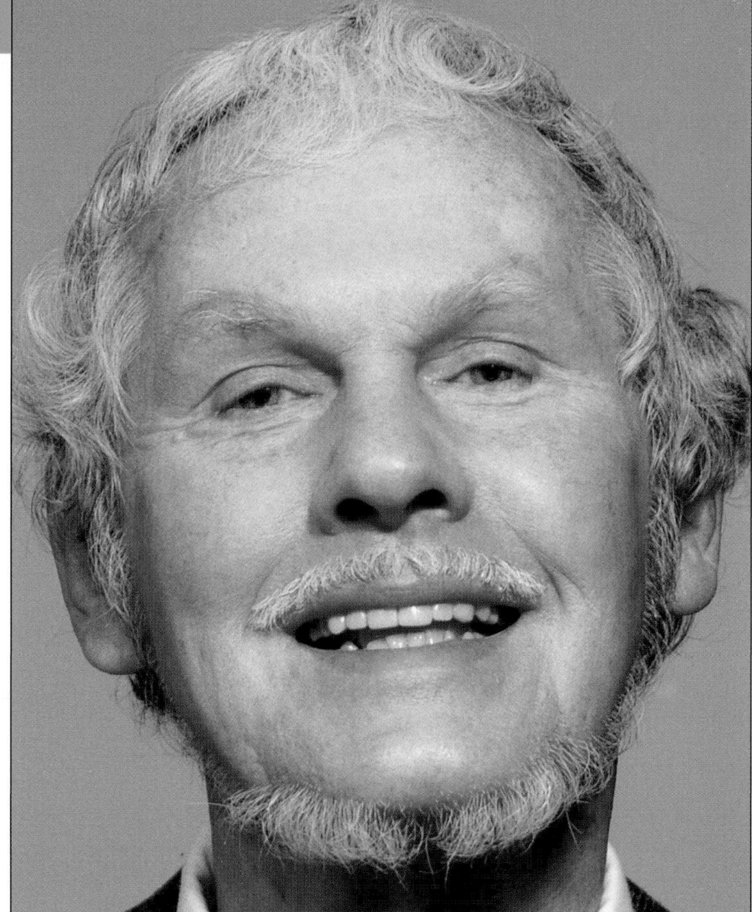

COMPOSITE RESIN BONDING AND COSMETIC CONTOURING

Two appointments were necessary for bonding and cosmetic contouring, which resulted in straighter teeth. A lighter shade of composite resin was selected, which contributed to a younger look.

Before

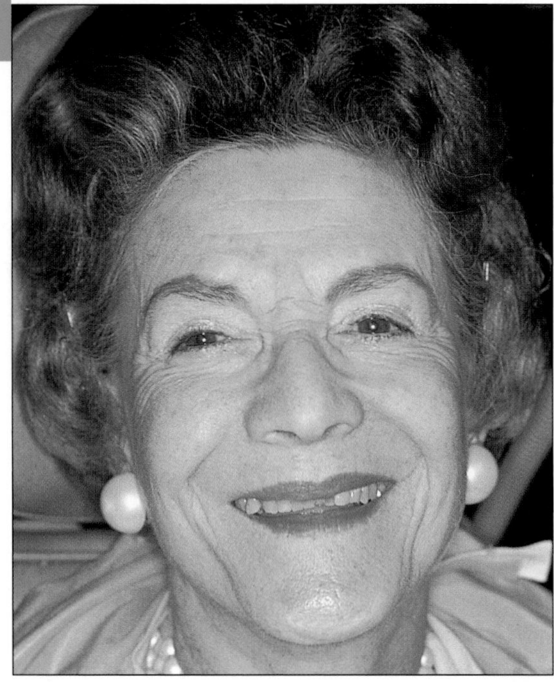

FAULTY AND DISCOLORED FILLINGS AND TOOTH WEAR

This woman's worn and discolored teeth had faulty fillings that spoiled an otherwise attractive smile. However, she did not want to have crowns on her "good" teeth if at all possible.

After

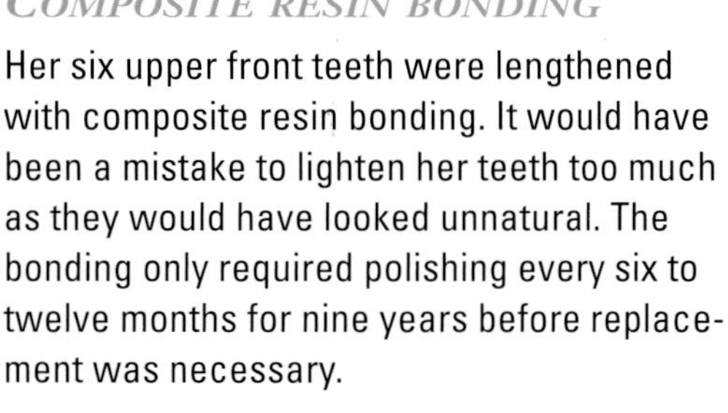

COMPOSITE RESIN BONDING

Her six upper front teeth were lengthened with composite resin bonding. It would have been a mistake to lighten her teeth too much as they would have looked unnatural. The bonding only required polishing every six to twelve months for nine years before replacement was necessary.

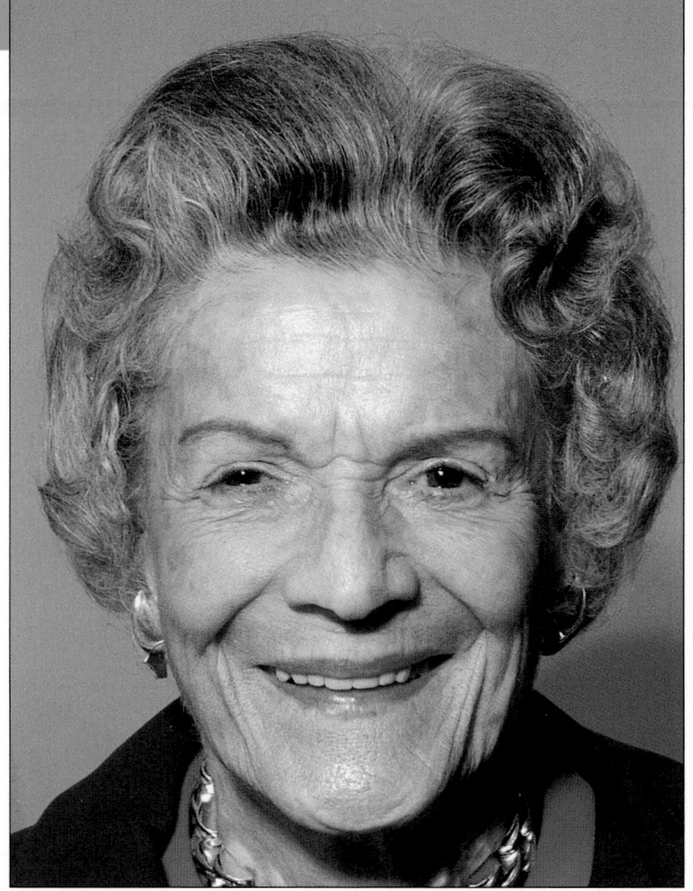

Before

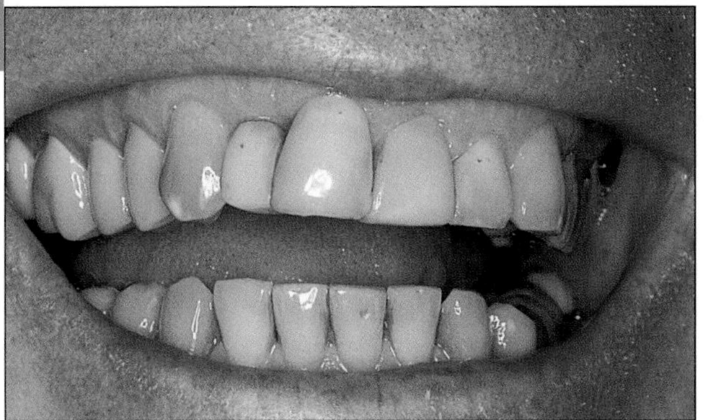

GUM ASYMMETRY AND WORN AND DISCOLORED TEETH

This CEO had discolored and worn teeth and irregular-looking gum tissue, resulting in an aged smile.

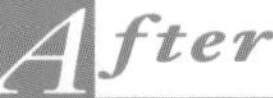

After

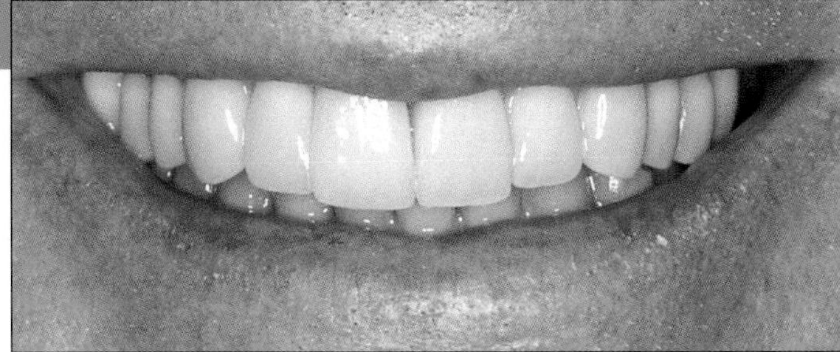

PORCELAIN LAMINATES PLUS GUM SURGERY

After the gums were cosmetically and functionally improved, five porcelain laminates were placed as were posterior crowns and inlays. The result was lighter teeth and improved tooth shape and arch alignment.

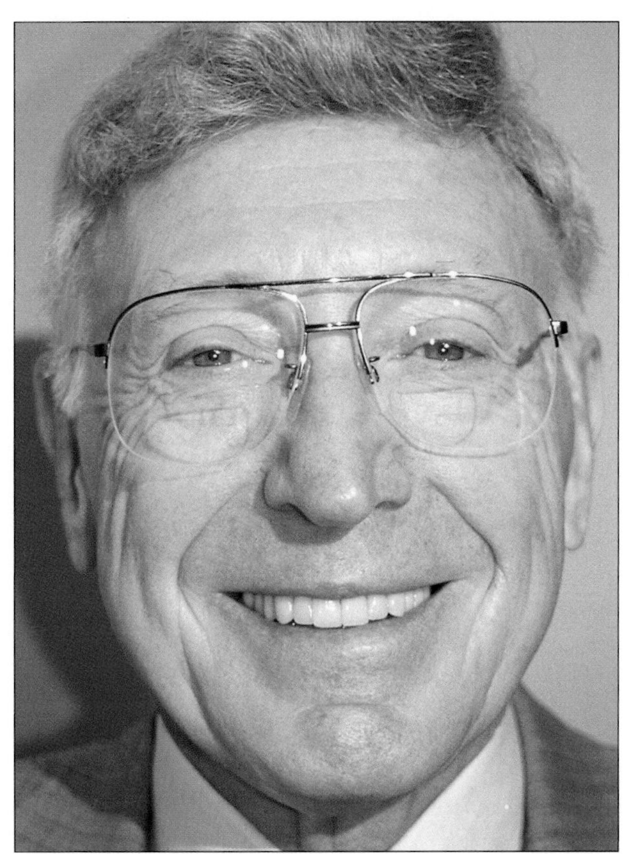

Crowning: A Good Solution for an Aging Smile

For patients with extensive tooth wear—regardless of the cause—maximum improvement is usually obtained with crowning. It may even be possible to restore your bite to its previous condition.

If your jaw has collapsed, the first step may involve wearing an acrylic or plastic bite appliance. If you can tolerate this appliance, the chances are excellent that you will be able to rebuild your bite with crowns or bridges.

The second step is to make plastic temporary crowns or bridges to replace the bite appliance. However, some dentists choose to proceed directly to this step without the use of an appliance. The last step involves replacing these temporary restorations with the final—and more durable—crowns or bridges.

The advantage of porcelain crowns is that they are made from a beautiful material that can completely mask staining. Crowns can also straighten and replace worn teeth simultaneously. On the other hand, crowning requires the reduction of the natural tooth. It is also more expensive than contouring or bonding, costing approximately $450 to $3000 per tooth.

Before

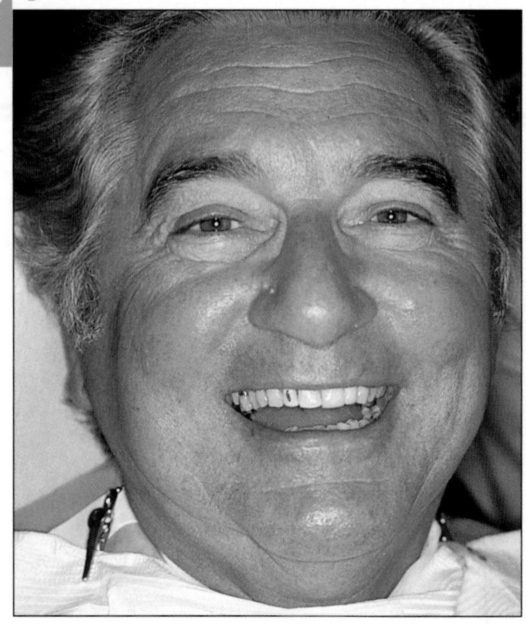

Worn and discolored plastic crowns

This businessman had so worn his front crowns that the gold beneath the acrylic veneer on the right front tooth showed. The other acrylic veneer crowns were discolored, making him look older than he was.

After

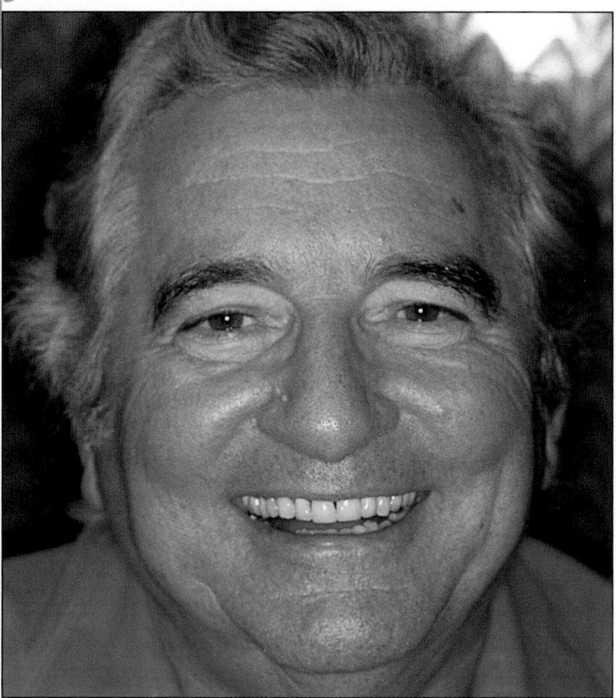

Full crowns

New porcelain crowns with a lighter and more youthful look combined to produce an attractive smile. Your smile can be the most expressive part of your face. When it looks good, so do you!

Before

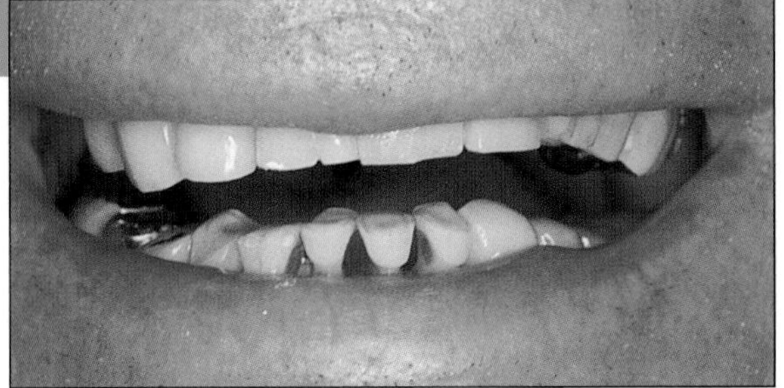

After

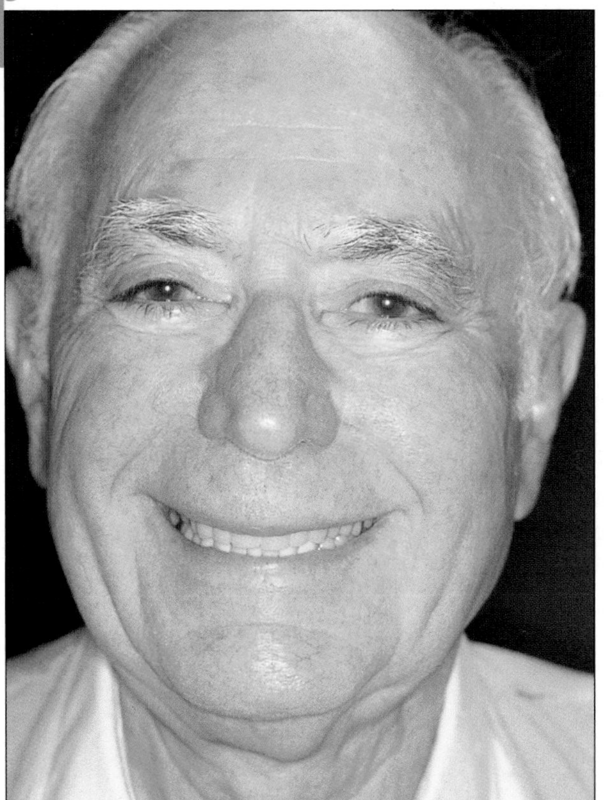

ADVANCED TOOTH WEAR AND BONE LOSS

This 75-year-old president of a large corporation had, over the years, worn down his upper and lower teeth.

CROWNS PLUS FIXED AND REMOVABLE BRIDGES

All of his remaining upper and lower teeth were crowned, and precision-attachment removable bridges were placed to rebuild his entire mouth. Notice how the new smile with longer front teeth makes for a more youthful and handsome appearance.

Before

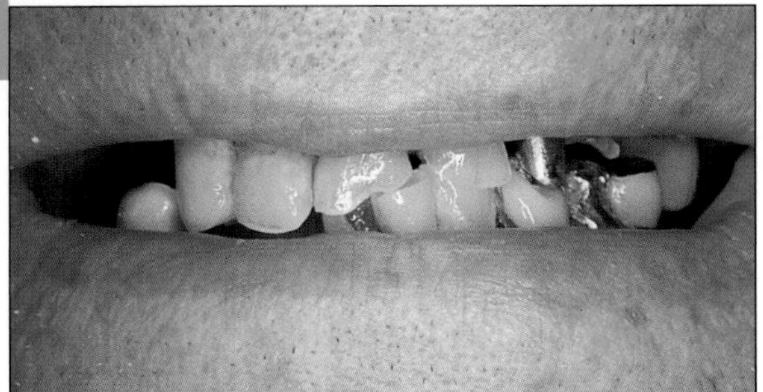

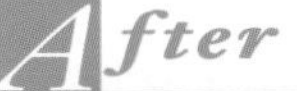

After

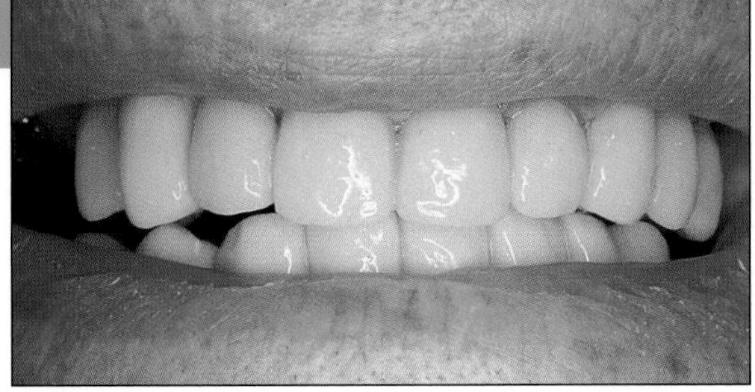

TOOTH DECAY AND BONE LOSS

Although this 69-year-old retired executive was in poor health, he wanted to improve the function of his teeth as well as his appearance. For patients who are ailing, a compromise treatment plan can improve their smile with a minimal investment of time and money.

TEMPORARY CROWNS AND BRIDGES

Temporary crowns and bridges on all the existing teeth were made in a lighter color to rebuild his teeth and improve his appearance. The patient was immediately satisfied with his good-looking smile.

Orthodontics: It's Never Too Late

During the past decade, the number of adults seeking orthodontic treatment has tripled. Clear plastic brackets and lingual braces that fit behind the teeth make it a more acceptable alternative than in years past.

If it takes tooth repositioning with orthodontics to improve your smile, do it if you can. You're never too old for tooth movement. Your bite will improve and so will your appearance.

Before

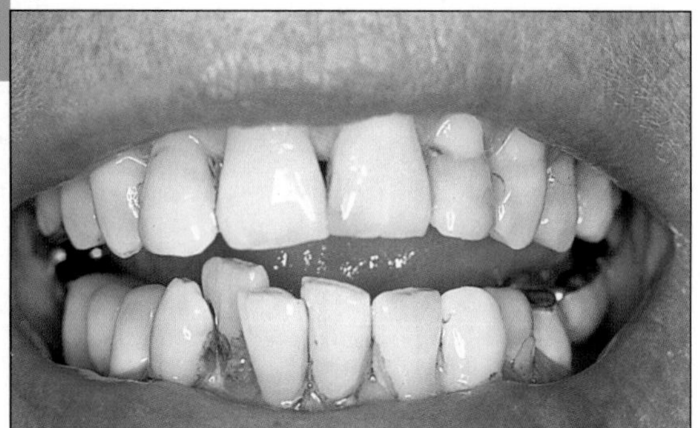

Crowded teeth

This 65-year-old woman's crowded and discolored teeth left her unhappy with her smile. She thought it made her look older than she felt.

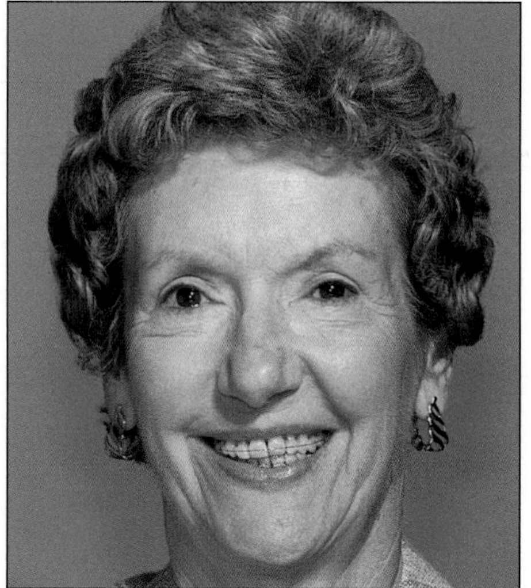

Orthodontic Treatment

Ten months of orthodontic treatment helped reposition her front teeth.

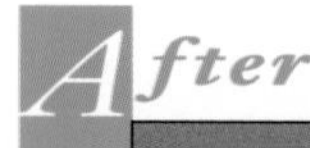

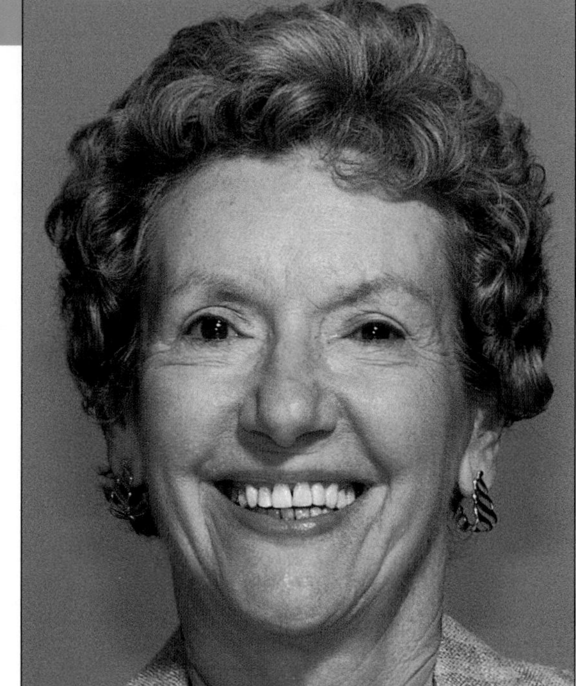

Orthodontics and composite resin bonding

After orthodontic treatment, bonding with composite resin lightened the teeth and helped mask the stained fillings. No one is too old to have teeth repositioned. Having straighter and lighter-looking teeth helps to make for a more youthful smile.

Before

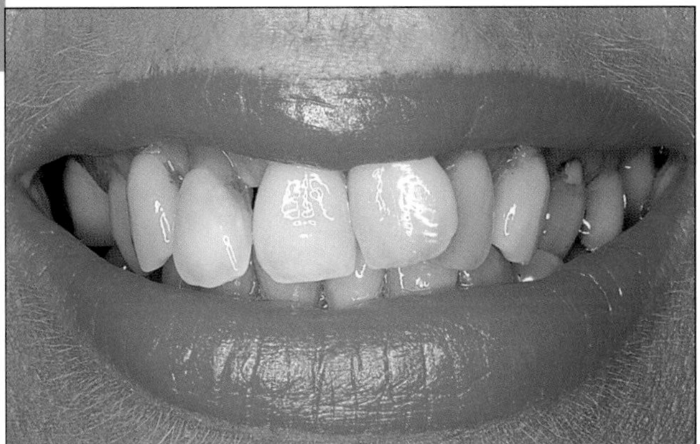

Crowded Teeth

This 56-year-old woman was health-conscious enough to want to properly correct her bad bite. Although she was prepared to have her teeth crowned if necessary, she chose the more time-consuming, but better, method of tooth movement.

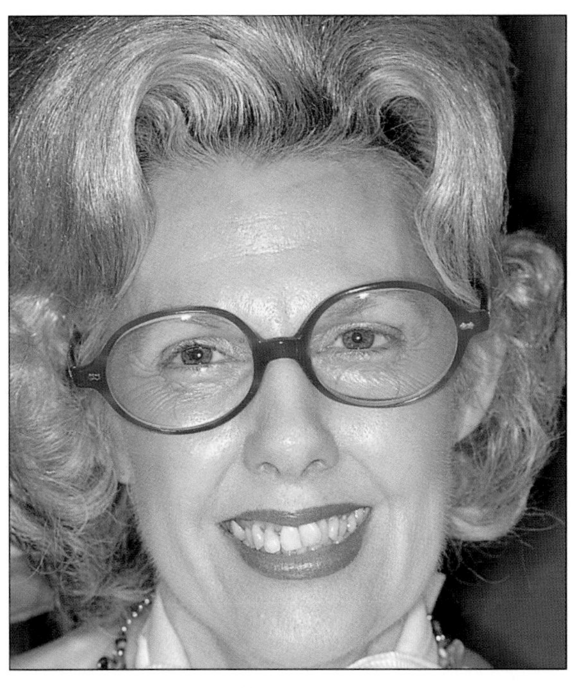

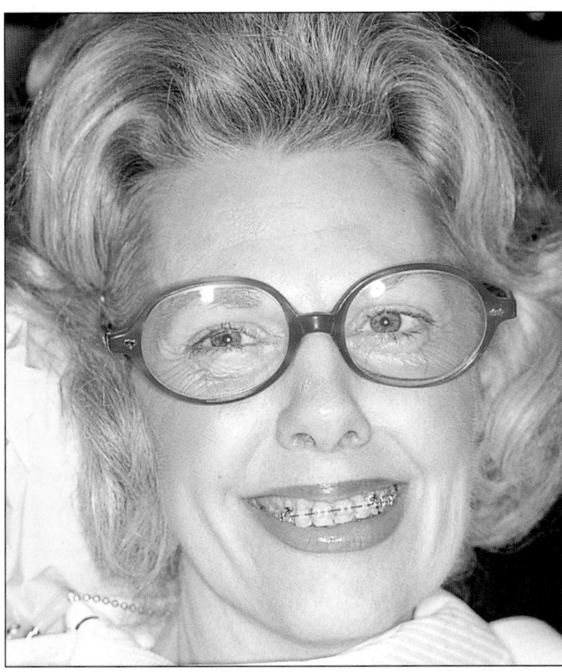

Orthodontics and Composite Resin Bonding

The patient opted for tooth-colored brackets, and the teeth were repositioned in 18 months. Composite resin bonding was then done to help her smile look more attractive.

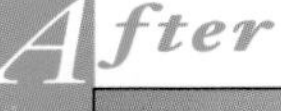

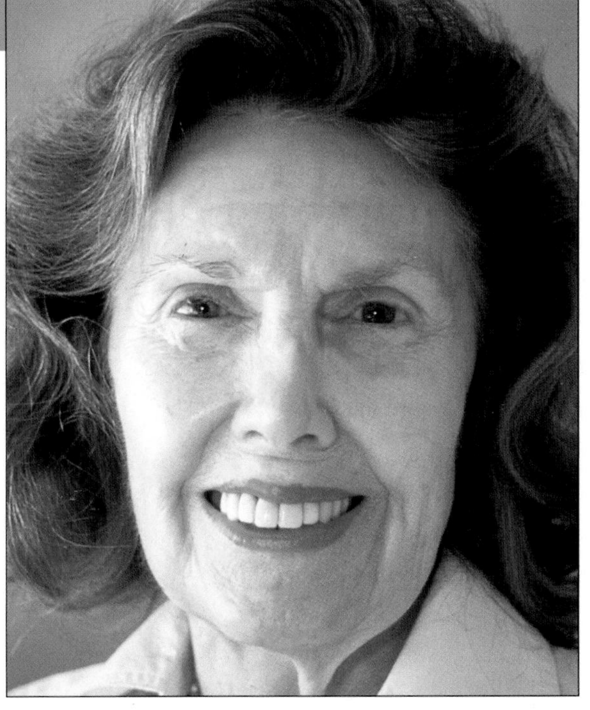

Orthodontics, a Lasting Result

Twenty-four years after orthodontic treatment, this lady's smile still looks good.

Implants: An Effective New Alternative

If you have lost certain teeth due to periodontal disease, it may be possible to replace them with dental implants. In fact, in certain instances, an implant can serve as *anchorage* for repositioning teeth (see Chapter 5 for more information).

Dentures: No One Has to Know You Have Them

Few people want to have their teeth extracted just to look better. But when restoring the teeth is impossible because there is simply not enough tooth structure left, dentures are an alternative.

It is important from a cosmetic standpoint, however, that you not allow too much time to lag between tooth loss and tooth replacement. Tooth loss causes the face to collapse and the mouth to sink in. At the same time, the nose appears to drop down toward the chin. Deep lines begin to form in the creases of this collapsed skin, adding years to the face.

Full dentures can make you look younger because there is almost no limit to what the dentist can create with them. There are basically four types of dentures.

Immediate dentures

Immediate dentures are measured for size with the natural teeth intact, and they are placed the same day as your remaining teeth are extracted. With this type of denture, you skip the try-in stages that accompany the fitting of other models. Because gums and bone tend to shrink after extraction, these dentures may become loose. However, an additional inner lining can be placed inside the dentures to make them fit. This means the replacement time for immediate dentures is often shorter than that for conventional models. It may also mean additional charges for adjustments and lining. Immediate dentures typically cost between $575 and $2500 for upper and lower dentures, plus appropriate surgical fees if required.

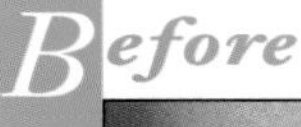

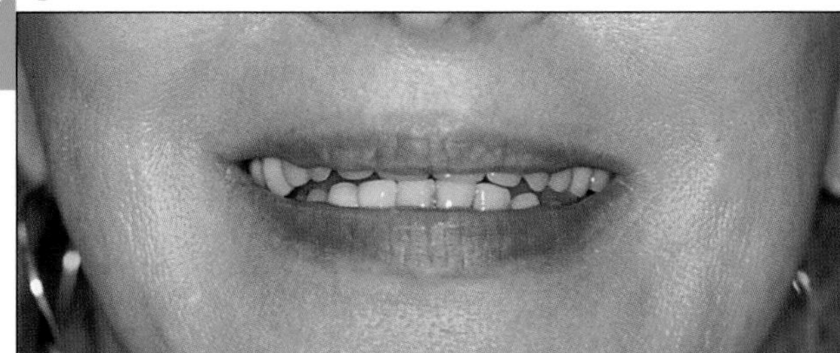

WORN TEETH ON UPPER DENTURE

Tooth wear combined with lack of proper lip support made this 48-year-old woman look older.

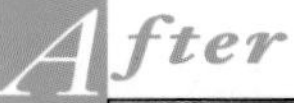

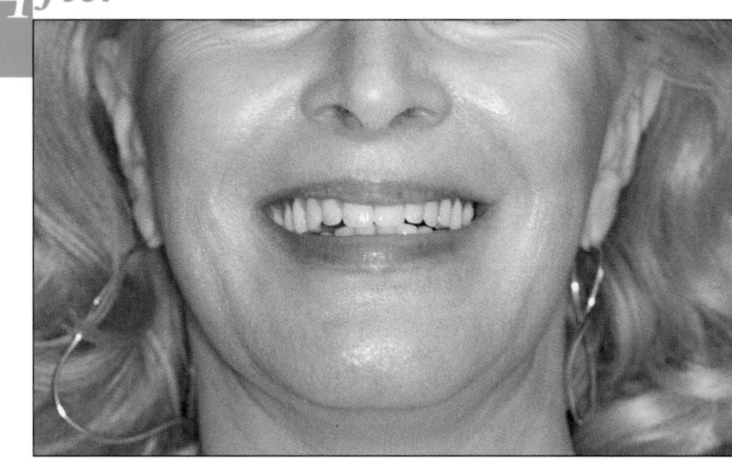

NEW UPPER FULL DENTURE

A new upper full denture provides increased lip support as well as a more youthful smileline.

Conventional dentures

Fitting conventional dentures typically requires three to six office visits after all of the teeth have been removed and the tissue has healed. It is up to you during these visits to pass judgment on the fit and look of the dentures. Your dentist will advise you on color, tooth type and lip position. If the color is too white, the dentures will look artificial.

Conventional dentures cost about the same as immediate dentures. Some dentists also include the cost of later adjustments in their fee.

Economy dentures

There are three types of economy dentures: the professional economy denture; the modular denture; and a denture that uses the basics of denture construction. The latter cost about 50 percent less than conventional dentures. For all practical purposes, they achieve basic function and adequate esthetics. Just don't look for much more than that.

The least desirable model is the "one size fits all," or modular, denture. Made of flexible plastic that molds to the mouth, these dentures are available in a limited number of sizes and are usually worn by people confined to institutions. Although the modular denture costs less than half of the economy denture, it should be used only when the latter cannot be made.

Custom-made dentures

Custom-made dentures have specially shaded teeth and gums, gold or silver fillings and other characteristics that duplicate natural teeth. Because of this, they cost more than other types of dentures, typically from $1500 to $6000.

Because dentures fracture and chip much more easily than natural teeth, you may want to have a spare set, particularly if you travel a lot. It's worth the extra cost to have teeth when you need a repair.

BECAUSE DENTURES FRACTURE AND CHIP MORE EASILY THAN NATURAL TEETH, YOU MAY WANT TO HAVE A SPARE SET

Some people may want an interchangeable spare set, which is a complete duplicate of the original. Although this can be expensive, it may be the best option if you require a perfect smile at all times.

Also remember that no dentures last forever. In fact, if the teeth are made of plastic—and most of them are—they may show wear within 3 to 6 years. If you grind your teeth, you can expect to show tooth wear in half that time. Therefore, be sure to have your dentures rebased, relined or remade when necessary so that your smile remains attractive.

PREVENTION: THE BEST WAY TO FIGHT THE YEARS

You can keep your smile intact for a lifetime. Good oral hygiene—including toothbrushing, flossing and regular visits to the dentist—will help keep teeth, gums and bone in good health.

Proper toothbrushing is one of the best ways to prevent tooth loss and other problems. If you're not sure that you're brushing correctly, ask your dentist to show you how. Although a loss of tooth structure due to mechanical wear is inevitable, incorrect toothbrushing often accelerates this process. You may also want to purchase chewable disclosing tablets that allow you to see the plaque you missed by revealing those areas in red.

You should also consider purchasing a rotary cleaning device with the advice of your dentist. Research has shown that many people can improve their tooth-cleaning ability with automatic tooth brushes.

Also choose a dentist who offers an aggressive program of preventive maintenance. This should include two to eight professional tooth cleanings per year, proper home care instruction, monitoring of plaque control and referral to specialists such as periodontists when needed.

Before

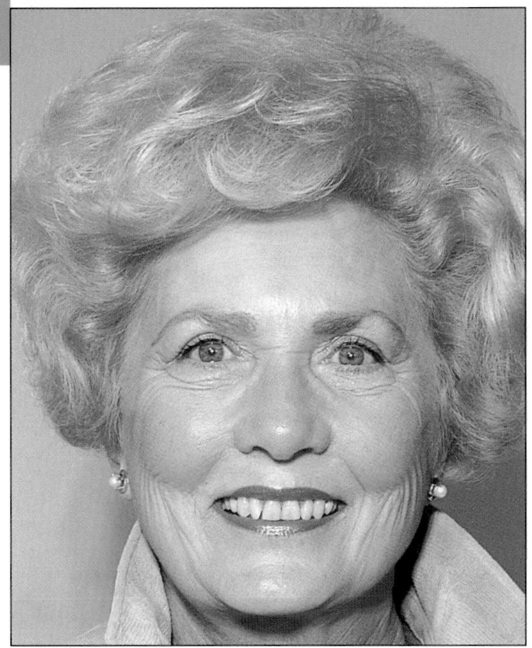

Twisted teeth

This woman was displeased about her discolored and twisted teeth. In addition, the sharp points of her teeth made it appear as if she had fangs.

After

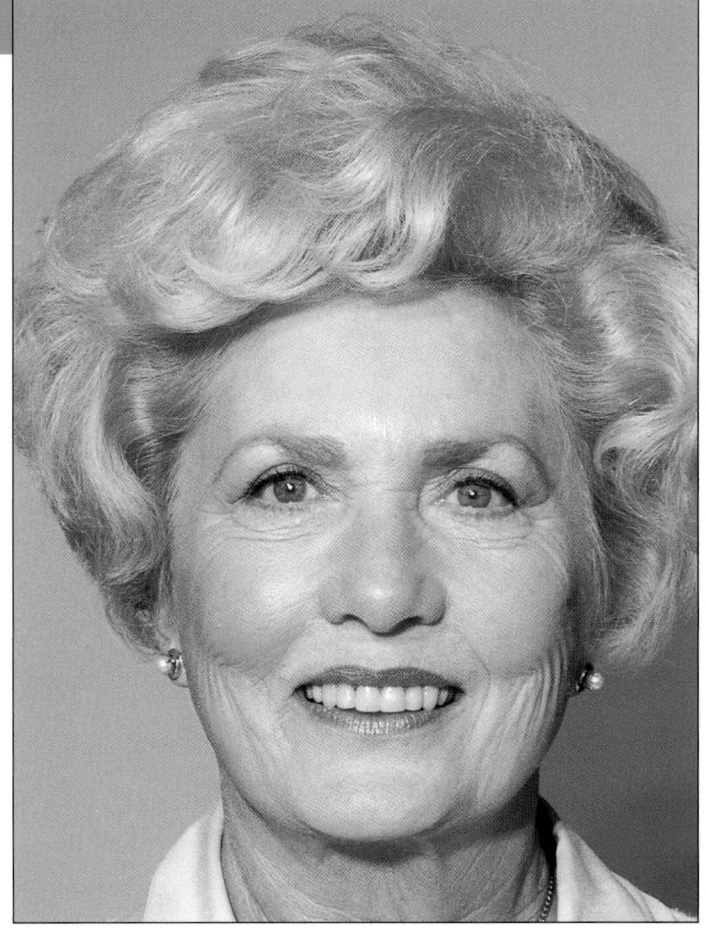

Composite resin bonding

Her six front teeth were first contoured and then bonded to make them appear straighter. Notice how a softer look was achieved just with contouring of the bonded teeth.

Finally, don't neglect to replace teeth that are lost. Failure to do so can result in more extensive—and expensive—dental treatment in the long run than replacing them. Leaving a space in the back of the mouth can lead to gum disease or throw off the bite by shifting chewing pressure to other teeth. This, in turn, can cause the front teeth to shift. In fact, newly developed spaces between front teeth are often the result of missing back teeth, so don't let it happen.

Never have your teeth extracted if there is sufficient bone to save them, even if only a root remains. You will chew better—and look better—if you restore, rather than replace your natural teeth.

If your bone is diseased, periodontal surgery can often allow you to save your teeth. And your own good roots are always better "implants" than artificial ones.

The Best Way to Look Younger

The best way to obtain a more youthful smile is by combining the advantages of cosmetic dentistry, plastic surgery and cosmetology—in that order.

First, improve your smile. Make sure it looks healthy and younger. Next, if you're concerned about sagging facial tissue, consider plastic surgery. And finally, don't forget that a new hairstyle and updated makeup can provide the finishing touches (see p. 297).

Never Stop Caring

With age, some people simply give up trying to look their best and stop taking proper care of themselves, including their teeth. As a result, their teeth become worn and discolored, fillings decay and gum disease sets in. If you're one of those people, remember that it's never too late to start taking care of yourself again. Many older persons today are seeking treatment to correct dental problems and improve their appearance. If you have friends or family members who no longer take an interest in their looks, share this book with them. Let them know how much better they can feel with a brand new smile. You could be a tremendous help in improving not only their appearance, but their outlook on life.

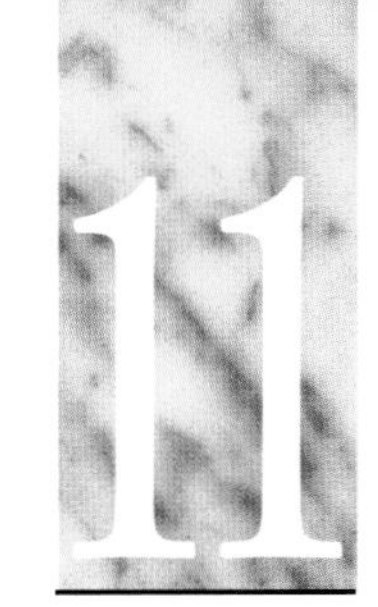

The Role of Plastic Surgery in Enhancing Your Smile

Foad Nahai, MD

Your face is like a picture frame that surrounds your smile. Plastic surgery can enhance your smile, just as beautiful teeth will complement the good results of cosmetic plastic surgery. A vast array of options is available to the patient considering facial plastic surgery today. The decision to choose plastic surgery involves several important considerations.

Selecting a Qualified Plastic Surgeon

Did you know that a doctor, any doctor, regardless of training, can call himself or herself a plastic surgeon? A medical license allows a doctor to practice in any specialty, including plastic surgery. To a certain degree, the only controls that exist are hospital admitting privileges where hospitals will allow a physician to practice only the specialty in which he or she is trained or board certified. However, because most plastic surgery procedures can be done as an outpatient in a doctor's office or ambulatory surgical center, these hospital admitting privileges don't necessarily protect you. Selecting a physician who is also able to perform your procedure in a hospital offers some reassurance.

Beware of slick advertisements where risks are ignored and results are guaranteed. It is your responsibility to select a qualified plastic surgeon. A qualified surgeon will be happy to answer your questions about his or her qualifications, which should always include Board Certification in Plastic Surgery.

Board certification means that your surgeon has had the prerequisite training in the specialty and has successfully passed certifying examinations. However, you should ascertain that your surgeon is certified by a board that is recognized by the American Board of Medical Specialists (ABMS). You should also make sure that your surgeon is certified by a board that specifically covers the surgical procedure that interests you.

WORD OF MOUTH IS AN IMPORTANT SOURCE OF INFORMATION

Next, ascertain that your surgeon is experienced in the particular procedure you are considering. Ask the surgeon how often he or she has performed this procedure within the last year. You will want to know that he or she is performing this procedure on a regular basis with good results.

Last but not least is reputation. If you know someone who has had cosmetic surgery, have seen the good results and know that they were happy with their doctor, ask for the doctor's name! Also, ask your dentist or other physicians for their recommendations. Word of mouth is an important source of information. You should have a short list of at least two or three surgeons, and you should consult at least two of them. Seek a second opinion and trust your instincts about which doctor you feel most comfortable with.

The More Informed You Are, the Happier You'll Be

Once you have selected your surgeon, feel free to ask to see before-and-after photos of previous patients. It is important to have realistic expectations about how your surgery may improve your appearance. It should be emphasized that plastic surgery, like any other form of surgery, carries certain risks and potential complications. Unfavorable results, though rare, are always a possibility. The complications and risks associated with anesthesia should also be discussed with your doctor.

By selecting an experienced and qualified surgeon, these risks are minimized and, when complications do occur, a good surgeon will know how to recognize and handle them.

Be Open to Your Surgeon's Suggestions

In most cases your surgeon will agree with your assessment about which of your facial features can be enhanced through plastic surgery. However, he or she may suggest a different approach than you had in mind for a more desirable result.

There is a wide variety of procedures available to enhance your smile and facial appearance. A thorough evaluation and consultation is essential to enable your surgeon to assess your particular needs, take into account your desires, and recommend which procedures and techniques will produce the best possible results. You may find his or her opinions very enlightening, as there are likely to be factors to consider and beneficial procedures that you did not know were available. In any case, you are half of the decision making team.

When you and your surgeon are in agreement, it is time to proceed. You have done your homework, you have been educated as to what is possible and reasonable, you have confidence in your surgeon, you understand the risks and you should look forward to your operation with an optimism based on your knowledge of all these factors.

When Is the Right Time to Have Plastic Surgery?

For correcting congenital deformities, age is not necessarily an issue. Cleft lip and palate should be corrected in infancy. An extremely large nose or other inherited features may be cosmetically corrected through plastic surgery at any time in the teen years, or later. However, for diminishing the negative signs of aging, "customizing over time" is recommended.

Customizing Over Time

Age is not the primary issue. Each patient is unique and individual. A woman in her forties may have her eyes done one year, followed by line removal and possibly liposuction of the neck or jawline at a later time.

You may wish to start early, in your twenties or thirties, with preventative or maintenance skin care using chemical treatments such a Retin A and alpha hydroxy acids. Over the years, as the need arises, you may wish to have an "eyelift" to remove excess fat from the area around the eyes. In the next year or so, you may choose liposuction of the neck, and so on, until finally a full face-lift is needed. By approaching cosmetic surgery in this manner, you will be subtly transforming the ravages of age as they occur on your own unique face. Each procedure will freshen your appearance gradually, making you the most attractive you can be at each age level.

The advantage of customizing over time is the subtlety of change. You don't want people to declare, "Look at that face-lift!" Tight facial skin is not believable when other parts of the body, such as the hands, look much older. The desirable result is a "freshening" in appearance. A subtle and gradual approach to cosmetic surgery elicits comments like, "You look wonderful" or "You look so well-rested."

Before

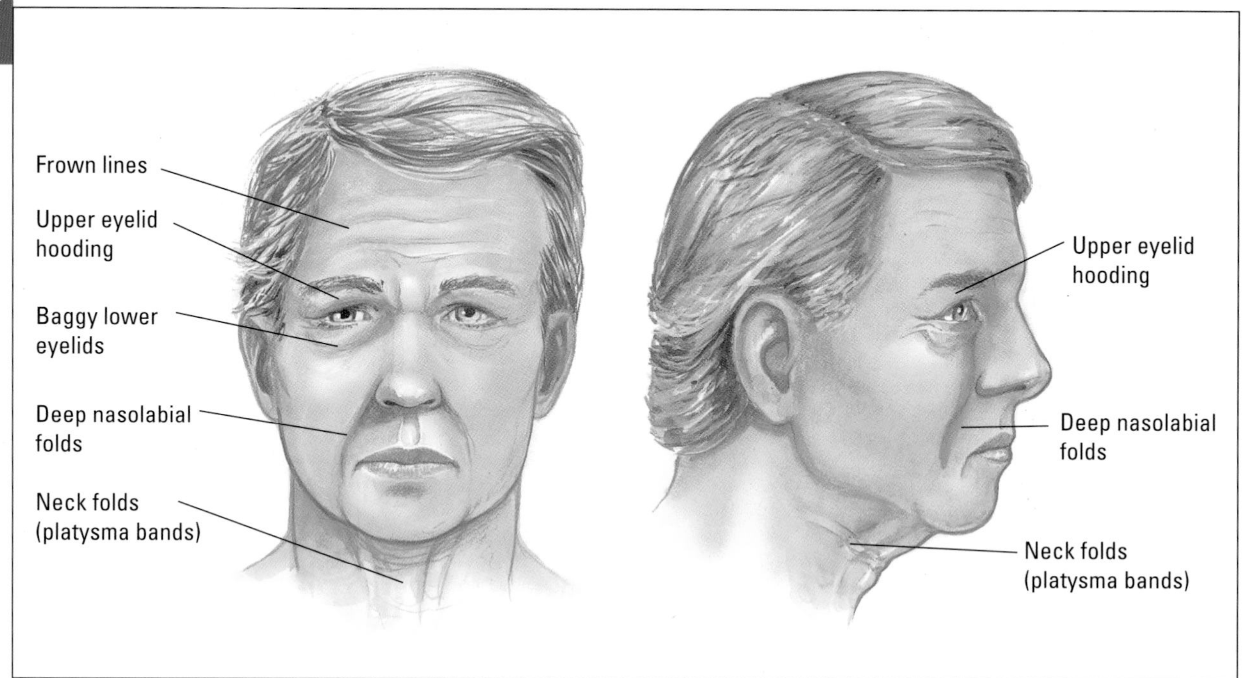

After

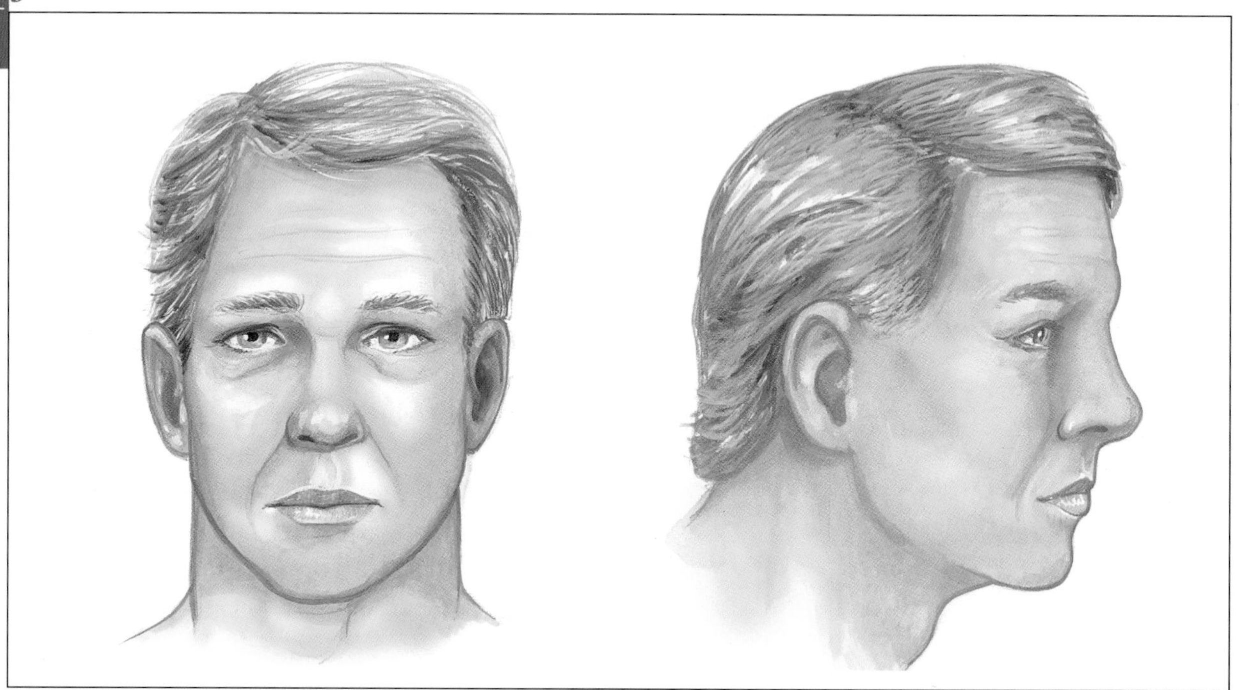

Note the frown lines, upper eyelid hooding, lower eyelid bags, nasolabial folds, and excess skin on the neck. A brow-lift removes the frown lines, and an upper and lower eyelid-lift removes bags and saggy skin around the eyes. A face-lift and neck-lift reduce the nasolabial folds and remove the excess skin on the neck, giving this man a more youthful appearance.

Before

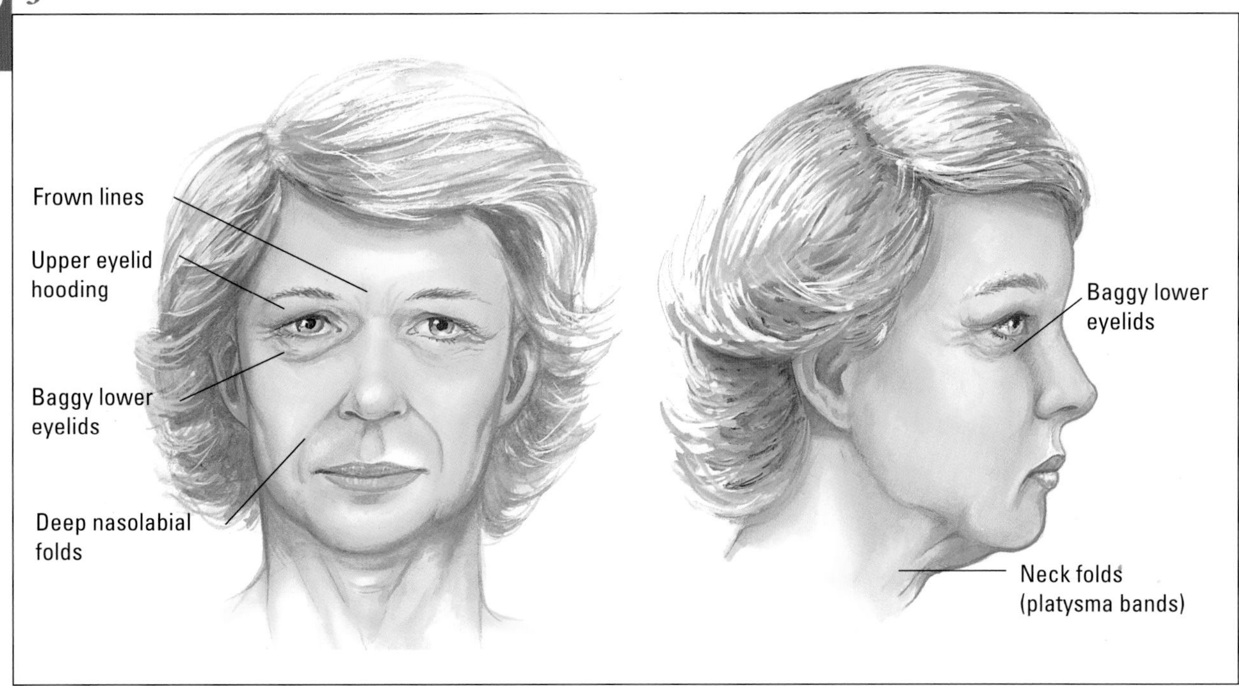

After

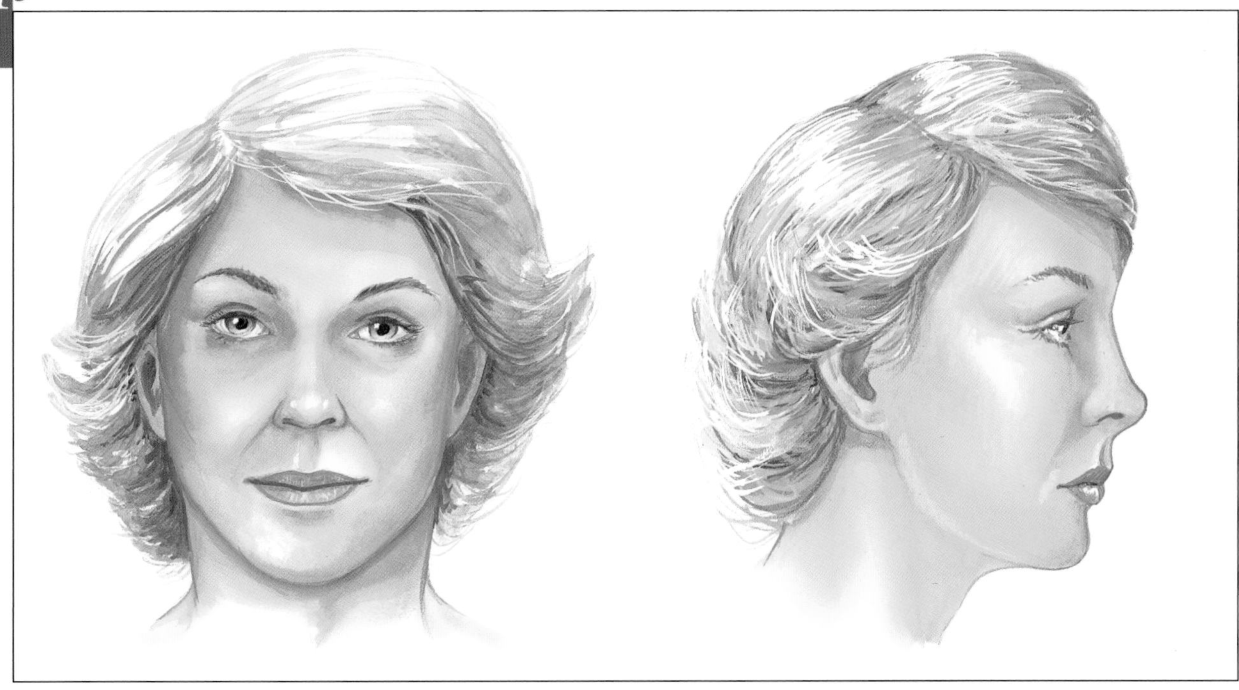

This woman reveals the same problems as the man on the previous page. With a brow-lift, face-lift and neck-lift, the same rejuvenating results are achieved.

Sometimes Less Is More

A radical change in facial appearance can cause a degree of psychological trauma. The most desirable results are achieved through subtle surgical correction. For example, with rhinoplasty, the nose need not be radically redesigned for the best results. The size and shape of the nose should be in proportion with the size and bone structure of the face.

Cosmetic Surgery Is Not for Women Only

Although it is much more common for women to have cosmetic surgery, this trend is changing. Currently only about 15 percent of cosmetic surgery is performed on men, but the number is increasing as it becomes more acceptable for men to actively improve their appearance.

Cosmetic surgery on men is more challenging. The scars are more difficult to conceal because of the shorter hair styles, and men generally don't feel comfortable using cosmetics to conceal scars. The surgical procedures are different as well for better placement of scars and for handling of the male tissues. As with women, proper rest, limited physical activity and smoking cessation are critical to avoid complications after surgery.

Despite the more challenging techniques required for cosmetic surgery for men, the patients are quite satisfied with the results and, like women, enjoy the emotional boost following surgery.

Are You a Candidate for Plastic Surgery?

Ask yourself two very important questions. Why do I want plastic surgery? What do I expect plastic surgery to do for me? There are right reasons and wrong reasons to have cosmetic dentistry or plastic surgery. Plastic surgery for the right reasons will be a satisfying experience. Plastic surgery for the wrong reasons will lead to dissatisfaction and disappointment.

Why change your appearance through plastic surgery?

Ask Yourself

Yes	No	
❑	❑	1. Do you think plastic surgery will add to your self-confidence?
❑	❑	2. Are you self-conscious about aging changes in your face?
❑	❑	3. Are you self-conscious about your nose?
❑	❑	4. Are you self-conscious about your chin?
❑	❑	5. Do you feel a more youthful appearance will be an asset in your job?
❑	❑	6. Do you think plastic surgery will bring about a significant change in your life?
❑	❑	7. Do you think plastic surgery will lead to a job promotion?
❑	❑	8. Do you think plastic surgery will alter a personal relationship?
❑	❑	9. Do you think plastic surgery will save a failing marriage?
❑	❑	10. Is your concern about the problems with your appearance out of proportion to what others think?
❑	❑	11. Are you looking for perfection?

Answering *yes* to questions 1–5 represents good reasons for having plastic surgery. Answering *yes* to questions 6–11 represents poor reasons for having plastic surgery.

A Very Personal Decision

Having a facial feature that varies from common standards of beauty is not reason enough to seek plastic surgery. A friend or loved one may suggest that you consider plastic surgery, but the ultimate decision rests with you. Remember, some of the most famous faces in the world have unconventional features, and yet these people (who could have easily afforded cosmetic surgery) decided against it.

Conversely, if you desire plastic surgery and a qualified surgeon has confirmed that your expectations are reasonable and attainable, don't allow others to dissuade you. The bottom line is that the decision to consider plastic surgery is a personal decision.

Sometimes No Surgery Is Better

The plastic surgeon is an advisor who helps patients make the right decisions. In some cases this will mean that a surgeon advises against surgery. Whatever else it may be, plastic surgery is not cure-all for depression or other problems.

Insecurity precipitates many people's desires for unwarranted plastic surgery. However, being advised against a specific cosmetic procedure may often provide a boost in self-esteem for the person who is told by an expert that his or her concern is unwarranted.

About Costs

The costs for plastic surgery will vary depending on whether you have a minor procedure (such as fat or collagen injections) or a full face-lift. You may desire a combination of several procedures, as decided by you and your surgeon. If deemed appropriate by your doctor, a modified face-lift may be all you require, which will be less costly than a more comprehensive procedure.

The costs for facial plastic surgery may range from $1,000 for a minor procedure such as fat or collagen injections, to around $14,000 for a full face-lift. In addition to these costs, you may also have to include the cost of the hospital or clinic's surgical facility, as well as the fee for the anesthesiologist. Costs will also depend on whether you undergo surgery in a city or smaller town. You should feel comfortable about inquiring about all of the costs before you decide to proceed.

You should feel comfortable inquiring about all costs

Cosmetic surgery is not covered by insurance, and it is usual and customary for the surgeon's fee to be paid in advance. The fees that are listed with each procedure under "Cost" are for the surgeon only. In addition to the surgeon's fee, there are hospital, clinic and anesthesia costs.

What You Should Know About Your Procedure

- What will it do for my smile?
- What are the risks?
- What is the recovery time?
- How long will the results last?
- What will it cost?

Ask your doctor to provide you with answers to these questions before you proceed.

The following outlines the most common problems and procedures. It is intended to give you a general idea about what to expect.

The Lips

The lips form the immediate frame around your smile. Overly thin or scarred lips may detract from your smile. The reshaping of the lips through plastic surgery can also correct other disproportions. Even if your teeth are straight and your smile is attractive, well proportioned and defined lips will not only enhance your smile, but make the nonsmiling, relaxed face more attractive.

For the purposes of plastic surgery, the lips may include the area above the lips to the bottom of the nose.

Treatment Summary

Thin Lips

Problem Thin lips.

Solution Lip augmentation using fat transfer or collagen injections.

Risks Insignificant with collagen, some bruising with fat transfer.

Recovery Time Overnight for collagen; three or four days with fat transfer.

Average Range of Treatment Life Expectancy Several months with collagen, longer with fat transfer.

Cost $1000 to $2000.

Treatment Summary

Wrinkled Lips and Lip Lines

Problem Wrinkled lips and lip lines.

Solution Chemical peels and/or dermabrasion or laser resurfacing.

Risks Include scarring and sun discoloration, but these are minimal with the lighter peel.

Recovery Time Depends on degree of treatment; two to three weeks.

Average Range of Treatment Life Expectancy Depends on the depth and degree of treatment.

Cost Chemical peels and/or dermabrasion, $500 to $1500; laser resurfacing, $1000 to $2000.

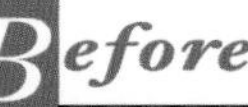

Before

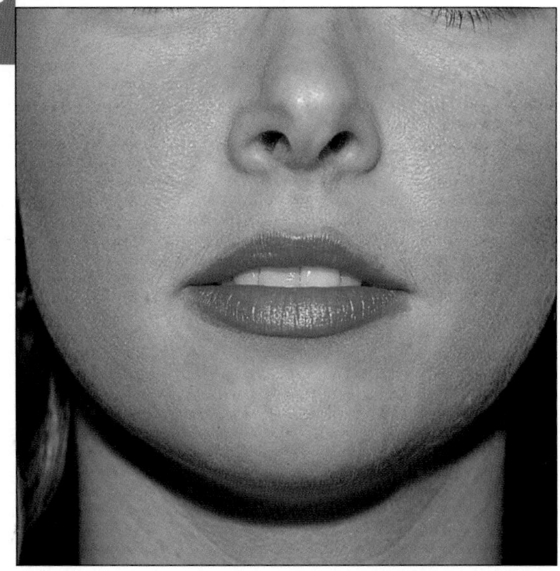

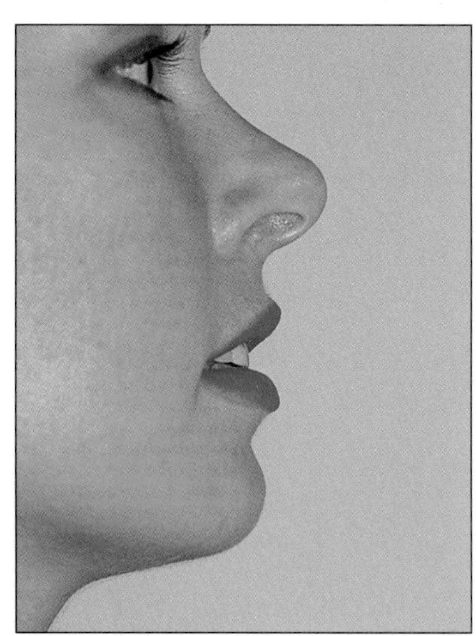

THIN, NARROW LIPS

This young woman wished to have fuller lips.

After

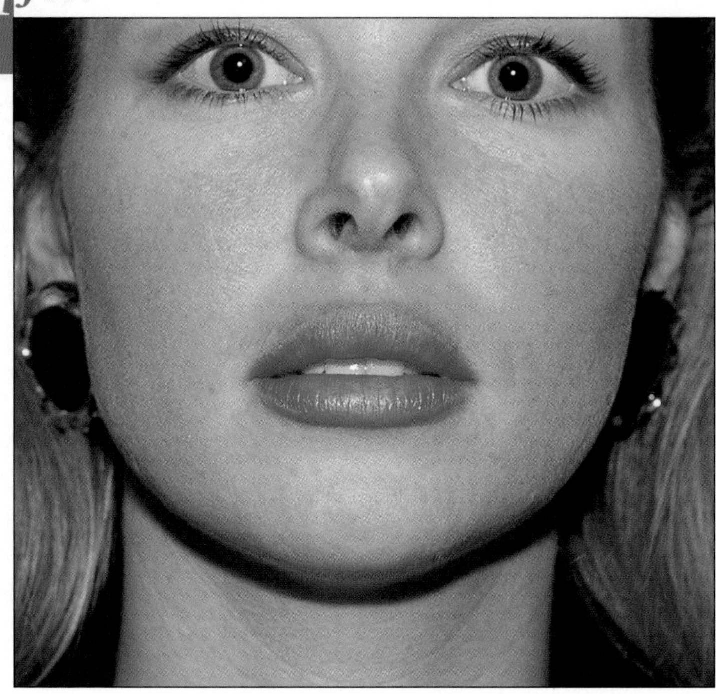

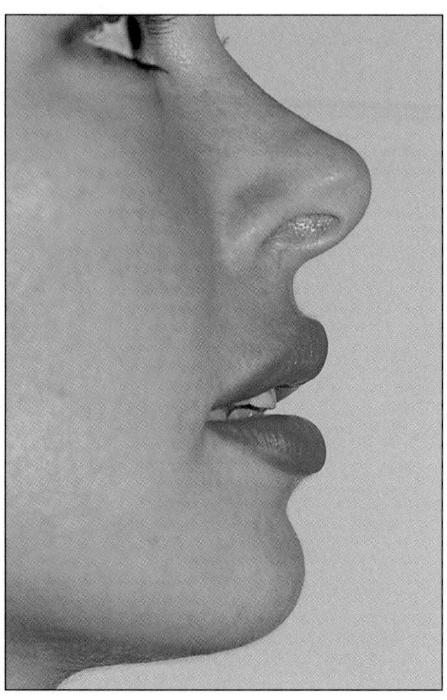

AUGMENTATION (ENLARGEMENT) OF LIP WITH COLLAGEN INJECTIONS

During a one-appointment procedure, collagen was injected into her upper and lower lips to add fullness.

The Cheeks

The cheeks affect the smile more than you might imagine. Heavy jowls and sagging facial tissue pull down the corners of the mouth, giving an unhappy appearance. The nasolabial fold (the line between the corner of the nose to the corner of the mouth) becomes deeper and more pronounced with age, and smiling may exaggerate this fold.

A face-lift supports the cheeks and corrects the drag on the corners of the mouth, making the smile more youthful.

Treatment Summary

Lax Cheeks, Heavy Cheeks or Wrinkled cheeks

Problems Prominent nasolabial fold (sagging in the cheeks with a marked fold line at the junction of cheek from side of nostril to lip corner and chin); laxity of cheeks and skin; heavy cheeks; wrinkled cheeks.

Solutions Face-lift (rhytidectomy); liposuction; buccal fat pad excision (for the "chubby" cheek, the buccal fat pad can be easily excised from inside the mouth, combined with a face-lift or alone).

Risks Complications are infrequent and usually minor. They can include hematoma (a collection of blood under the skin that must be surgically removed), injury to nerves that control facial muscles (rarely permanent), infection and reactions to anesthesia. Poor healing is more likely to affect smokers.

Recovery Time Recovery is in stages. You may go back to work in two weeks, and in four weeks you'll be looking and feeling much better, with bruises fading.

Average Range of Treatment Life Expectancy Although your face will continue to age, the effects of the face-lift are everlasting. Even years later, you'll continue to look better than if you'd never had a face-lift. You may want to repeat the procedure or certain aspects of a total face-lift several times over the years. The lasting effects to a large degree depend on you; avoiding sun and stress and maintaining good health are all important.

Cost Full face-lift, $8000 to $14,000; liposuction of cheeks, $1000 to $2000; buccal fat pad removal, $1000 to $2000.

Before

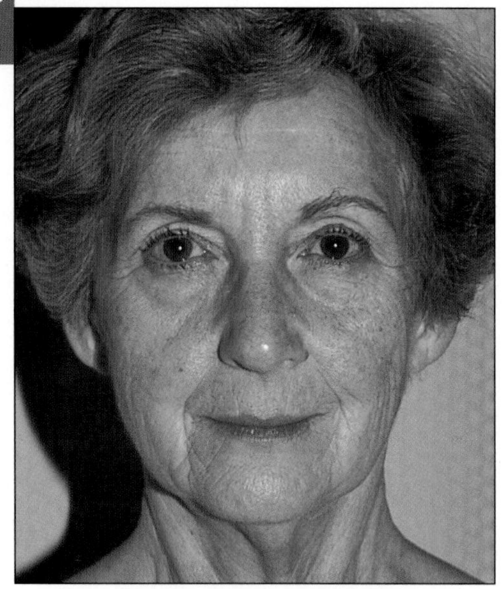

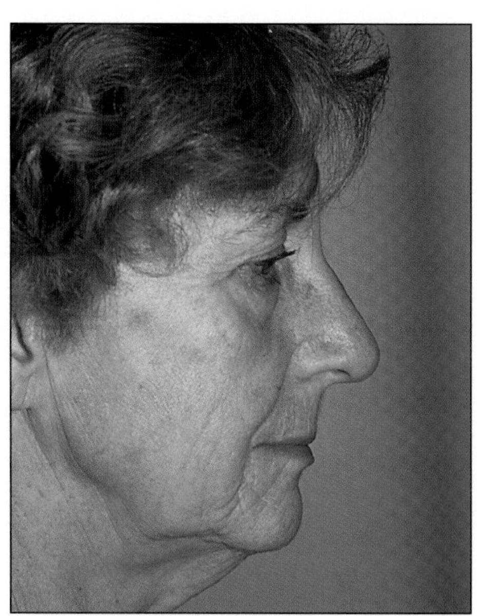

FOREHEAD LINES, LAXITY OF CHEEK, NECK AND JOWLS AND HEAVY EYELIDS

This sixty-year-old woman complained about the lines on her forehead, and the laxity of her cheek, neck and jowls. She also disliked her baggy eyelids.

After

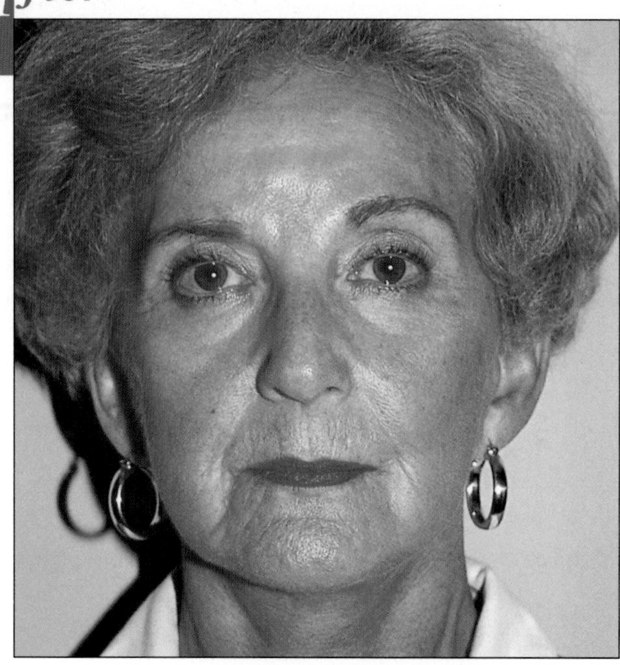

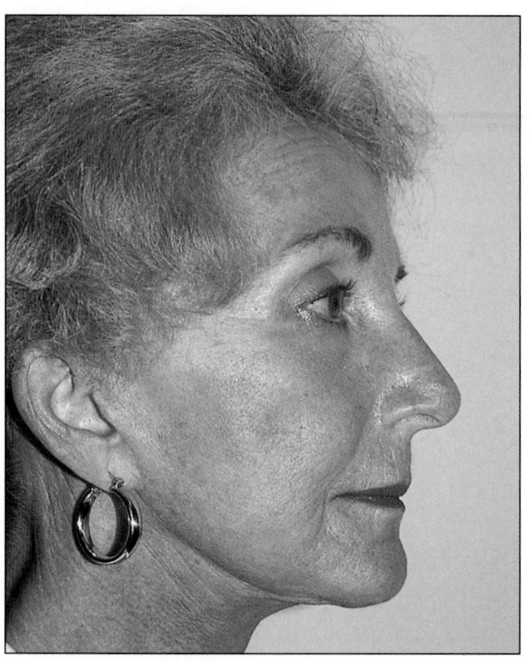

FOREHEAD-LIFT, FACE-LIFT, NECK-LIFT, AND UPPER AND LOWER EYELID-LIFTS

In a single outpatient operation, an endoscopic forehead-lift was performed along with a neck-lift and face-lift. (See p. 271 for more information on endoscopy.) The patient also had upper and lower eyelid-lifts, which resulted in a refreshed, natural look. Note her well-defined neck and jawline.

The Nose

The nose is the face's central and most prominent feature; its contour, character and size have a considerable effect on the smile. If too large or not well shaped, it may shadow and obscure the smile. An overhanging tip of the nose can partially hide the upper lip. A nose that is too wide may appear out of proportion with the smile. Correction of the nose may completely change the smile, making it softer and more natural by improving the proportions of the entire face.

Before

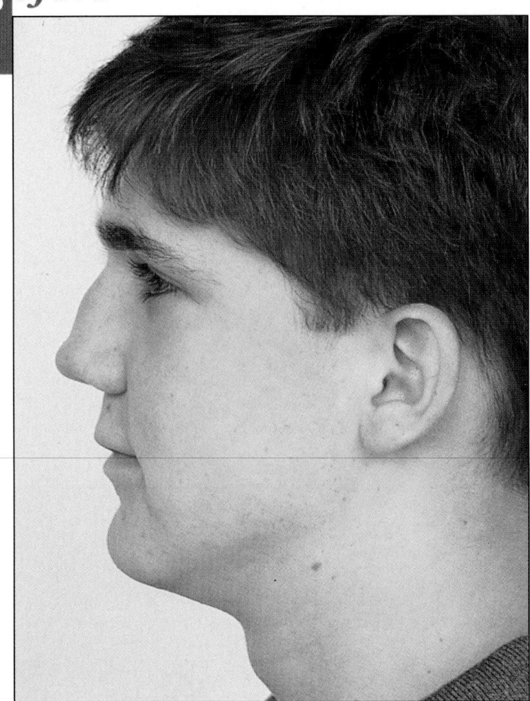

Crooked Nose

This young man's nose was broken in a sports activity, resulting in a crooked nose and difficulty in breathing. A previous operation had failed to correct the problem.

After

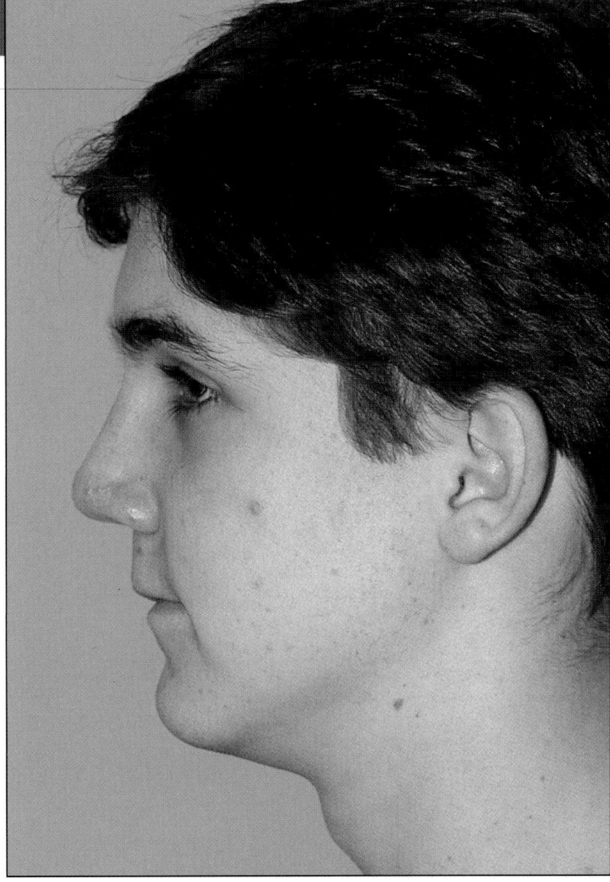

Rhinoplasty (Nose Surgery)

In one outpatient operation, the patient's breathing problem was corrected and the appearance of his nose was greatly improved.

TREATMENT SUMMARY

NOSE TOO BIG, TOO LONG

Problems Nose too big, too long.

Solution Rhinoplasty (surgery to reshape the nose), which can reduce or increase the size of your nose or change its shape or angle. It may, in some cases, even help relieve some breathing problems.

Risks Complications are infrequent and usually minor, although possibilities of infection, nosebleed or reaction to anesthesia do exist. There is also the possibility that small burst blood vessels may appear as tiny red spots on the skin's surface. These are usually minor, but may be permanent. In about one of ten cases, a second procedure may be required. Corrective surgery in these unpredictable cases is usually minor.

Recovery Time Two to three weeks for most of the swelling and bruising. You may go back to work in seven to ten days, but limit strenuous physical activity for three weeks.

Average Range of Treatment Life Expectancy Results are permanent.

Costs $2000 to $5000.

THE CHIN

The chin, like the forehead, nose and lips, contributes to the contour of both the full face and the profile.

The receding chin is more common than the protruding chin. It can be improved dramatically with a surgical implant. With chin reduction, reshaping of bone is performed surgically. In either case, correcting a poorly proportioned chin can dramatically enhance a smile by creating a proper esthetic balance to the face as a whole.

TREATMENT SUMMARY

PROTRUDING CHIN

Problem Protruding chin.

Solution Chin reduction.

Risks Bleeding, scarring and nerve damage.

Recovery Time Two to three weeks if bone is involved.

Average Range of Treatment Life Expectancy Results are permanent.

Cost $2000 to $5000.

Before

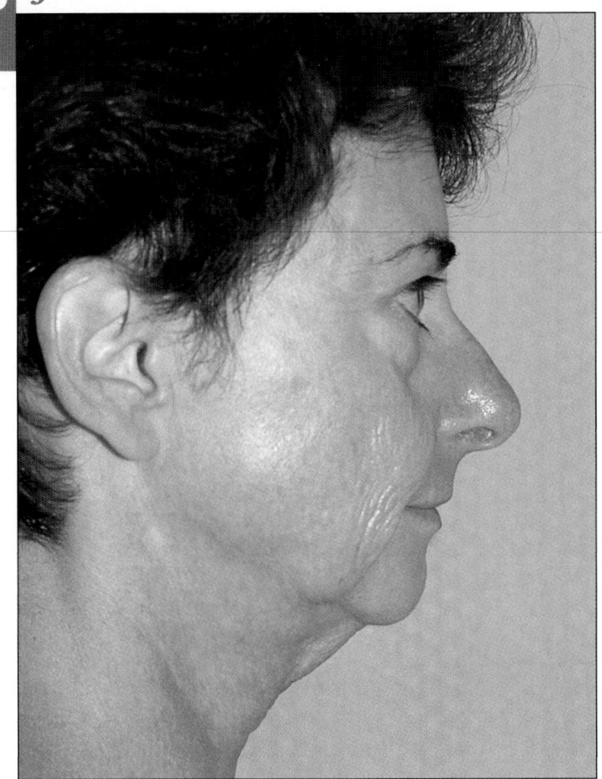

LAXITY OF NECK AND JOWLS WITH EXCESS SKIN

This woman has a soft fleshy appearance, with little distinction between her chin and neck.

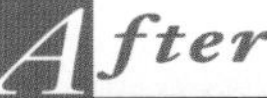

After

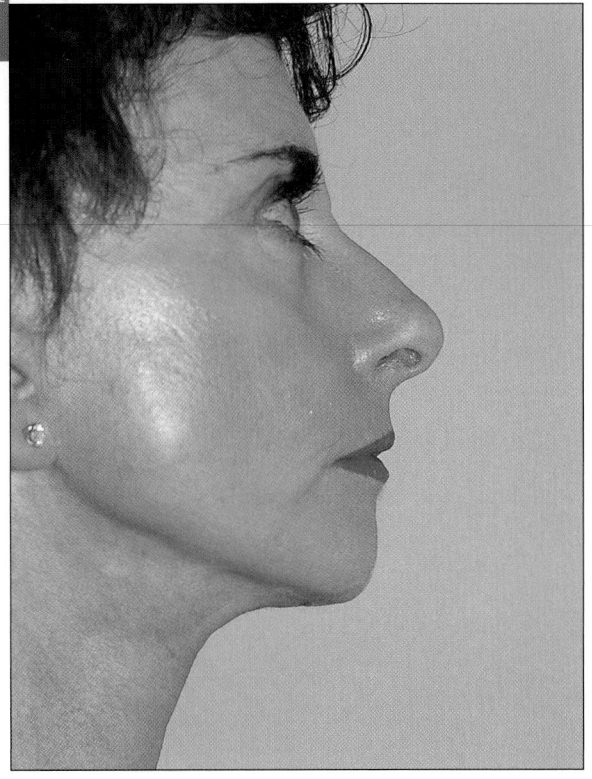

FACE-LIFT, NECK-LIFT AND REMOVAL OF EXCESS SKIN

The combined therapy of removing the excess skin coupled with a face-lift and neck-lift improved the contour of her jawline and gave her a well-defined chin.

THE EYES

The most common early signs of aging appear around the eyes. Sagging upper and lower eyelids can detract from even the most attractive smile by making you look tired and old.

Tiny lines and wrinkles around the corners of the eyes also age a face. Blepharoplasty can correct these problems on the upper and/or lower eyelids. A chemical peel may enhance the surgeon's results by eliminating certain fine lines and wrinkles. The overall effect is a "freshening" of the eyes. You will appear well rested, alert and younger when you smile.

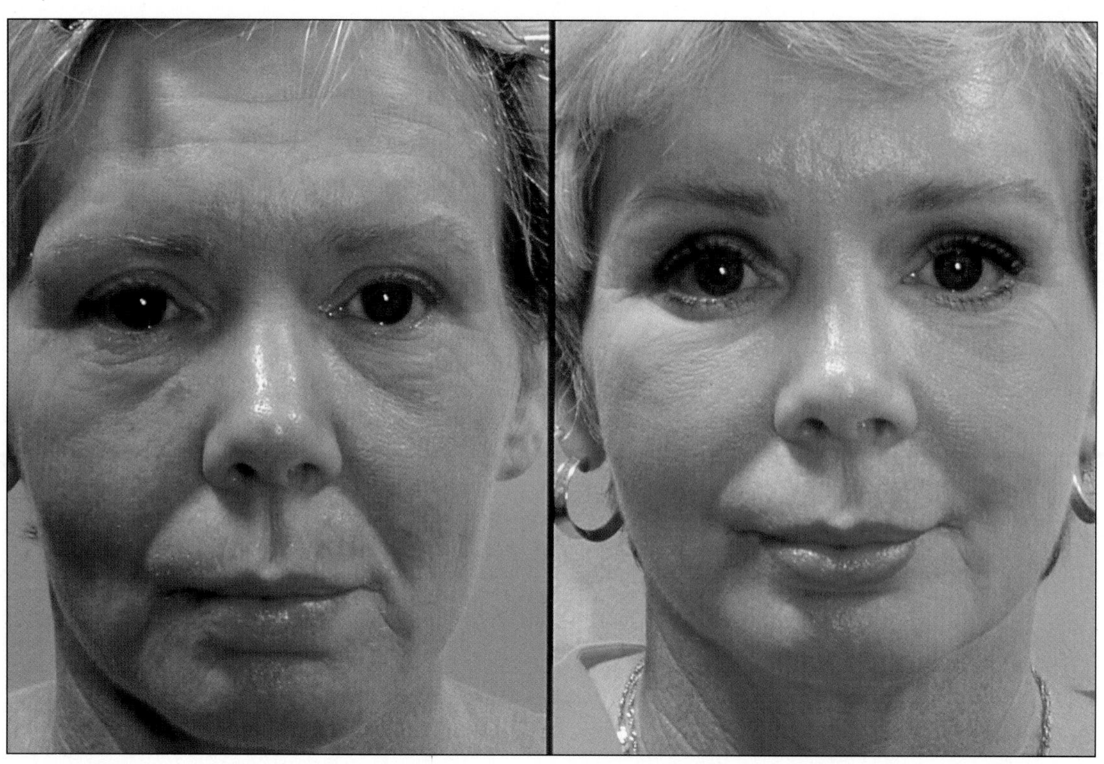

FOREHEAD LINES AND HEAVINESS OF BROW

This woman complained of frown lines and heavy, tired-looking eyes.

ENDOSCOPIC FOREHEAD-LIFT AND LOWER EYELID-LIFT

During a one-appointment procedure with local anesthesia, a forehead-lift was done to remove the frown lines and an eyelid-lift was done for a fresher look around the eyes.

TREATMENT SUMMARY

BAGGY UPPER AND LOWER EYELIDS

Problem Baggy upper and lower eyelids.

Solution Blepharoplasty (eye-lift). Eyelid surgery can correct drooping upper lids and puffy bags below your eyes, features that make you look old and tired and that may interfere with vision.

Risks Risks and complications are infrequent and usually minor. Possibilities include infection or reaction to anesthesia, double or blurred vision for a few days, temporary swelling, and a slight asymmetry in healing. Tiny whiteheads may appear following removal of stitches. Rare complications include an inability to close your eyes when you sleep. Again, these complications are rare and easily treated by a qualified surgeon.

Recovery Time A week to ten days to go out in public. Depending your rate of healing, you may be able to conceal remaining bruises with make-up at that time. Avoid strenuous activity for three to four weeks until complete healing occurs.

Average Range of Treatment Life Expectancy Results will give you a more alert and youthful appearance that will last for many years. For many people, these results are permanent.

Cost Both upper and lower eyelids, $3000 to $6000; upper or lower eyelids only, $2000 to $4000.

THE NECK

Some people develop "double chins" or "turkey necks" as they age. This can detract from your smile by weighing down your face and detracting from your appearance both in full face or profile. A sagging or overly full neck can make you look older and chubby in the face.

A neck-lift can correct the problem of excessive or baggy skin on the neck. Liposuction is appropriate in younger patients who have good elasticity and will achieve similar results. A slender, tighter neck lifts the appearance of the face and the smile and improves the profile dramatically.

Before

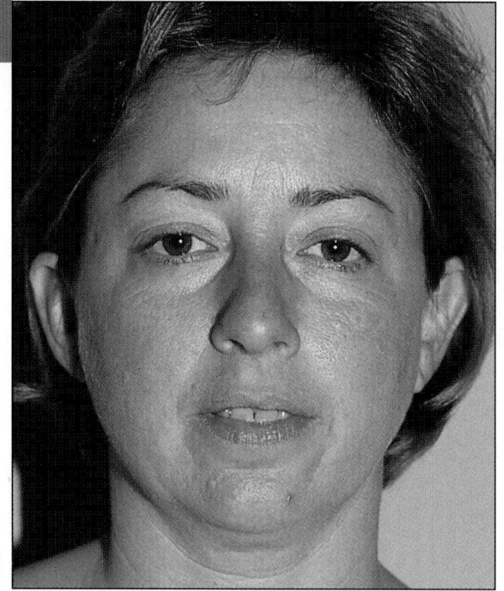

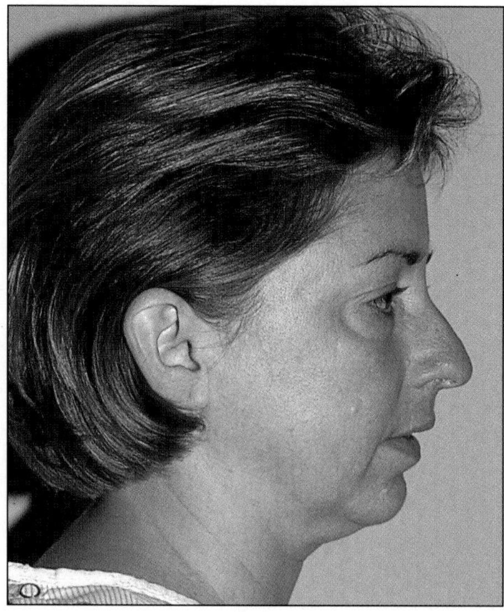

DROOPY EYES, SAGGY NECK AND LACK OF JAWLINE

This woman had a tired, heavy look around her eyes and a saggy neck and indistinct jawline.

After

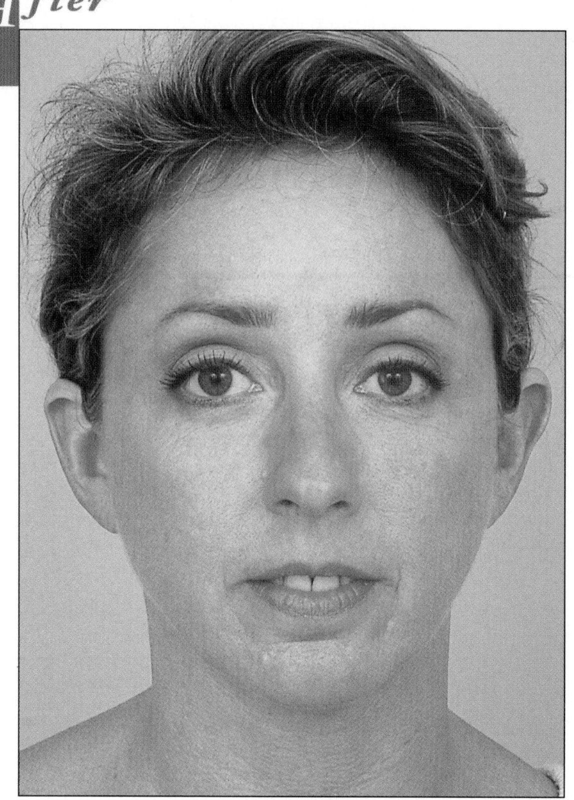

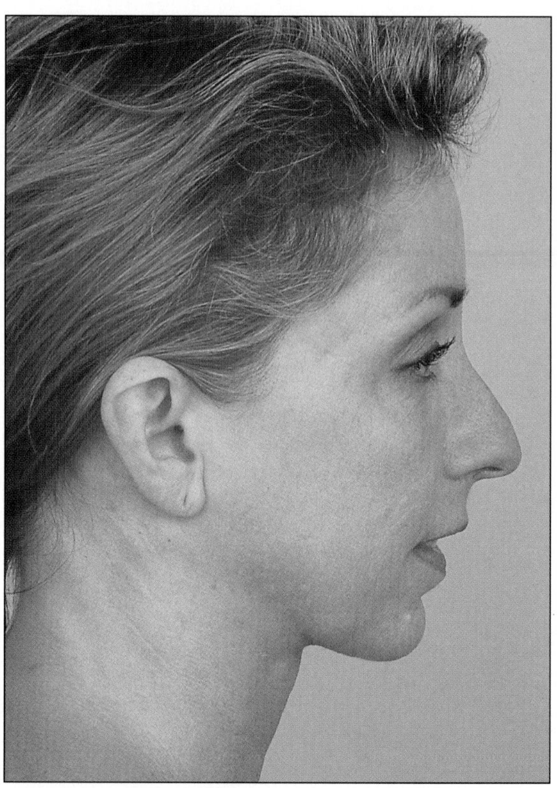

FOREHEAD-LIFT, NECK-LIFT, AND UPPER AND LOWER EYELID-LIFT

In one outpatient operation under general anesthesia, she underwent an endoscopic forehead-lift and neck-lift. There are no visible scars from this endoscopic face-lift, which is best suited to the younger patient with minimal skin excess. She also underwent an upper and lower eyelid-lift. She now has an open, fresher appearance, a thinner neck and a well-defined jawline.

TREATMENT SUMMARY

LOOSE SKIN, EXTRA SKIN OR FAT

Problems Loose skin, extra skin or fat.

Solutions Neck-lift and/or liposuction. An older patient with loose skin without elasticity will require a lifting and excision of skin (neck-lift). If the patient is young with good skin elasticity, liposuction may be all that is required to achieve good results.

Risks Hematoma and minor skin irregularities, which can be easily smoothed out.

Recovery Time For liposuction, minimal; for neck-lift, several weeks.

Average Range of Treatment Life Expectancy Results will be permanent if weight and health are maintained. Drastic weight gains and losses can result in loosening of the skin as will normal aging after a number of years.

Cost Neck-lift, $3500 to $5000; liposuction of neck, $1200 to $2500.

Endoscopy

The endoscope is a hollow instrument a quarter of an inch or less in diameter and up to ten inches in length. A light is attached to the far end, and the near end is attached to a camera. When placed under the skin, if transmits images onto a video screen. The surgeon watches the video screen and, with instruments introduced through tiny incisions in the skin, manipulates and modifies the underlying tissues. Endoscopy has changed the way brow-lifts and some face- and neck-lifts are performed. Instead of making long incisions up to twelve inches in length to perform a brow-lift, or twenty inches or so for a face- and neck-lift, the surgeon can with the endoscope work with incisions of three inches or less.

While almost everyone is a candidate for the endoscopic brow-lift, not everyone is a candidate for the endoscopic face-lift or neck-lift. If your neck or face has a lot of excess skin, then longer incisions will be necessary so that the excess skin can be excised. Only minimal amounts of excess skin can be handled by endoscopic techniques.

The Brow

Your forehead and eyebrows contribute greatly to your smile. Sagging eyebrows give you a tired, unhappy appearance, especially when the droop is in the outer portion. If there is more droop in the inner portion of the eyebrows, it can result in an angry appearance, especially when there are also vertical wrinkles between the eyebrows. If the eyes smile while the brow appears angry, the result is a quizzical look.

Treatment Summary

Frown Lines, Laxity and Drooping Brow

Problems Frown lines, laxity and drooping of the brow.

Solution Brow-lift. This procedure has been radically improved by the development of the endoscopic surgical technique. Whereas the procedure previously required an ear-to-ear incision behind the hairline, it can now be done with three tiny incisions and the endoscopic procedure. Trauma, swelling and healing time have been dramatically reduced.

Risks Your ability to raise your eyebrow may be altered on one or both sides. This may require additional surgery to minimize this complication.

Recovery Time Two to three weeks, traditional method; one week to 10 days, endoscopic method.

Average Range of Treatment Life Expectancy 10 to 15 years.

Costs Brow-lift, $3500 to $5000.

Before

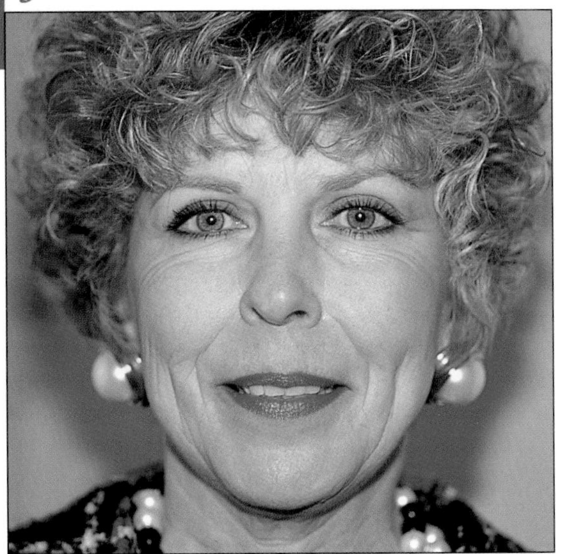

Heavy brow, lines on cheek and neck

This woman has a heavy, tired-looking brow and lines along her cheeks and mouth.

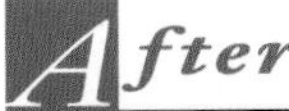

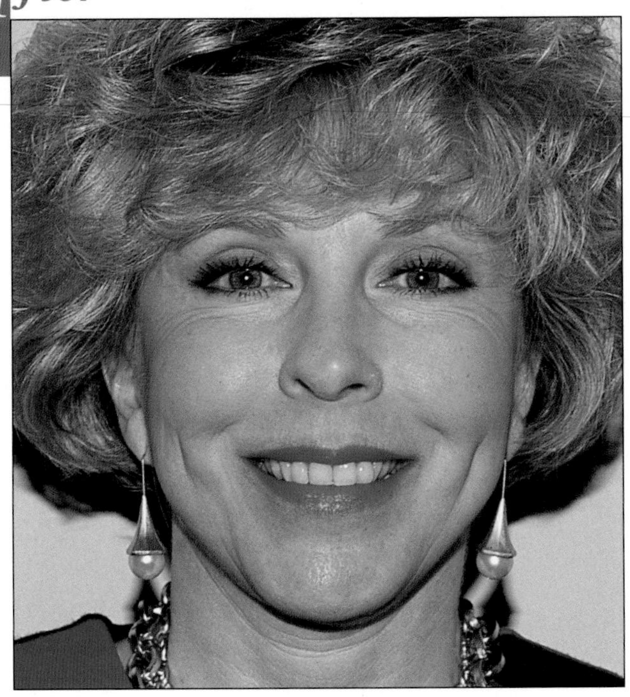

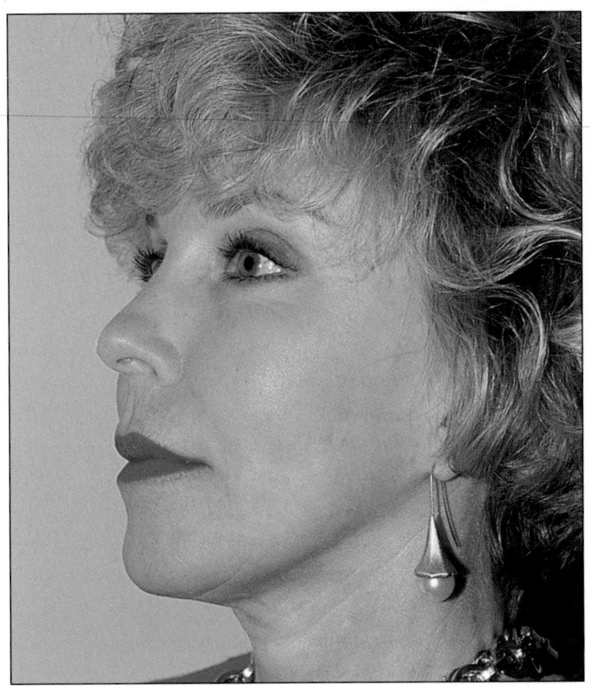

Brow-lift, full face-lift and fat injections into nasolabial folds

A face-lift improved this woman's cheeks, a brow-lift and upper and lower eyelid-lift enhanced the area around her eyes, and fat injections into the nasolabial folds softened the lines around her nose.

Skin

Chemical Peel

Snug, youthful skin graciously tolerates both the smile and the frown, but as aging or sun-damaged skin begins to sag, it develops wrinkles, creases, and enlarged veins. Prolonged sun exposure also promotes age spots and creates a network of fine wrinkles. Improvement of the smile on a very wrinkled face is usually best accomplished by chemical peel, dermabrasion, laser resurfacing or one of these processes combined with a face-lift.

Treatment Summary

Flawed Facial Skin

Problems Wrinkled, blemished, unevenly pigmented, sun-damaged facial skin.

Solutions One of several chemical solutions to peel away the skin's top layers, resulting in the formation of new cells, which produces a smoother, firmer skin surface.

Risks Risks are nominal when surgery is performed by a qualified surgeon. Complications, which are extremely rare, include infection, numbness and scarring. Heart irregularities during phenol peel are also possible, though very rare. Patients should be carefully monitored during the procedure.

Recovery Time With the phenol peel, you may return to work in two to three weeks; full healing may take three to six months. With the TCA (glycolic acid) peel, improvement is less dramatic but the recovery time is much quicker.

Average Range of Treatment Life Expectancy Results are longer lasting with the phenol peel, less so with the TCA peel, which can be repeated if desired.

Cost TCA and phenol peels: full face, $1000 to $3000; regional (around eyes or mouth only) $500 to $1500. Glycolic acid and other alpha hydroxy acids, $500 to $1500.

Lasers for Facial Resurfacing

Lasers have been used by plastic surgeons for a variety of problems, including cutting tissue, treatment of birthmarks and tattoos, removal or "vaporization" of certain tumors and most recently for the improvement of facial lines and wrinkles, "facial resurfacing."

There are several different types of lasers, each suited to a particular purpose. For example, the yellow-light laser for (vascular) red/birthmarks and the carbon dioxide (CO_2) laser for facial resurfacing. The CO_2 laser has proven particularly effective for the lines or wrinkles that develop around the mouth, forehead, the lower eyelids and particularly around the outer part of the eyelids referred to as "crows feet." These lines or wrinkles are not always effectively treated by surgical procedures, such as face-lifts and eyelid-lifts, and until recently they have been treated by chemical peels and dermabrasion.

THERE ARE SEVERAL DIFFERENT TYPES OF LASERS, EACH SUITED TO A PARTICULAR PURPOSE

The chemical peel might be described as a "burning" process, and the dermabrasion a type of "scraping" or "sanding." On the other hand, the CO_2 laser works on wrinkles by "vaporizing" the outer layers of the skin, while being rapid enough to limit heat damage to the underlying tissues.

Laser resurfacing is an outpatient procedure performed under local or general anesthesia. During the procedure, the teeth and the eyes are protected from laser injury. The procedure takes anywhere from thirty minutes to an hour and a half depending on the extent of the areas to be treated. Typically, treatment around the mouth or eyes will take only thirty minutes whereas a full face will take an hour and a half. There is swelling, redness and oozing for a few days after the treatment. It may take ten days to two weeks before make-up can be applied to cover the reddened skin, and it may take several more weeks before all the redness resolves.

Laser resurfacing is relatively new but has already proven to be safe and effective. Though rare, there is a small chance of complications including scarring and skin discoloration.

The cost of laser resurfacing depends on the extent of the areas treated and will vary from $500 for small areas up to $5000 for full face.

Giving Informed Consent

When it comes to cosmetic surgery, the best surprise is no surprise. Forget the word "cosmetic" and remember the word "surgery" . . . because it is surgery with the risks normally associated with any surgery.

Before your surgery, you will be asked to sign a form generally called "Informed Consent." This form will clearly state the general risks involved in any surgery (not just plastic surgery). Whenever anesthesia is used, there are certain dangers; you will see words like "death, cardiac arrest, brain damage, disfiguring scar, paraplegia, quadriplegia, paralysis," etc. These tragic events are extremely rare in plastic surgery, but it is required that, regardless of the remoteness of these occurrences, you understand that they exist.

In addition to the general risks associated with all surgery, your "informed consent" will detail the specific risks that may be associated with your particular operation. It will also detail certain other information, which may include likelihood of success, practical alternatives and prognosis if surgery is rejected.

Rest assured that if you have done your homework and selected a qualified surgeon, he or she will recognize any complications that may occur and be prepared to handle them successfully.

Cosmetic Claims That Seem Too Good to Be True Usually Are!

There have always been a wide variety of products and treatments on the market that make extraordinary claims that are simply not true. The confusing issue for the consumer is that many of these products are widely advertised and slickly promoted, which tends to make them convincing. The best way to ascertain the credibility of such products is to verify their effectiveness with a qualified medical professional. One of the most widely promoted of these fraudulent products is breast enlargement cream.

There are claims made for a variety of miraculous results from using certain topical creams and lotions. Ranging from nonsurgical face-lifts to the elimination of wrinkles, claims of this nature should be verified by a qualified doctor before you invest your time and money. While some of the product claims are justified, some are questionable and some are fraudulent.

It is important to emphasize that while alpha hydroxy acids and Retin-A are effective in reducing fine lines and the general appearance of the skin, they cannot eliminate established deep wrinkles, and they are in no way a substitute for a surgical face-lift. Electrical stimulation of facial muscles may produce temporary improvements, but again it is no substitute for surgery.

Topical Treatments That Are Beneficial

There is no question that moisturizing creams can improve, smooth and protect the skin. Proper cleansing and daily skin care maintenance will enhance the good results of plastic surgery. Facial masks for deep cleansing may also be helpful. A plastic surgeon and a qualified skin care specialist should work together to prepare your skin for surgery and to maintain the good results following surgery.

The Latest Advances in Plastic Surgery

The most exciting high-tech advance in plastic surgery is the endoscopic technique (see p. 271). Because the least invasive surgical techniques are always the most desirable, the new developments in endoscopic plastic surgery are a significant breakthrough.

THE MOST EXCITING HIGH-TECH ADVANCE IS ENDOSCOPIC SURGERY

Computer imaging is another important advance. The surgeon can alter your face on the computer screen to help you see what improvements may be possible with plastic surgery. While computer imaging can be useful in giving you an idea about what can be done, the video image cannot guarantee an exact result.

The latest technology in surgical lasers is another advance in esthetic surgery. Lasers can be useful as a substitute for the knife to minimize tissue trauma and early postoperative swelling. However, the main contribution of laser technology is in the removal of pigmented defects and wrinkles in the skin. Available are lasers for both red and brown spot removal, including tiny spider veins, birthmarks, freckles, age spots and moles.

The Future of Plastic Surgery

The goal of plastic surgery has always been to correct or improve an esthetic physical problem with the least invasive surgical or medical treatment possible. Whether treatment is reconstructive or cosmetic, the best solution has always been to produce the best possible result while minimizing risk and trauma. New techniques and treatments are evolving with these goals in mind. Developments in "growth factors," which encourage the body's own rejuvenating powers, are currently being studied.

In selecting your plastic surgeon, you should determine that he or she is diligent in acquiring the knowledge and skills on the latest developments in plastic surgery. There are very few surgical approaches that have not undergone revolutionary advances in the last ten years. The more current your doctor is in this rapidly evolving science, the better your surgery will be.

If you are fortunate enough to live in an area of the country where there are major medical centers, you should be able to research not only who the leading plastic surgeons are, but preferably which doctors are responsible for the research and development of the latest advances in their field.*

Portions of this chapter were taken from a series originally published in the health and beauty section of Presenting the Season *magazine in 1993. Dr. Nahai was the prime source of information in this award-winning editorial series, produced by Eileen Gould Freeman, originally titled "The Human Image" Parts I, II and III.*

*For the name of a qualified plastic surgeon in your community, call the information line of the American Society of Plastic and Reconstructive Surgeons, Inc., 800 635-0635.

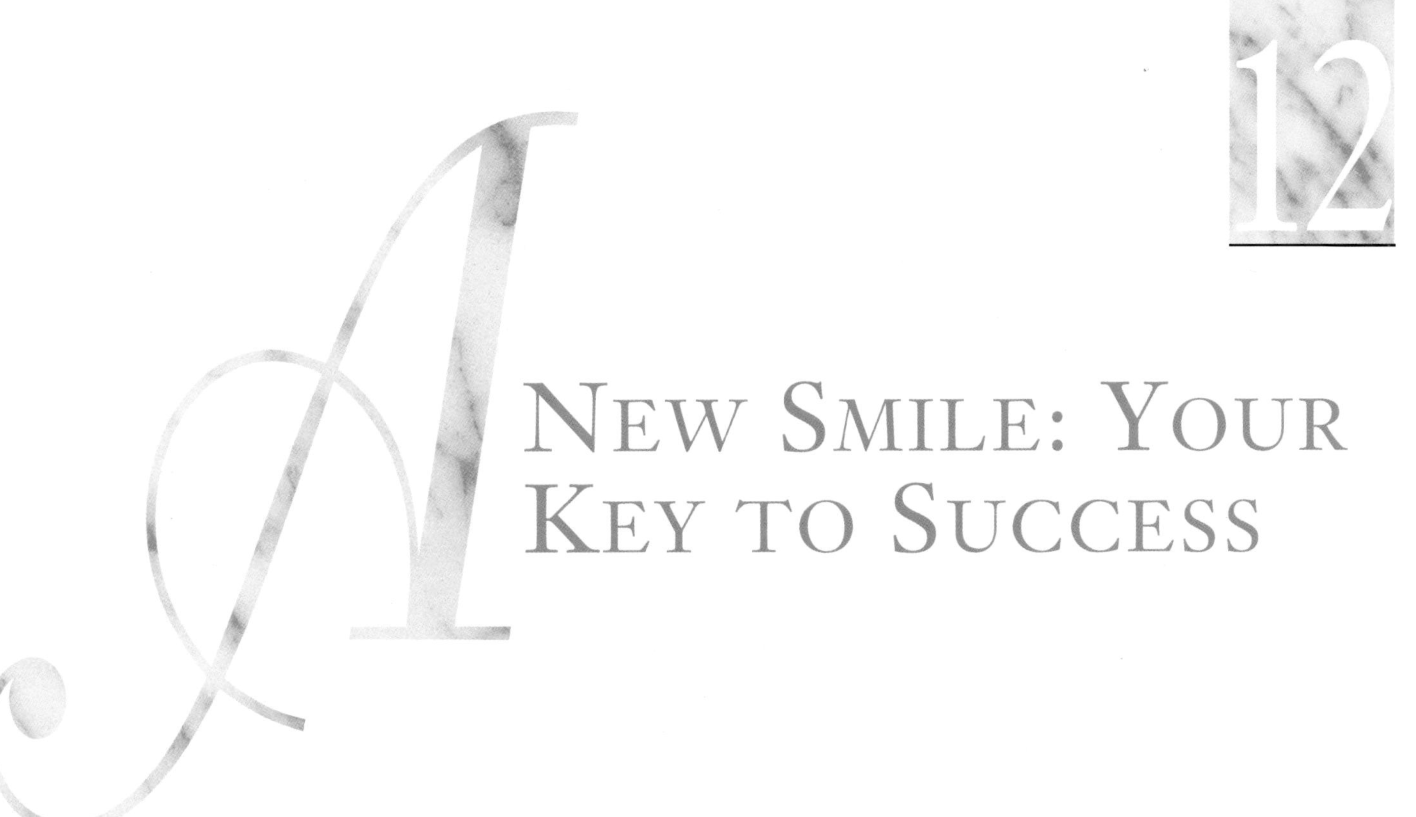

12 A New Smile: Your Key to Success

Although dental researchers are working hard to develop tooth-colored materials that will not wear or break, none yet exist. Understanding this before seeking dental treatment will spare you disappointment when your restorations need to be repaired or replaced.

Most restorations remain in place long after they begin to fail. It is often difficult for dentists—and virtually impossible for patients—to spot failure in its early stages. And, when failure does become apparent, many patients grudgingly accept the resulting discoloration and loss of tooth contour as inevitable.

Planning for Long-Term Esthetics

Repair or replace your worn restorations before they become the source of new problems. Ask your dentist at every checkup if any of your restorations are showing signs of wear. If they are, do something about it sooner rather than later.

Although restorations have limited lifespans, you want them to function and look good for as long as possible. Your treatment plan, therefore, should include two basic considerations:

• **Selection of a restorative material.** This choice should be based on your functional and esthetic needs, the life expectancy you desire from the material and your economic situation.

• **Need for maximum preservation of your natural tooth.** It is always best to treat your teeth in ways that leave as much of the natural enamel intact as possible. Such techniques not only conserve your tooth structure, but usually enhance esthetic results.

Also, because restorations have limited lifespans, recognize that it is necessary to replace them periodically. Each time this is done, a little more tooth structure may be lost. For this reason, conservative treatment is encouraged early on, particularly in young people.

When to Replace Your Old Restorations

1. They have discolored and you find them esthetically unappealing
2. The metal is breaking down; cracks or chips occur and the remaining tooth structure is not protected
3. The junction between tooth and filling is no longer fitting well or is "leaking"
4. Your fillings are showing signs of wear (if too much wear appears, filling material will no longer support the enamel)
5. Sensitivity occurs; it may be the cement has washed out or the margins are faulty
6. Your dentist tells you that the restoration is not compatible with your gum tissue

Function and Beauty: You Can Have Both

As people have become more aware of the impact that looking good can have on their lives, they also have become aware of the significance of an esthetically pleasing smile.

Fortunately, good dental health does not require sacrificing beauty for function. For example, gold is considered a superior restorative material because of its long life expectancy. Yet, most people prefer not to use it in the front of the mouth because of its color. For those patients who like the longevity of a gold filling or crown but do not like its appearance, there are alternatives. The gold can be dulled or muted. Or, it can be used as a base beneath a tooth-colored material such as porcelain. Such restorations provide excellent strength as well as outstanding esthetics.

Before

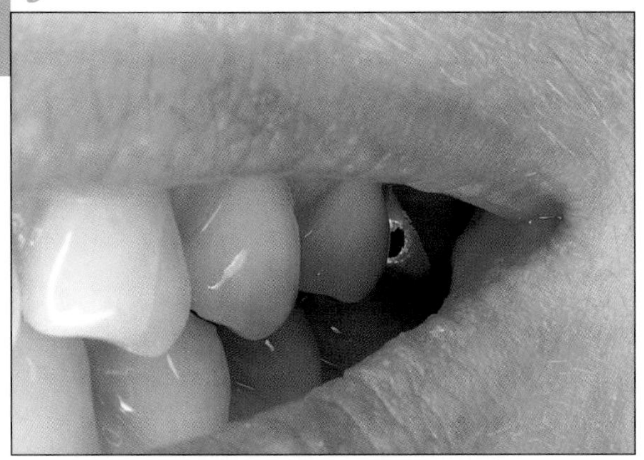

GOLD SHOWING DURING SMILING

This 43-year-old woman wanted her gold restoration replaced because it reflected too much light.

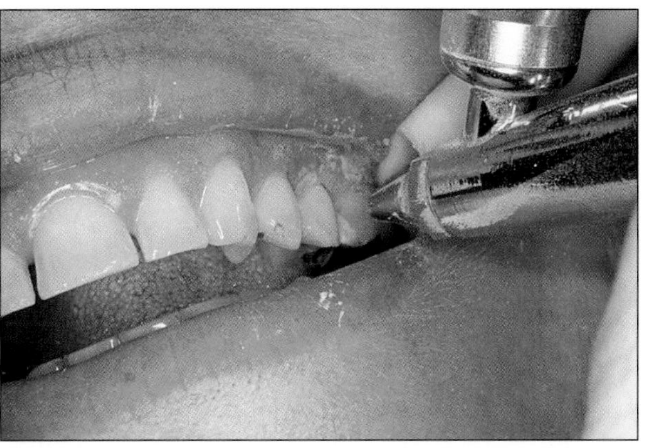

Since the restoration fit so well, it was decided to dull the finish with a special type of "air eraser." This abrasive sanding takes only a few minutes to accomplish.

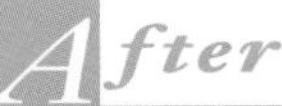

After

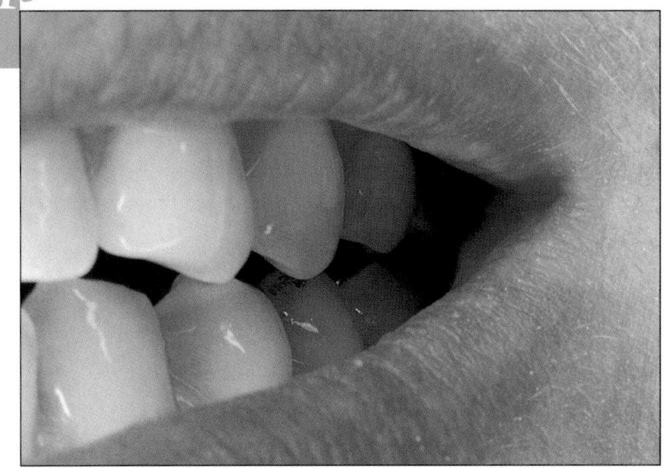

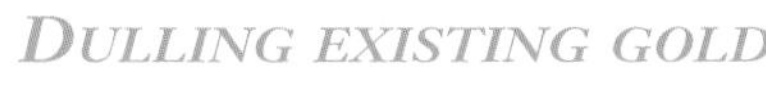

DULLING EXISTING GOLD

This procedure can be done again as often as necessary, since it is relatively easy to do. Because the gold restoration is the longest lasting and best fitting of all dental restorations, dulling the finish is preferable to replacing the gold.

You Are What You Eat

Ultimately, beauty emanates from good health. And, good health begins with proper nutrition.

Be sure your diet includes a proper mix of fruits, vegetables and grains, and drink eight to ten glasses of water daily. What you put into your body is reflected in your skin tone, your nails, your hair, your tooth structure and in your overall sense of well-being.

Eating Disorders Are Dangerous

Overeating can cause obesity, which can cause a change in the shape of your face. This, in turn, can alter the proportion of your tooth size to your face, thereby affecting your smile.

Sometimes, emotional problems are reflected in our eating habits. Psychological stress or trauma can cause people to overeat or develop such eating disorders as anorexia nervosa and bulimia.

These conditions not only wreak havoc on emotional and physical health, but may also cause neglect of oral care. This neglect, in turn, often results in gum disease or decay. Additionally, bulimia can cause severe dental erosion, destroying the beauty of teeth. If not stopped early enough, so much tooth structure can be lost that it becomes difficult to even restore a tooth.

If you have an eating disorder, no amount of cosmetic dentistry or plastic surgery will correct it. Seek professional help for the underlying problem. Gaining determination and confidence can have a tremendous impact on your self-image.

You can then turn your attention to your appearance, and do what it takes to keep your smile looking its best.

Before

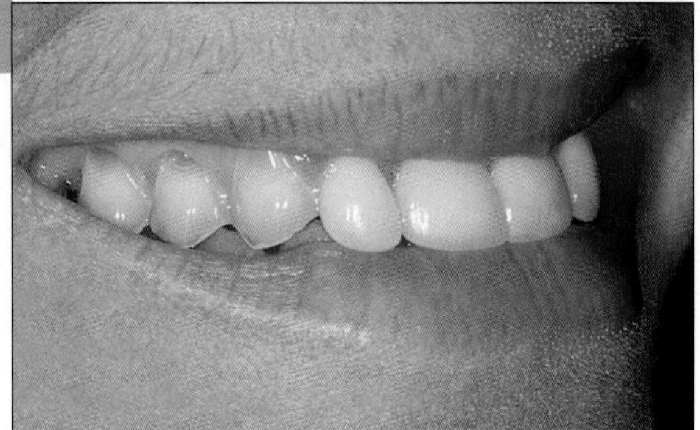

Erosion caused by bulimia

This 34-year-old interior designer suffered from bulimia for 15 years, causing severe erosion and tooth sensitivity. After two years in therapy to control her eating disorder, she wanted to correct her severely eroded teeth.

After

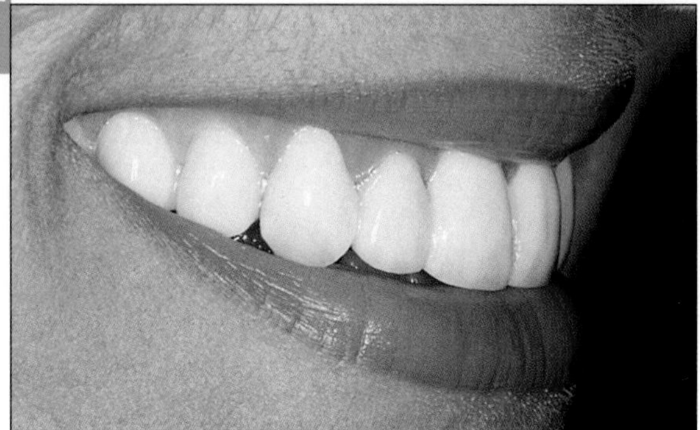

Temporary full crowns

Temporary acrylic crowns were made as an interim procedure to help relieve tooth sensitivity and enhance the patient's smile. Eventually final ceramic crowns will be made.

Before

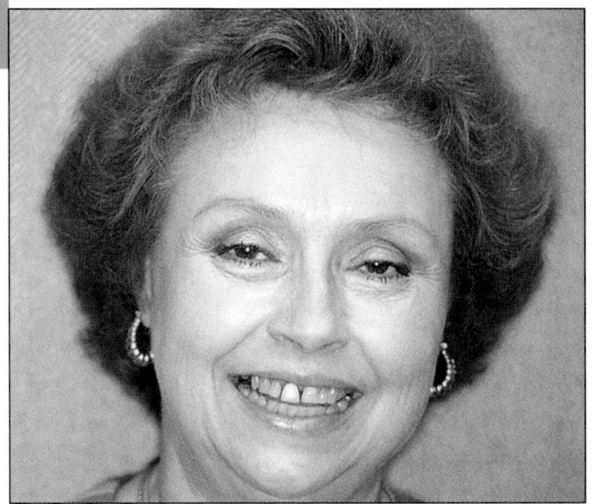

DISCOLORED, SPACED AND MISSING TEETH

A smile can be affected by weight change as shown by this patient who gained considerable weight due to stress.

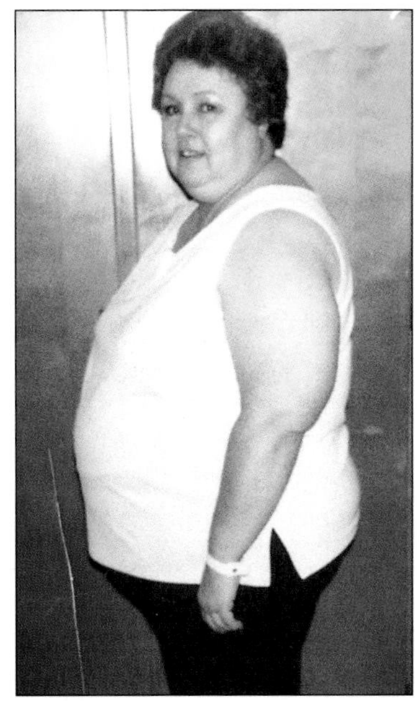

Psychological stress that causes people to overeat can also contribute to neglect in oral care and thereby destroy a beautiful smile with gum disease or decay.

After

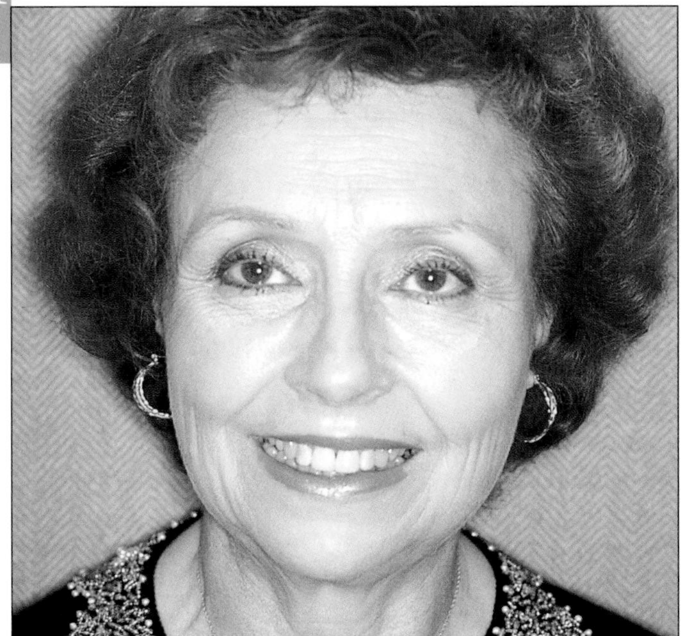

COSMETIC CONTOURING, BONDING, CROWN AND BRIDGE

This woman undertook a weight-loss program. Her facial shape changed, but a new smile was achieved through cosmetic contouring, bonding, crowning and a new fixed bridge.

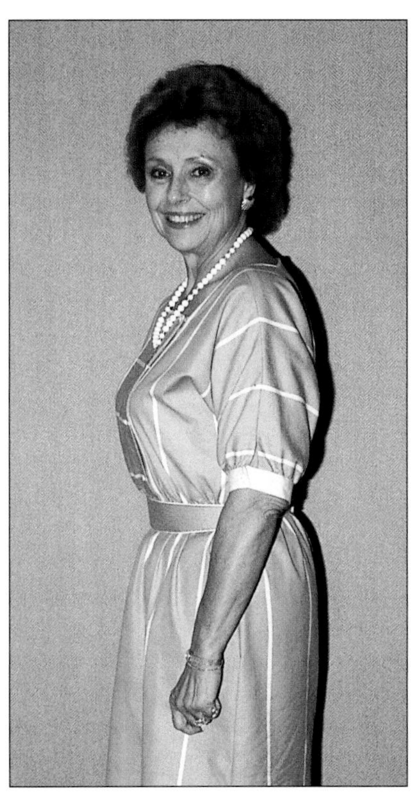

Considerable weight loss combined with a new smile gave this patient renewed confidence and a better self-image.

Bad Habits Cost Money and Time

Your dentist can provide the treatment that gives you an attractive smile, but it is up to you to provide proper maintenance. The following questionnaire will help you identify bad habits that can cost you time, money and tooth structure!

Does Your Habit Affect Your Smile?

Do you now or did you ever:

Yes No

❑ ❑ 1. Chew your lips or cheeks?
❑ ❑ 2. Suck your fingers or thumb?
❑ ❑ 3. Chew ice?
❑ ❑ 4. Bite your fingernails?
❑ ❑ 5. Hold pins or needles in your mouth?
❑ ❑ 6. Chew pencils or pens?
❑ ❑ 7. Chew or hold your glasses in your mouth?
❑ ❑ 8. Crack nuts with your teeth?
❑ ❑ 9. Play a musical instrument that requires you to hold the instrument with your teeth?
❑ ❑ 10. Smoke a pipe, cigar or cigarettes, or use chewing tobacco?
❑ ❑ 11. Bite or suck your lips?
❑ ❑ 12. Use toothpicks or similar wood or plastic cleaning devices?
❑ ❑ 13. Keep your tongue pressed against the upper teeth?
❑ ❑ 14. Place your tongue in a space between your teeth?
❑ ❑ 15. Grind or clench your teeth?

If you answered *yes* to one of these above questions, you may have a habit problem. Ask your dentist to see if your habit or habits are causing potential damage to your teeth.

Recognizing Your Bad Habits

Are you guilty of one or more of the bad habits listed in the questionnaire? Most of us are, including me! Unfortunately, we sometimes pay the price with unnecessary tooth loss.

It is easy to see how many bad habits can ruin a beautiful smile. Smoking, for instance, stains the teeth, as does drinking coffee and tea. Chewing pencils or pens or holding hard objects like a pipe or a pair of glasses between the teeth can wear down the enamel and cause spaces to develop. Chewing ice or cracking nuts with the teeth can actually cause them to chip or fracture. Although these fractures are often undetectable to the eye, they are large enough to permit staining. The end result is an overall dingy appearance.

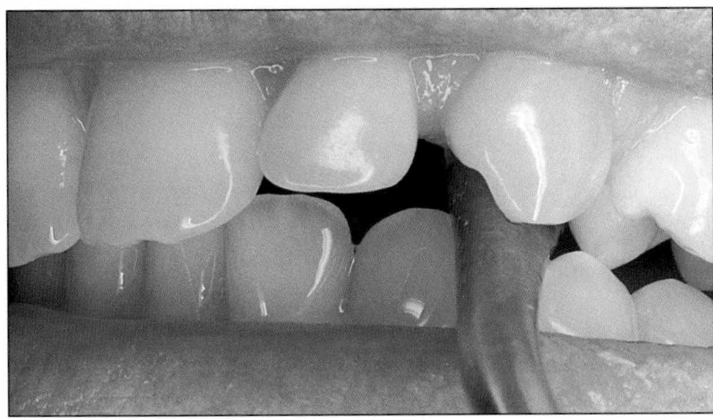

This restaurant owner habitually held his eyeglasses with his teeth. Since he always held them in the same position, he caused the left cuspid to flare out, creating an unattractive and unnecessary space between his front teeth. Don't hold objects between your teeth!

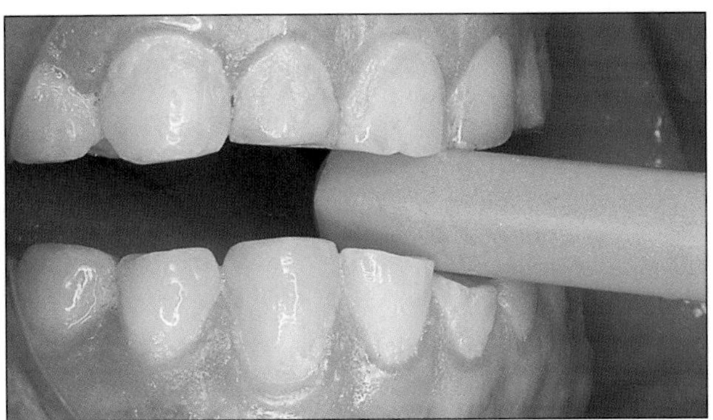

This young man's habit of twisting pencils between his teeth resulted in severe wear of his front teeth.

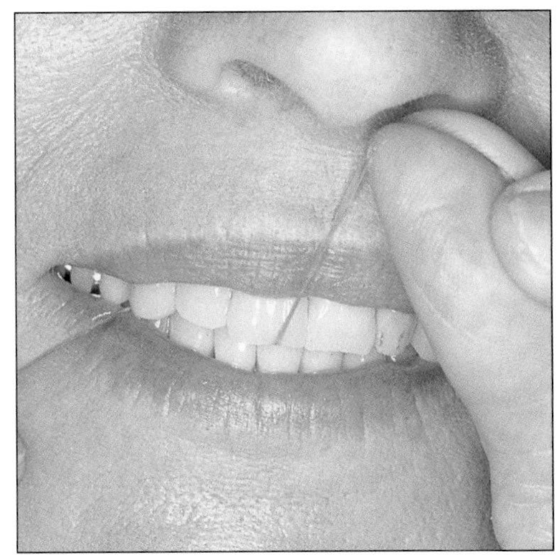

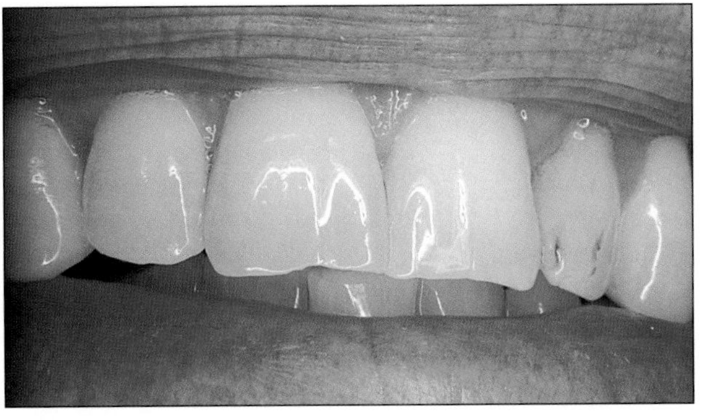

This housewife had a habit of using her teeth to cut sewing thread, resulting in wear and a V-notch in the right central incisor.

Biting, sucking or chewing on your lips or cheeks not only damages tissue, but may cause abnormalities in the arrangement of your teeth. Constant tongue thrusting or placing your fingernails between your front teeth can also cause irregular spaces.

Other harmful oral habits may appear benign—or even helpful—on the surface. For example, do you frequently use toothpicks? Or do you have some other favorite device for cleaning your teeth and massaging your gums? Although such tools can be helpful when used properly, they can cause damage to gum tissues when handled incorrectly. Review your technique with your dentist or hygienist periodically to make sure you are not causing irritation or even permanent damage to your gum tissue.

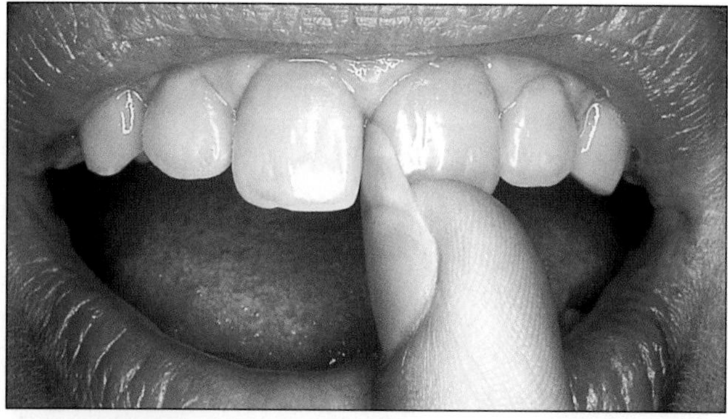

This woman had a habit of forcing her fingernails between two teeth, causing this space. Use dental tape or floss, rather than a fingernail, to remove food caught between teeth to help avoid unnecessary spaces.

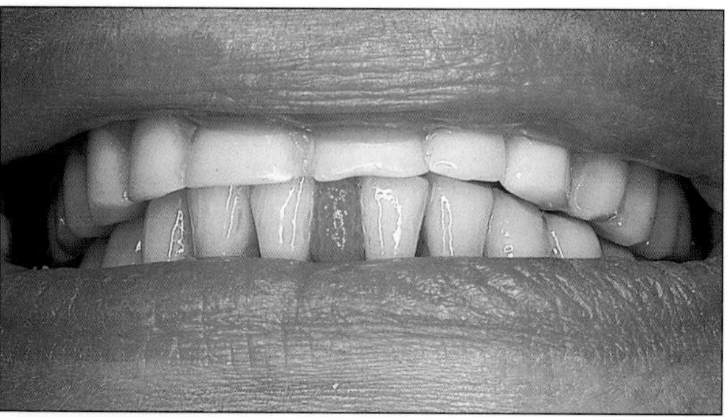

This elderly lady had a habit over many years of placing her tongue between her teeth. Her tongue thrust actually created a huge space between the lower incisors, which she made worse by continuing the habit. Again, orthodontics is the best solution to close unwanted spaces.

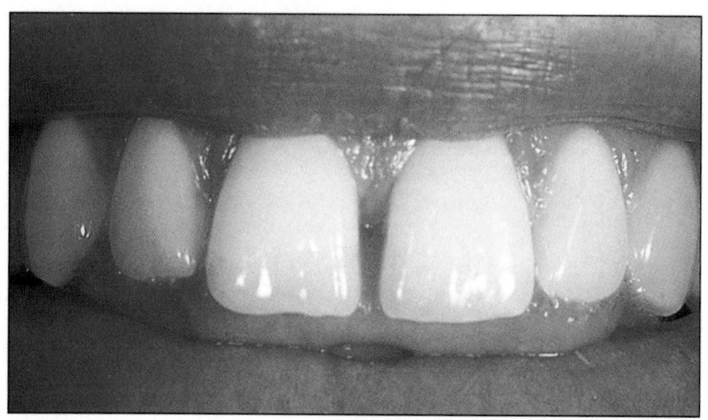

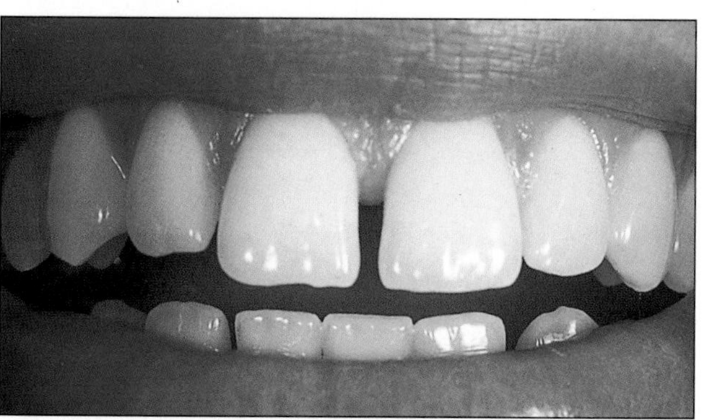

This young businesswoman and former model tried to obscure the spaces between her teeth by placing her tongue against the inside surfaces of the front teeth. (Many people subconsciously realize that the spaces are less noticeable if they do this.) Note how dark the spaces appear when the tongue is in a relaxed position. Unfortunately this tongue thrusting results in undue pressure on the front teeth, creating even greater spaces.

Some of us are not even aware of our bad oral habits, which makes them difficult to diagnose. Many people have harmful habits that began in childhood. Others experience bruxism, or grinding of the teeth (usually at night).

Plastic mouth appliances are sometimes used to help break bad habits like bruxism. These devices are typically worn at night and may be abandoned if the habit is broken. However, even if the problem is not eliminated—as is often the case with bruxism—the use of an appliance can spare the front teeth from accelerated wear.

Prevention, of course, is the best way to eliminate most dental problems. Proper brushing and flossing, combined with regular visits to the dentist, means less decay. This, in turn, means fewer restorations and eliminates at least one cause of esthetic treatment—replacement of stained restorations.

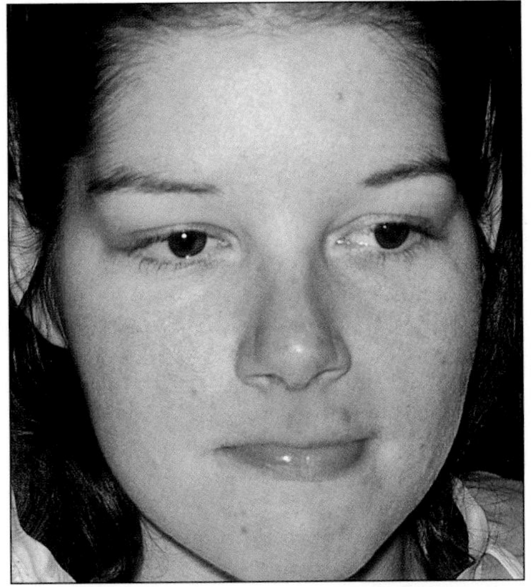

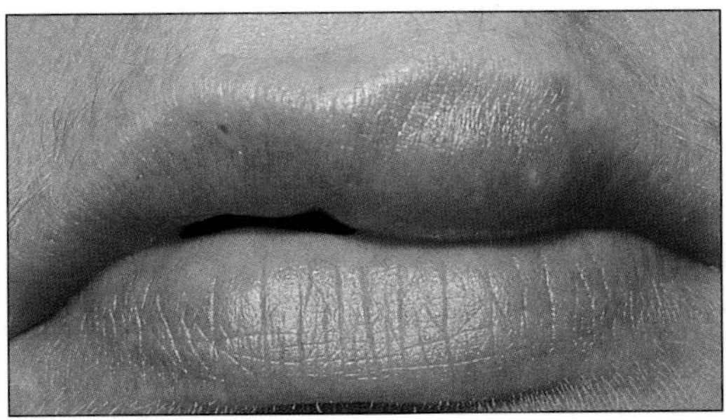

This woman had an unconscious habit of sucking her upper lip. Because she feared permanent damage, she sought assistance in breaking the habit.

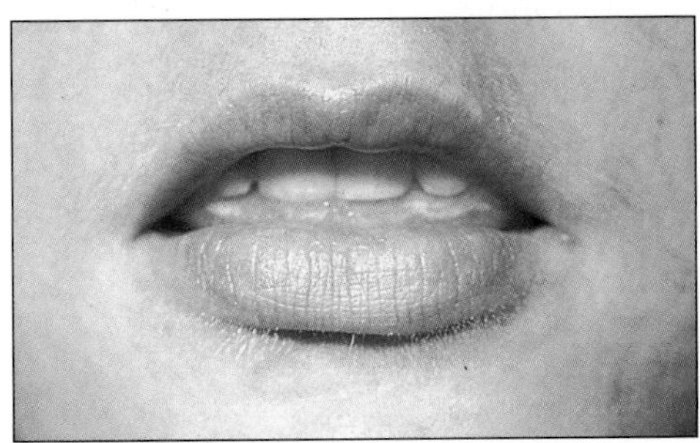

An appliance that prevented her from closing her mouth sufficiently to suck her lip was constructed. Within four weeks the habit was broken and the lip returned to normal size.

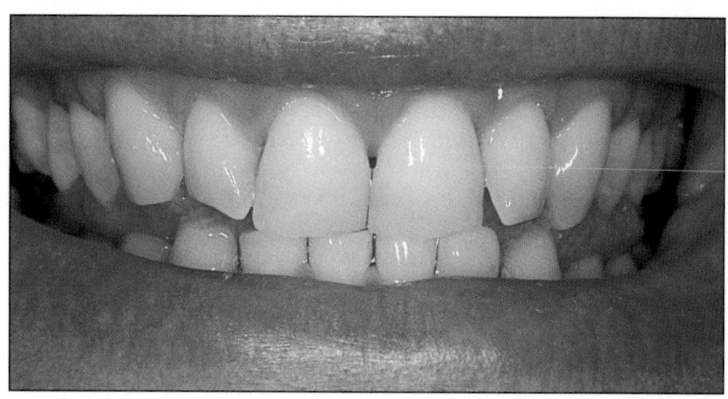

Note the unnatural wear on this young businessman's right lateral incisor.

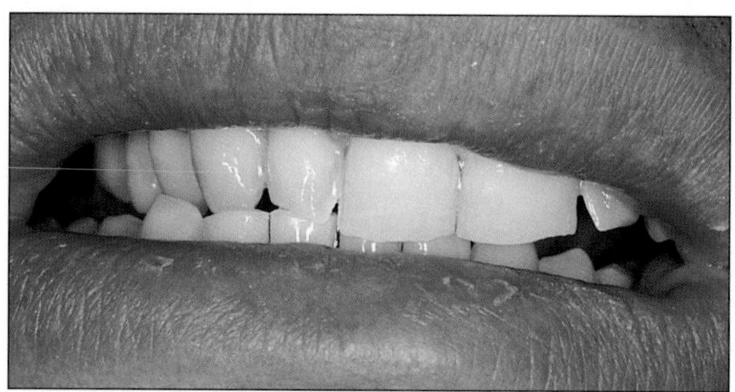

He created this wear by grinding his teeth in an abnormal position. Usual treatment for this condition is wearing a bite appliance to help control or eliminate the grinding, followed by repair of the deformed teeth.

Preventing Esthetic Problems in Your Children

If you're a parent, you can help ensure good oral health and dental esthetics for your children's teeth.

In general, children should receive periodic dental exams beginning at two and one half to three years of age. However, if at any time you see a spot on a tooth that you cannot clean, consult your child's dentist. Early intervention can prevent problems from developing later in life.

Every effort should be made to preserve all your child's teeth until they are to be lost naturally. The natural tooth is the best space maintainer. If your child suffers an injury to his or her teeth, and if any tooth is fractured, loosened, displaced or completely knocked out, consult your dentist immediately. If you notice a primary tooth suddenly turning dark, consult your dentist. It is probably a sign of nerve damage as a result of an injury of which you were not aware.

If your child has a permanent tooth knocked out, try to find it and contact your dentist immediately. If you cannot get in touch with your dentist, do one of the following:

1. Clean the tooth in running water, avoiding touching the roots, and place the tooth back into the socket.
2. If this is not possible, have your child hold the tooth inside his or her cheek.
3. Obtain Save-a-Tooth™ from a pharmacy; it can store the tooth until your child can see a dentist.
4. Place the tooth in milk (or water, if milk is not available).

Most importantly, try to position the tooth in the socket within a two-hour period.

Tips on Preventing Esthetic Problems During Childhood

1. Avoid taking tetracycline antibiotics for any extended period during pregnancy and giving it to your child before eight years of age. It can cause staining of primary and permanent teeth that may be impossible to remove and difficult to cover.
2. If your water supply is properly fluoridated, it is not necessary to give your child vitamins containing fluoride.
3. Avoid foods high in calories and junk foods, such as candy, which may promote decay.
4. Watch out for telltale signs of clenching or grinding. Have your child's dentist look for signs of wear on the teeth surfaces. Also, pay attention to headaches, backaches and neckaches, which can be associated with clenching or grinding.
5. If the teeth are crowded, consult your child's dentist. An early orthodontic appointment may be useful. If you see a permanent tooth erupting where the baby tooth has not yet been lost, consult your child's dentist.
6. If orthodontic treatment is required, make certain careful oral hygiene and regular visits to your child's dentist are observed and avoid refined sugars. Such foods can cause hidden discoloration and cavities of the teeth, which may be evident after the bands or brackets are removed.
7. Learn about restorations ("fillings"), which can be gold, plastic, silver, etc. Learn how long restorations may be expected to last and what type of materials could or should be used to give your child the most appropriate treatment.
8. A slight chip or fracture of front teeth can usually be bonded. In cases of severe decay or fractures of primary teeth, a crown may be needed. For back teeth, this could be a silver-colored or stainless-steel crown. For a front tooth, a plastic or composite tooth-colored crown may be used.
9. If it can be saved, don't have a tooth extracted. It's better to maintain a tooth in health. If a primary or baby tooth is prematurely lost or removed, ask your dentist if space maintenance (to preserve room for the permanent tooth) is needed. Loss of space can often lead to the need for orthodontic treatment later on.

Tips for Models, Actors and Actresses

If you are in a business that requires you to be photographed often, such as modeling or acting, you probably have a greater need for cosmetic dentistry than the general public.

Bright lights create shadows and emphasize discoloration, spaces, crowded teeth and other defects. Photographs may also appear larger than life. Because you are in a profession where your appearance can make the difference between getting a job or not, maximize your odds with a terrific smile! Do not, however, automatically think, as some do, that crowning your teeth is the best option.

Your smile can probably be improved with cosmetic contouring. In fact, in a two-year study I conducted on beauty contestants, I found that 95 percent of them could have been helped with cosmetic contouring alone.

Before

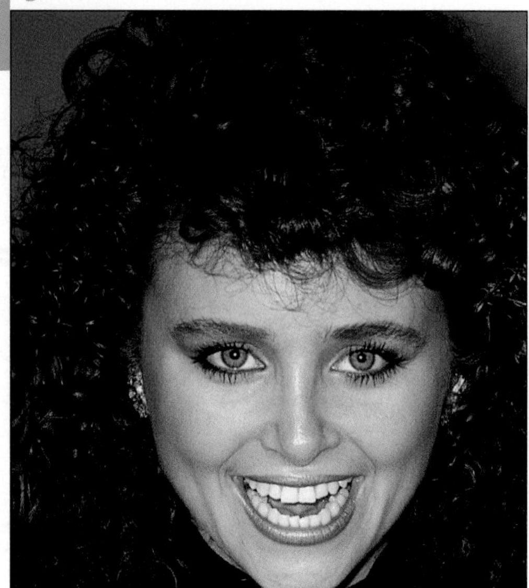

Crowded and Worn Teeth

The only problem with this woman's smile was her crowded and worn anterior teeth.

After

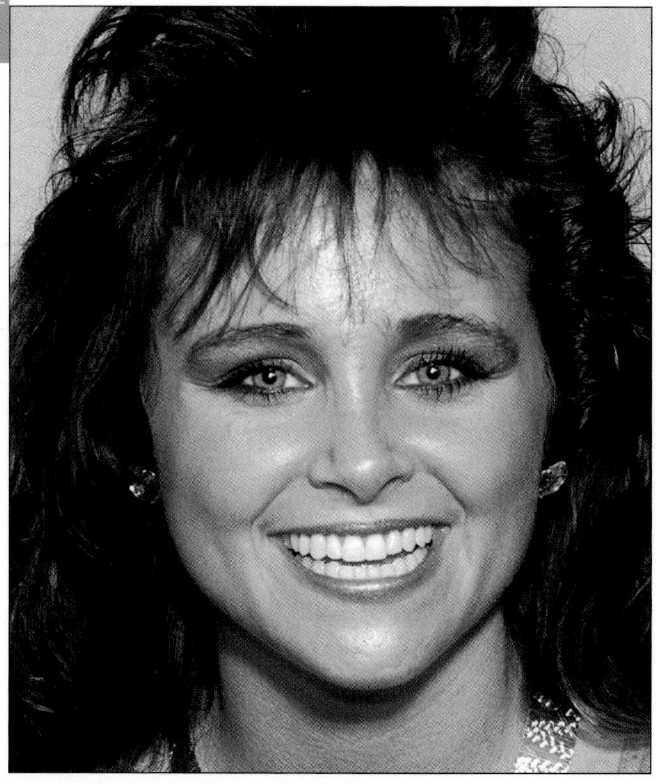

Cosmetic Contouring

Although orthodontics would have been the ideal treatment for her, this woman elected a compromise for a straighter and less-jagged look. It took only one appointment to create a better-looking smile through cosmetic contouring. This procedure helped to give her teeth a softer, more feminine look.

Every model should have a smile analysis to see if cosmetic contouring could improve his or her smile.

Before

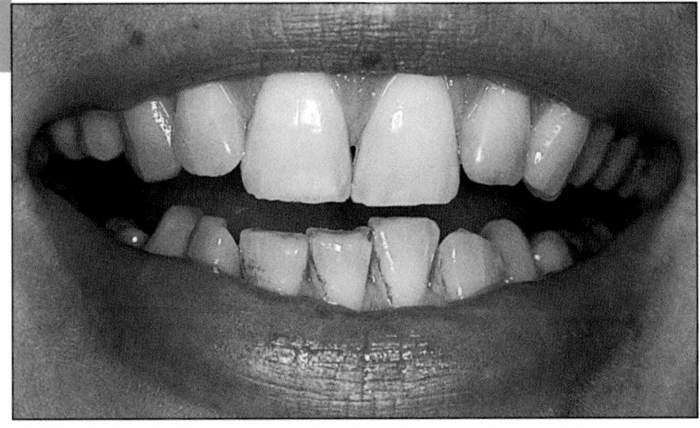

CROWDED AND DISCOLORED TEETH

This model was good at "closed mouth" modeling, but she wanted a more attractive smile, especially for television.

After

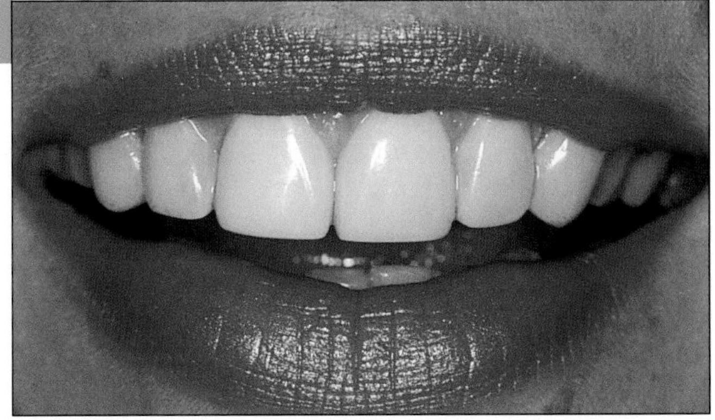

COMPOSITE RESIN BONDING AND COSMETIC CONTOURING

After her six upper teeth were bonded, she underwent cosmetic contouring to reduce the irregularities of her teeth. Notice her improved smile.

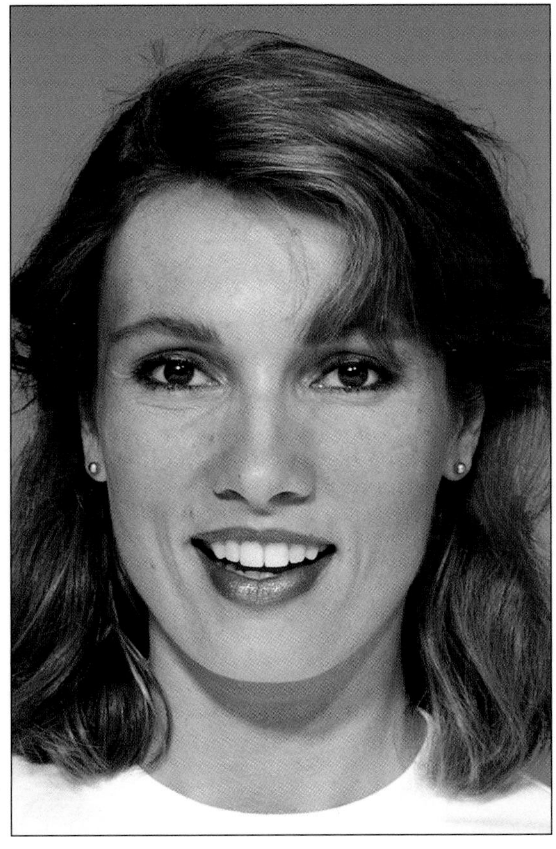

Before

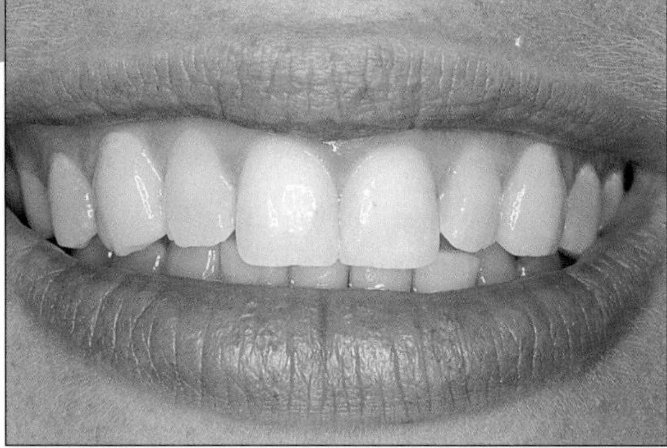

This beauty-pageant winner wanted to perfect her already-winning smile.

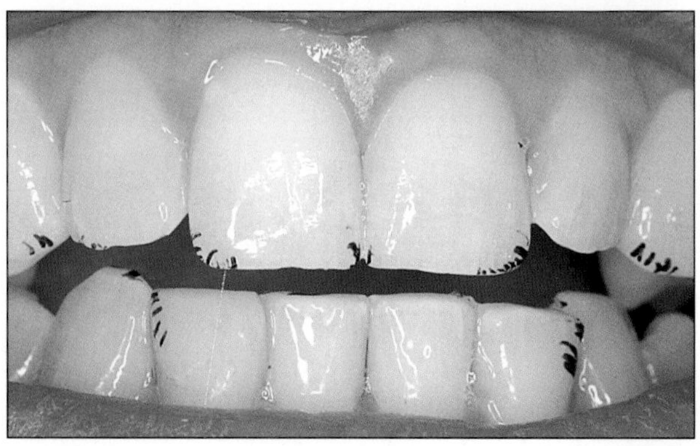

The black marks indicate areas where her teeth will be reduced by cosmetic contouring for improved tooth shape and the illusion of more straightness.

After

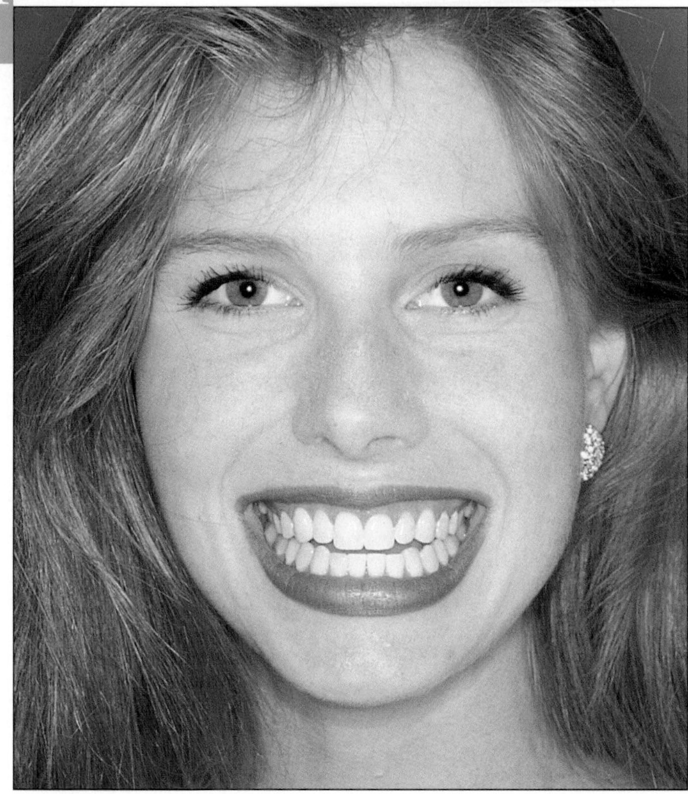

Note the prettier shapes and more attractive smile accomplished in a single appointment of cosmetic contouring.

INSTANT FACIAL SHAPE CHANGE

You can sometimes alter the shape of your face by changing the way you smile. Stand in front of a mirror and observe your facial shape while smiling normally and broadly. Can you see the difference a more open smile has on your facial outline?

A square face, for example, can appear longer or more oval when the mouth is in a more open position. If your face is round, practice smiling with your mouth open and teeth showing. Chances are, both your facial profile and smile will improve.

When smiling, also make sure the bottom biting edges of your upper teeth are visible. Again, opening the mouth a bit more may keep the lower lip from covering the edges and prevent the teeth from looking like a row of Chicklets gum.

If these tips work for you, practice them in front of a mirror so you will remember just how much to open you lips when smiling. This procedure is especially effective for photographic purposes.

Before

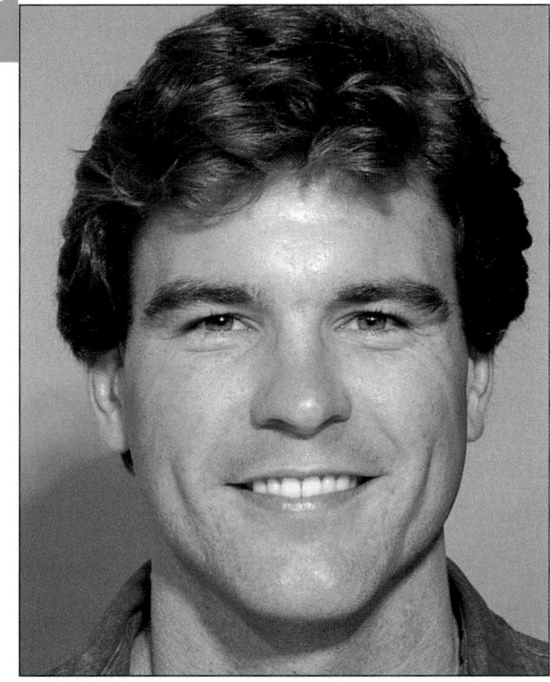

THE CHICKLETS SMILE

A smile that shows only the surfaces of your teeth is not as appealing as a more open smile.

After

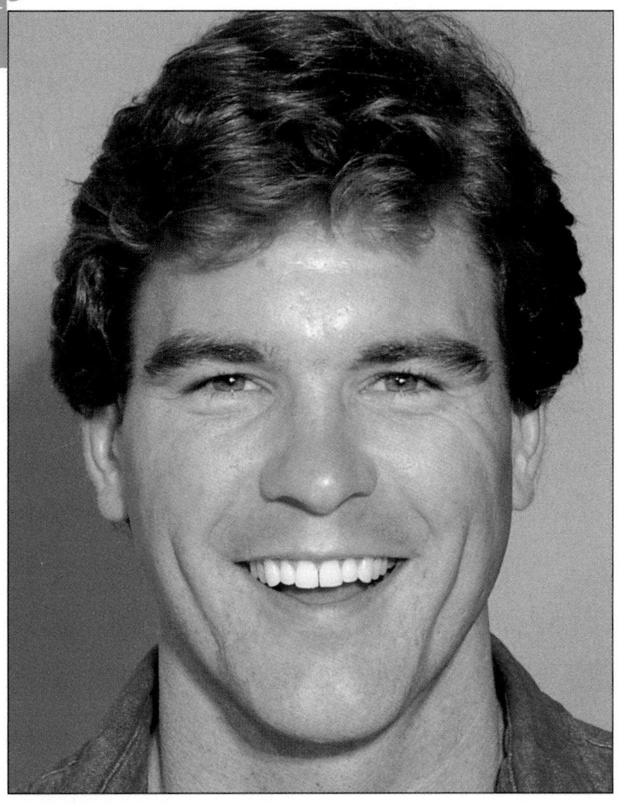

SHOW THE EDGES OF YOUR TEETH!

Note how this man's smile appears more attractive with the edges of his upper teeth revealed. Smiling this way takes conscious effort, however, and practice before it becomes second nature.

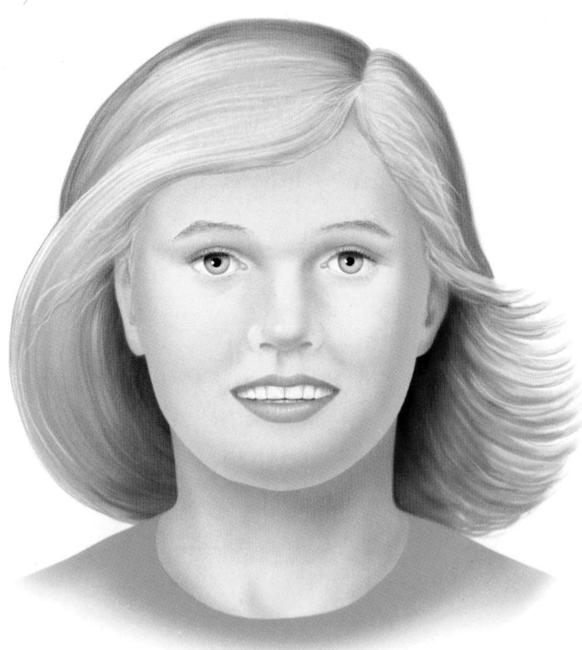

If you have a round face and teeth that are flat or straight-across because of wear, your face may appear much wider than it really is.

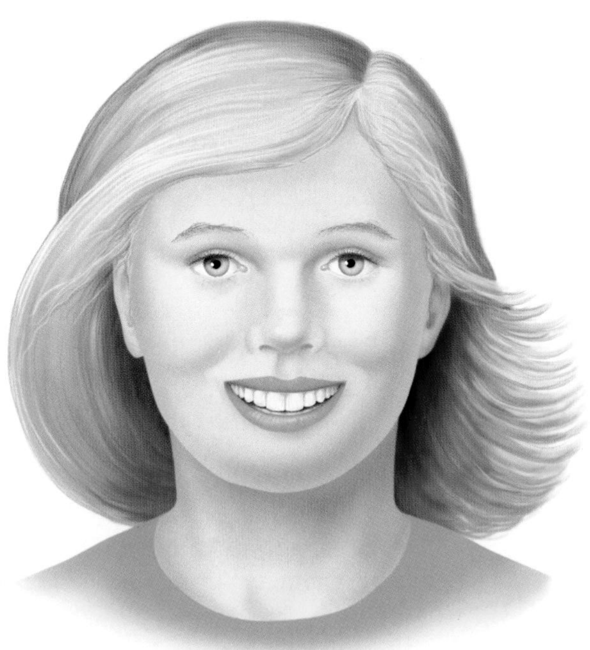

Consider having your central incisors slightly longer (or your lateral incisors shortened) to break up the straight-across front smileline for a better look.

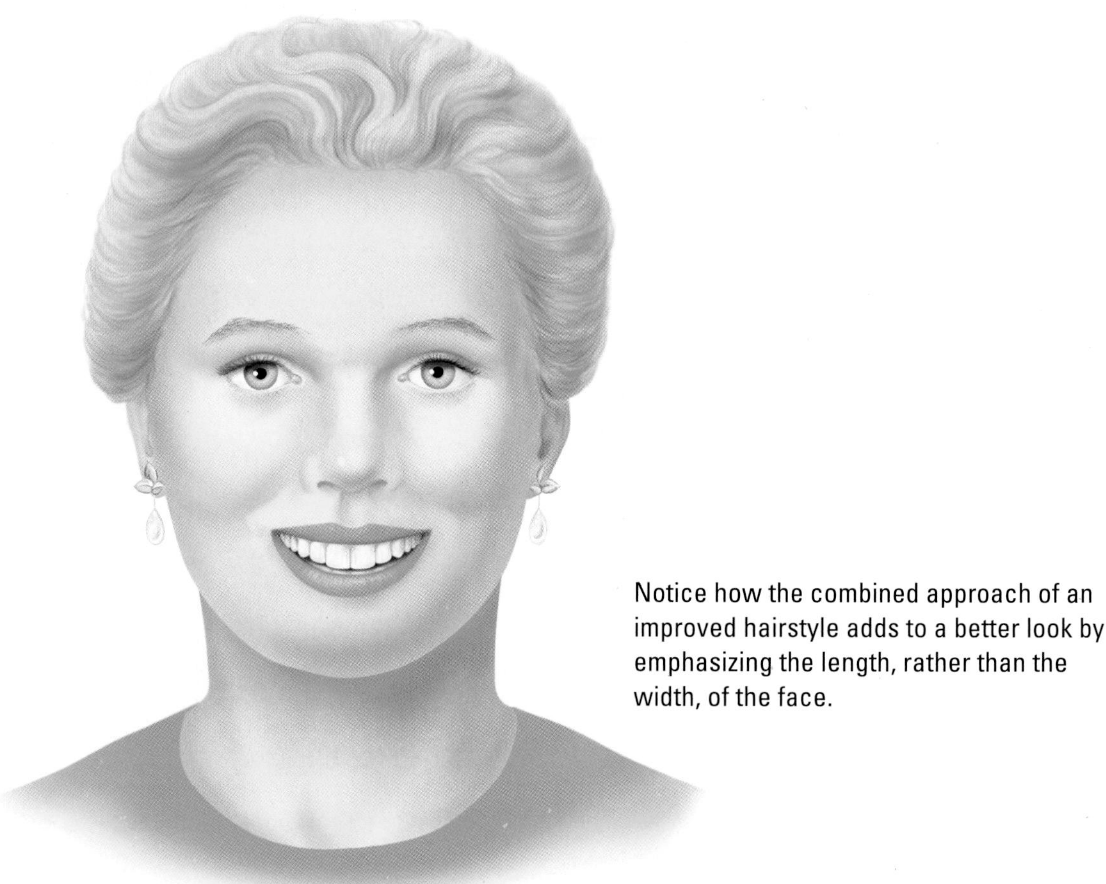

Notice how the combined approach of an improved hairstyle adds to a better look by emphasizing the length, rather than the width, of the face.

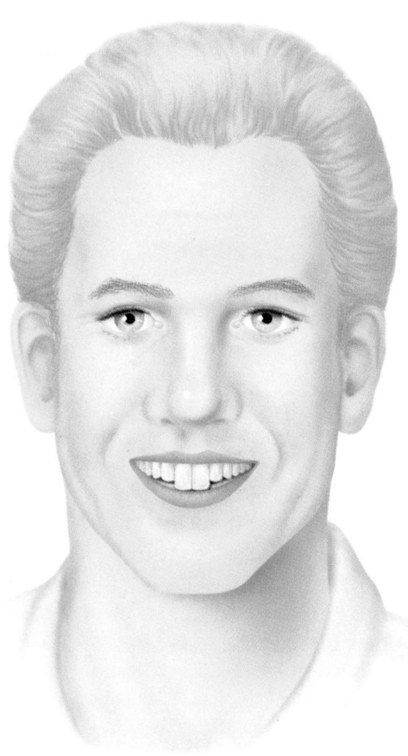

If you have a long face, be aware that long front teeth emphasize its length.

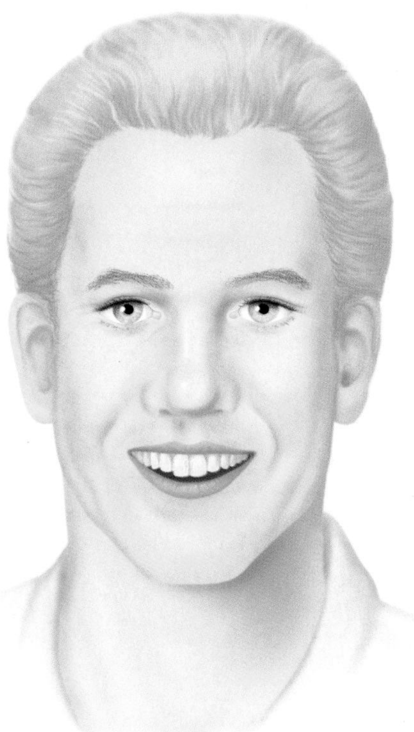

Consider cosmetic contouring to reshape the teeth.

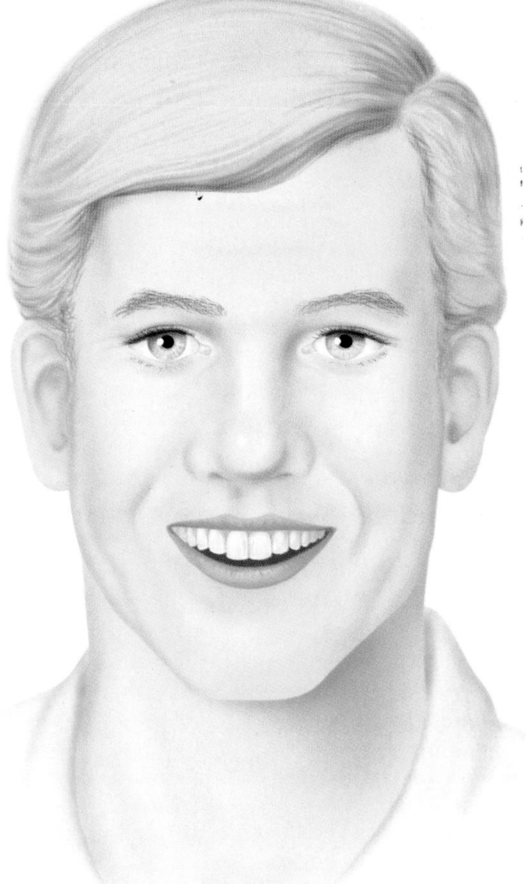

A new hairstyle combined with recontoured teeth can give the illusion of a different facial shape.

Ten Tips Before and After the Camera

1. Ask your dentist to contour your teeth so that their shape is as attractive as possible. The cost is reasonable, and it may well be the best investment you've ever made. Remember, tooth shape is just as important as tooth color.
2. Ask your dentist if your teeth can be effectively bleached. Don't waste your time or money on over-the-counter bleaching kits that may not work.
3. **Do not request upper teeth that are "perfectly straight-across." They will look worn and give you an older appearance.**
4. If you need a crown, inlay or filling, make sure you understand how much of the restoration will show when you speak, smile and laugh. If you object to having any metal show, tell your dentist before treatment begins.

And if you are being professionally photographed . . .

5. If you have a chipped tooth or a space you want to hide, correct the defect before your photographic session.
6. If you cannot correct a defect permanently, ask your dentist to temporarily camouflage it with moldable wax or bonding. Even unsightly gum loss between your teeth can be disguised with pink wax or bonding.
7. **If you are being photographed up close, make sure your gums as well as your teeth look good. But do not wait until the last minute to do something. It takes time for swollen and inflamed gums to heal, so begin treatment at least 30 days before your photo session. Often, a professional tooth cleaning is all it takes to make gums look healthy and attractive.**
8. Ask your dentist to repair or replace discolored tooth-colored fillings. You may find the discoloration more noticeable in photographs than in the mirror.
9. If you have metal fillings or crowns, alert the photographer. He or she may be able to photograph you from an angle that will not reveal them. If not, don't despair. Negatives can often be touched up so that metal does not show. **If the show of metal bothers you, your dentist can dull the shine in less than a minute with an instrument that works like a miniature sandblaster.**
10. The way you hold your head can change the appearance of your front teeth. Remember that your teeth are shadowed most of the time by your lips. When you lean your head down, your upper teeth generally appear longer than they really are. If your is head is tilted back, your upper teeth appear shorter.

Hairstyle and Makeup Provide a Frame for Your Smile

A new smile is like a painting. It takes the proper frame to show it off to its best advantage. Once you have your beautiful new smile, analyze your other facial features and use hairstyle and makeup to either accentuate or downplay them.

For example, if your brow is broad and square, a hairstyle that dips over the opposing corners can be flattering because it rounds off the right angles. If your eyes are small, light colors of eye shadow can make them appear larger. Creamy matte foundations help hide skin imperfections.

Just remember that the purpose of any cosmetic is to enhance your appearance and create an illusion of beauty. When makeup is applied too heavily it can give you a harsh or theatrical look. Also, keep in mind that whatever is dark will recede and whatever is light will look more prominent.

Proper makeup application is an art that can be learned. The trick lies in making the most of your own facial shape and features by accentuating your good points and minimizing or disguising your weaker points.

Before

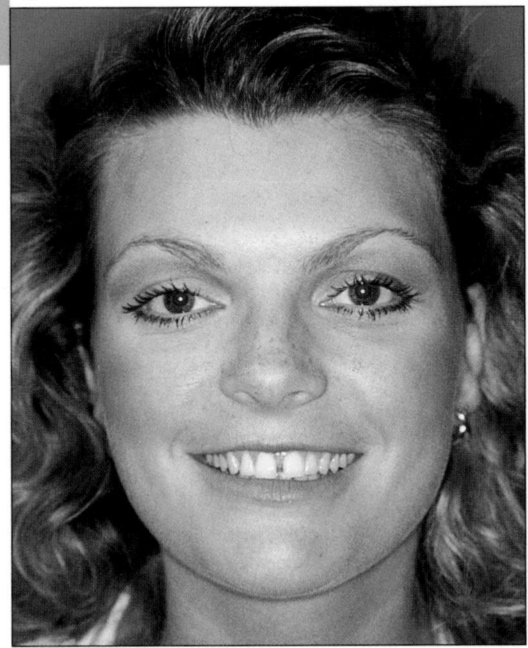

Diastema

This young lady was unhappy with the space between her front teeth.

After

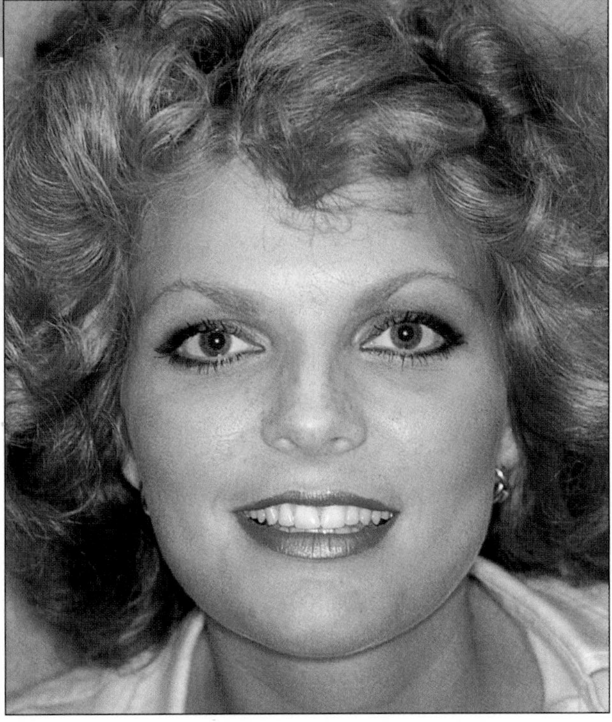

Composite Resin Bonding Plus Makeover

Composite resin bonding on her two front teeth helped create a new smileline by closing the space between her central incisors. With new makeup and hairstyle, the squareness of her face was de-emphasized.

Before

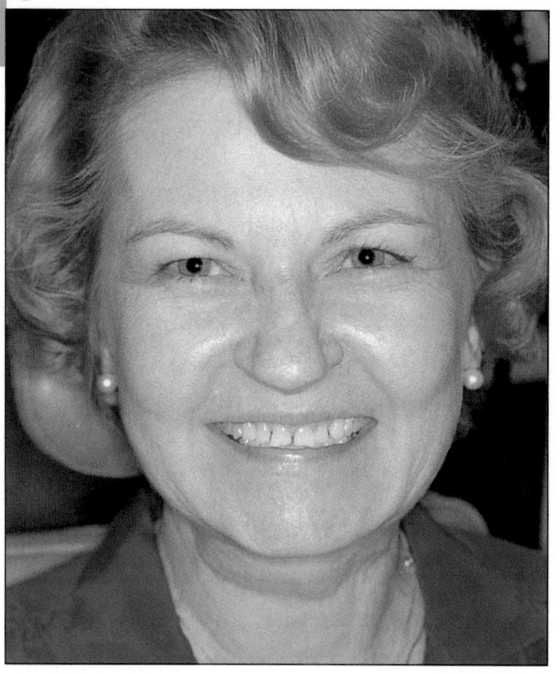

ADVANCED TOOTH WEAR AND COLLAPSED BITE

This woman looked older than her years because of advancing tooth wear and a collapsed bite. She was determined to improve her appearance. Cosmetic dentistry, plastic surgery and cosmetology were planned to produce a whole new look.

After

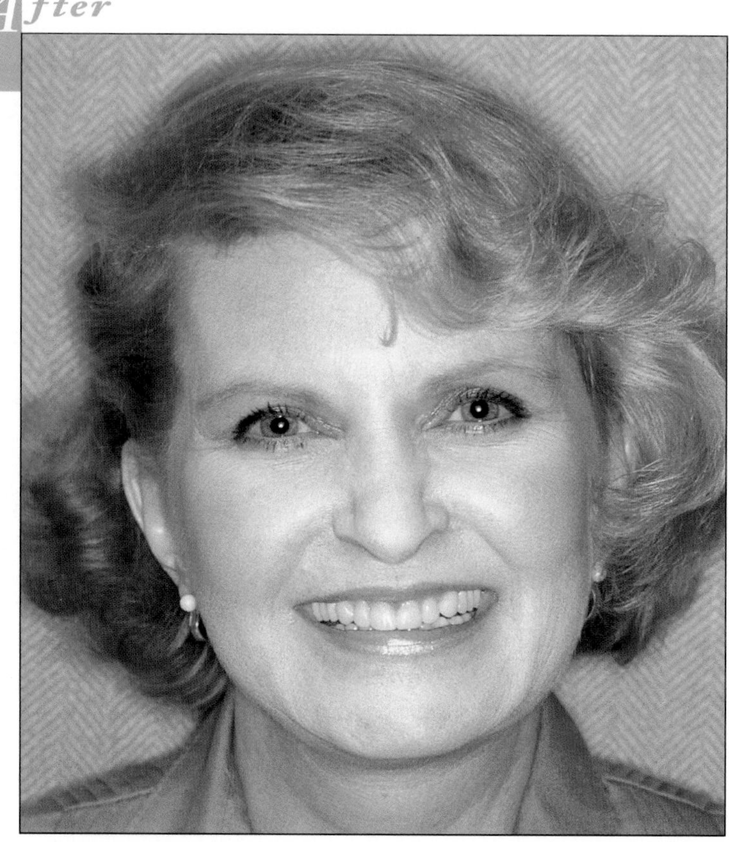

FULL CROWNS, COMPOSITE RESIN BONDING, PLASTIC SURGERY AND COSMETOLOGY

Her bite was corrected with full crowns on all the back teeth. The front teeth were bonded with composite resin to lengthen them, helping create a younger smileline. Note the improvement in the total appearance after a new smile, plastic surgery, new hair color and style, plus makeup. This total new look is the epitome of what cosmetic dentistry combined with the field of plastic surgery and cosmetology can do for those who want to look their best.

Before

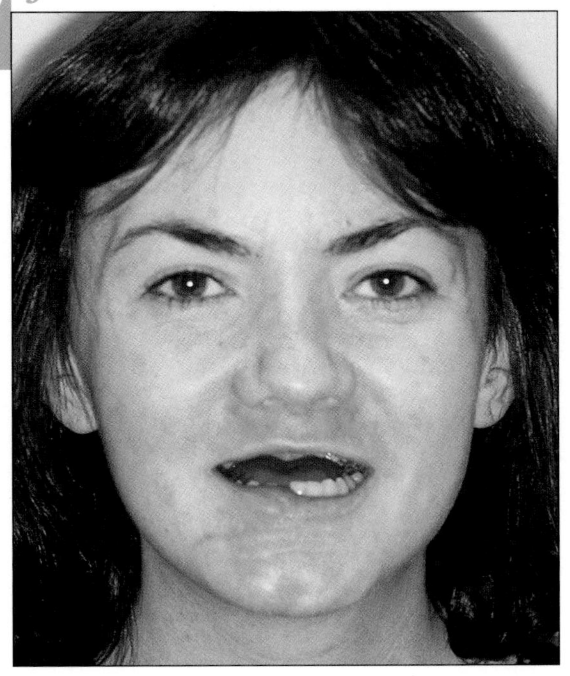

Tooth loss affecting facial esthetics

A terrible car accident causing the loss of four front teeth marred the beauty of this 24-year-old student. It took the combined efforts of oral surgery, plastic surgery, cosmetic dentistry and cosmetology to recreate the beauty that was once there.

After

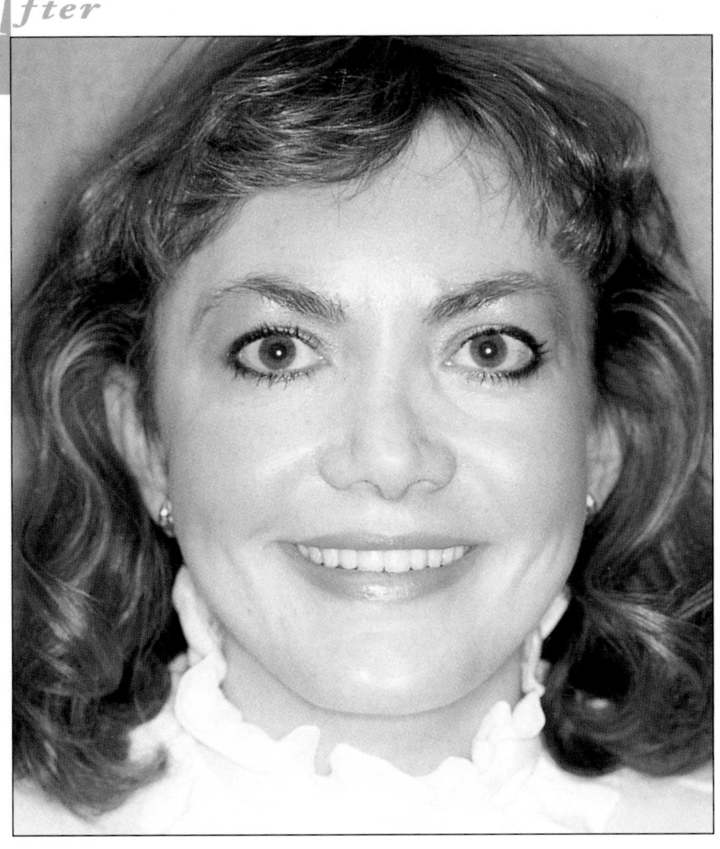

Cosmetic dentistry, plastic surgery and cosmetology

Severe accidents can not only destroy outward beauty, but diminish self-confidence. After plastic surgery and oral surgery to extract what teeth had to be removed and stabilize those that remained, new fixed bridges replaced the missing teeth to help recreate a pretty smile. The total improvement in facial appearance can be seen following the combined treatment of all the specialties.

Before

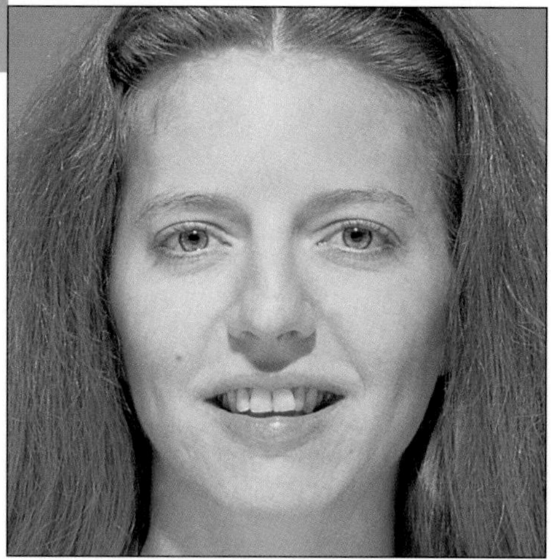

Open bite and crowned and discolored teeth

This 30-year-old statistical analyst was dissatisfied with her overall appearance. She was willing to undergo combined treatment necessary to achieve a better look.

After

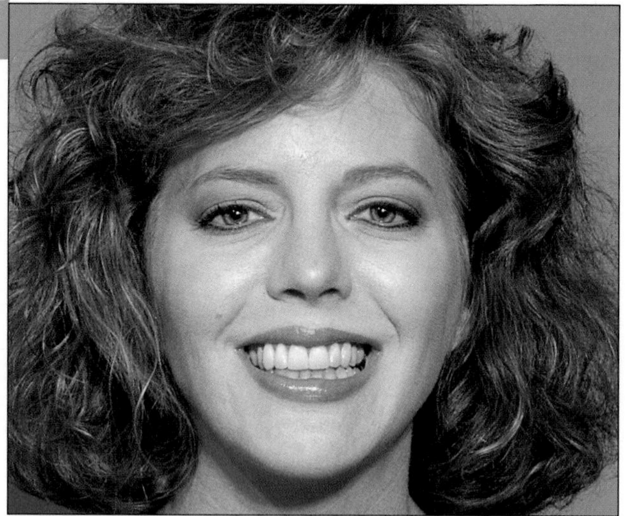

Orthodontics, orthognathic surgery, bleaching, porcelain laminates, porcelain crowns, plastic surgery and a makeover

A complete new look, as well as the ability to function better, was the result of two years of combined therapy. Often it takes a combination of treatments to give you the results you desire.

Before

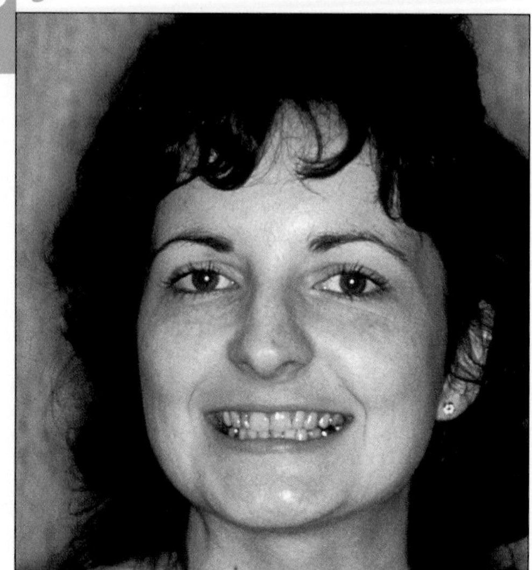

Discolored teeth

This 36-year-old writer felt her dark teeth were unattractive. She did not, however, want an unnatural look.

After

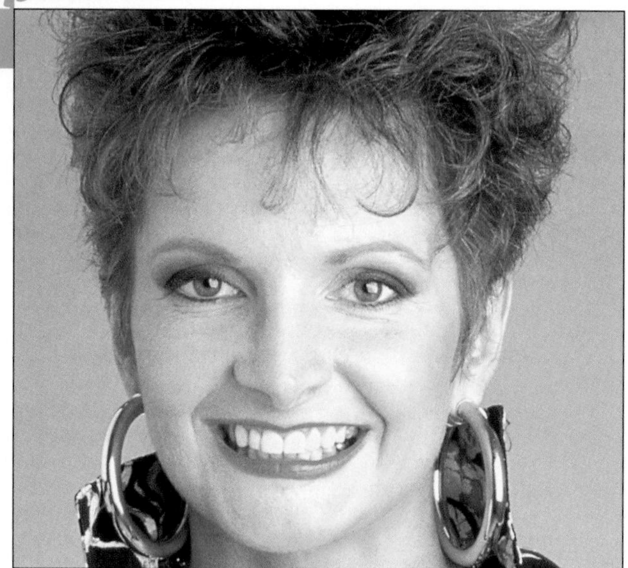

Composite resin bonding

Ten teeth were bonded with a lighter shade of composite resin to help brighten her smile. Finally, a makeover helped to create a new image to go with her new smile.

Tooth Shape Makes a Difference, Too

The shapes of your teeth also play a key role in your overall appearance. For example, if you have a square face, you don't want square-looking teeth.

A space between the front teeth also emphasizes the horizontal plane and the squareness of the jaw. Although this feature can be quite becoming, it tends to give a masculine appearance.

If your face is round and your teeth are worn, your face may appear heavier than it really is. In such cases, the teeth can be contoured or lengthened through bonding or laminates to give you a more attractive smileline.

If you have a long, angular face, your two front teeth should be just slightly longer than the ones next to them. If they are too long, your face will look droopy and thin.

Before

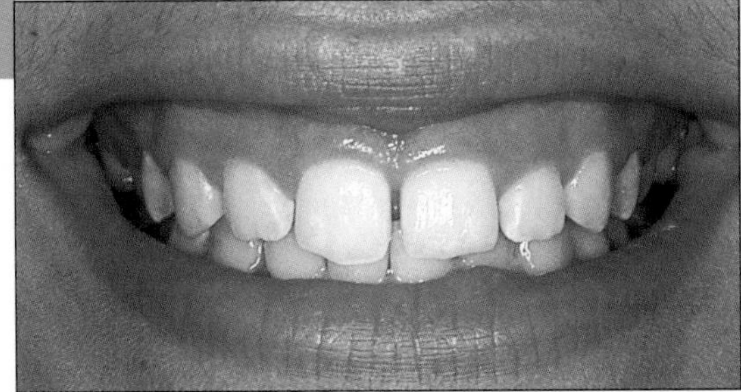

Spaces and High Lipline

This former beauty queen was dissatisfied with her smile. She was unhappy with the show of so much gum tissue as well as the spaces between her front teeth.

After

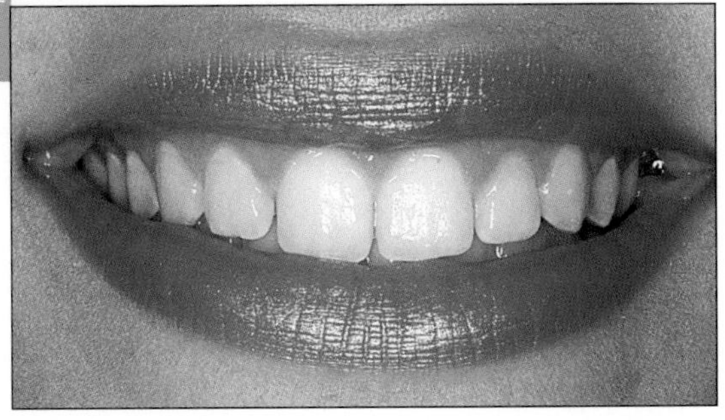

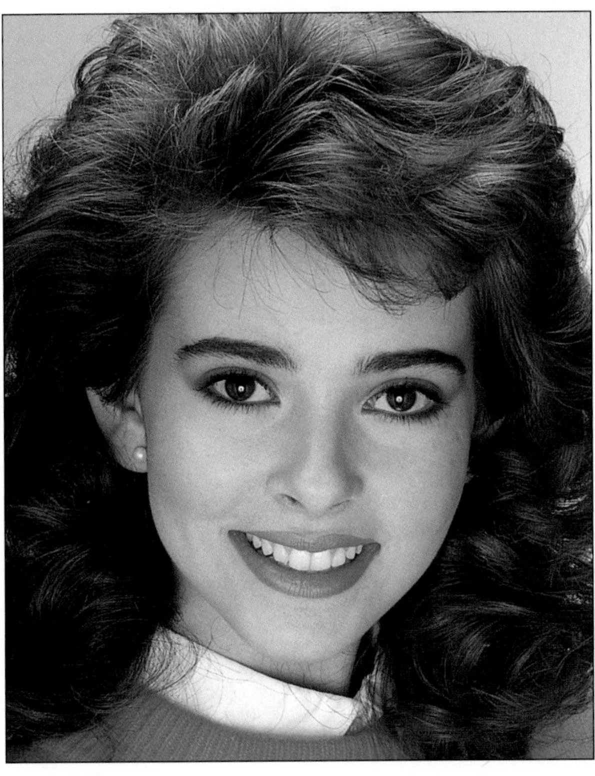

Gum Repositioning Surgery and Orthodontics

An important part of helping improve this woman's smileline was repositioning the gum tissue through cosmetic surgery. After this procedure, the spaces between the teeth were closed with clear plastic brackets. Note how the new smile helps improve the overall facial appearance of this beautiful young model. (Courtesy of Andrew O. Wilson.)

Before

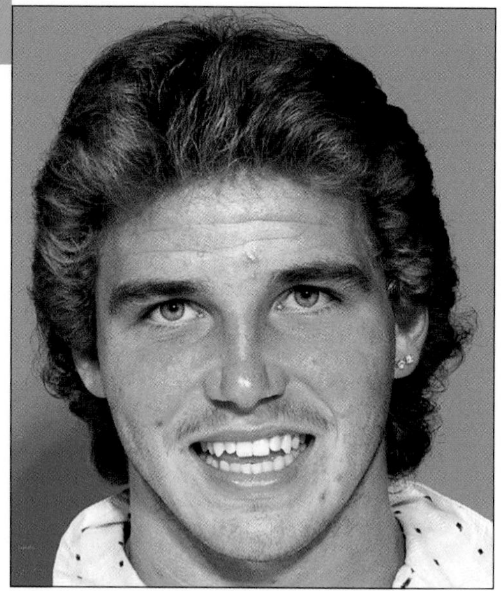

TOO-LONG, IRREGULAR TEETH

This 20-year-old salesman did not like his "vampire" teeth.

After

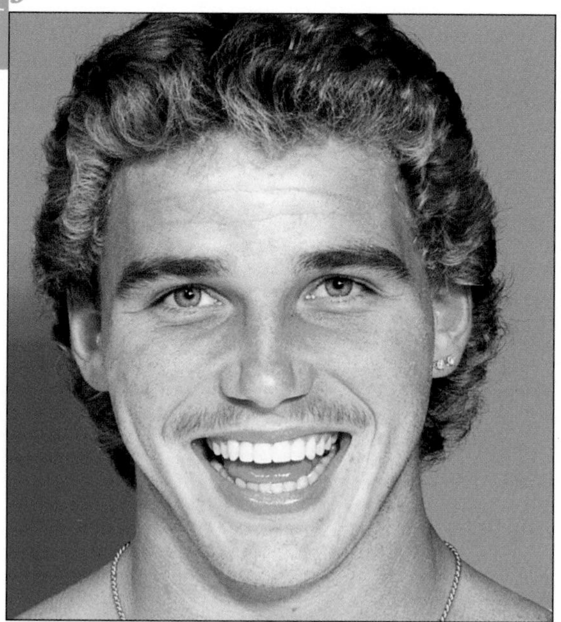

COSMETIC CONTOURING AND COMPOSITE RESIN BONDING

A new look was created by simply contouring and bonding the front teeth. Notice how much his new smile enhances the total facial look.

Before

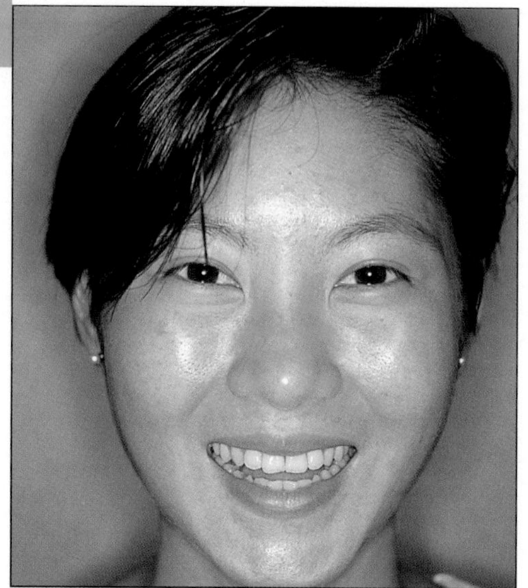

CROWDED FRONT TEETH

This young model wanted straighter teeth but didn't want to undergo lengthy orthodontic treatment.

After

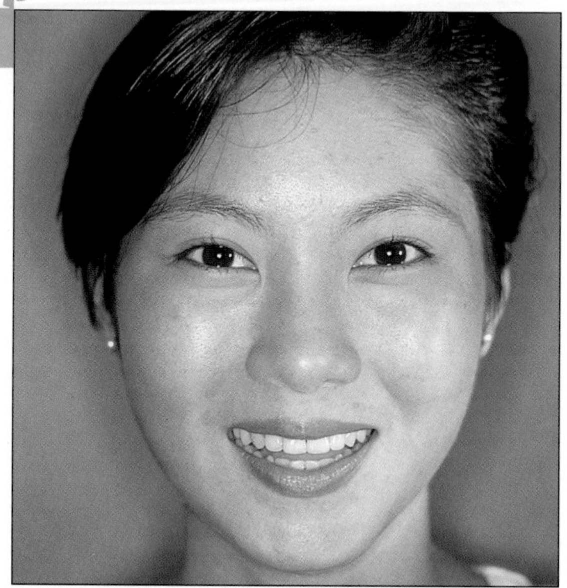

COSMETIC CONTOURING

A smile with straighter-appearing teeth was the result of cosmetic contouring. This one-appointment procedure helped to make her face look more symmetrical.

For Men Only

If you have a receding chin or if the lower part of your face is asymmetrical, think about growing a beard to help balance out these irregularities.

If tooth extraction or an upper facial deformity have caused your upper lip to collapse, consider growing a mustache for the illusion of better facial proportions.

Keep in mind that a mustache accentuates the shadow that the lip creates over the teeth, causing the teeth to look even darker. If you're undergoing restorative treatment and have facial hair and plan to keep it, ask your dentist for a slightly lighter tooth shade to offset the shadow effect.

To Compromise or Not to Compromise

We all make compromises every day. Although we'd prefer to have our way all the time, sooner or later we learn that life has its trade-offs. The same holds true for your dental treatment.

Before you begin treatment, ask yourself what you are willing to sacrifice for a more attractive smile. How much of a perfectionist are you? What demands will you make on your dentist? If you want the best, are you willing to pay for it? If orthodontic treatment is suggested, can you live with a lengthy treatment plan? Or would you prefer a more immediate solution such as bonding, knowing that it may have to be redone in a few years?

Also think long-term as you evaluate your esthetic needs. It will help you put things in perspective.

Give yourself the best whenever you can. Don't look for a quick fix when you need extensive treatment. In the long run, you'll save time and money if treatment doesn't have to be redone or repeated so often.

Before

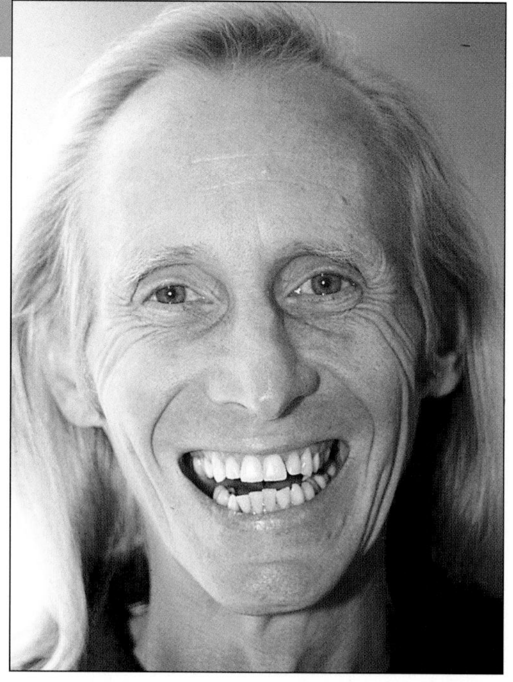

SPACED UPPER TEETH AND CROWDED LOWER TEETH

This hair stylist was dissatisfied with his smile and wanted to enhance his appearance.

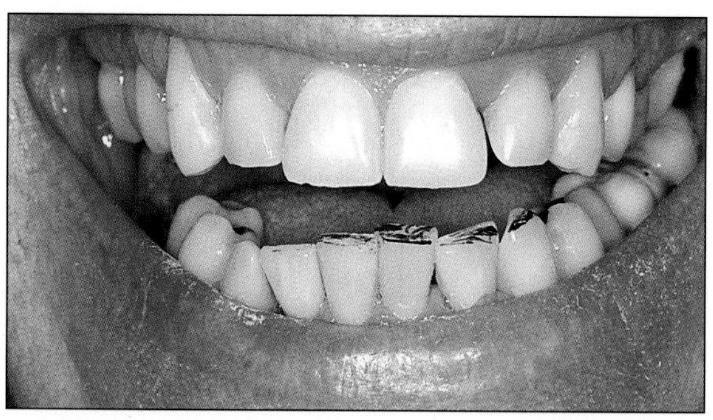

COSMETIC CONTOURING

The teeth have been marked to show where cosmetic contouring will be performed.

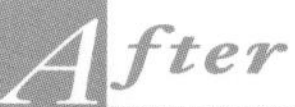

After

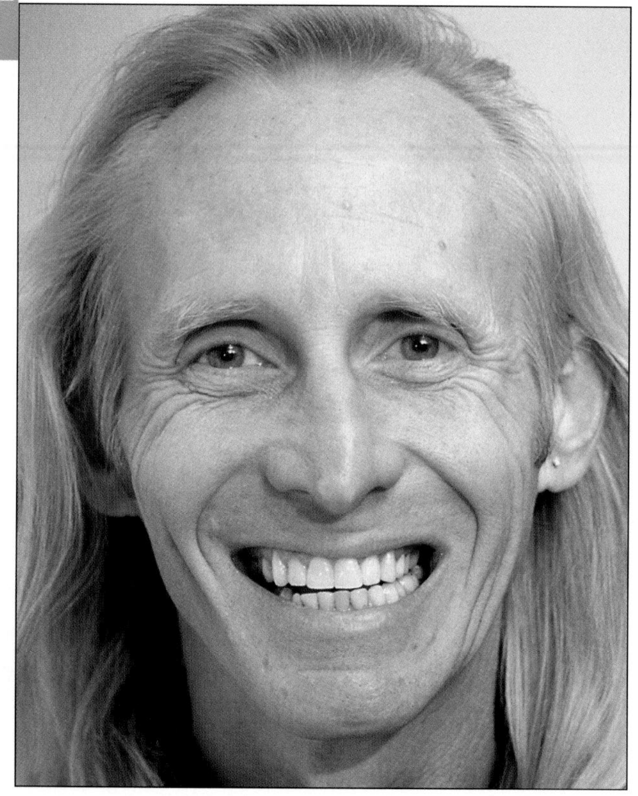

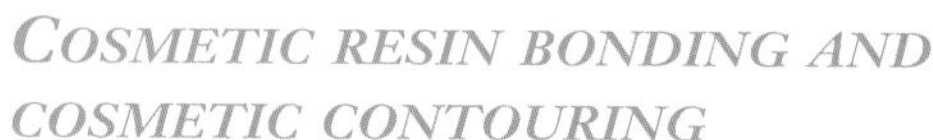

COSMETIC RESIN BONDING AND COSMETIC CONTOURING

Cosmetic resin bonding combined with cosmetic contouring resulted in a more pleasing smile.

Before

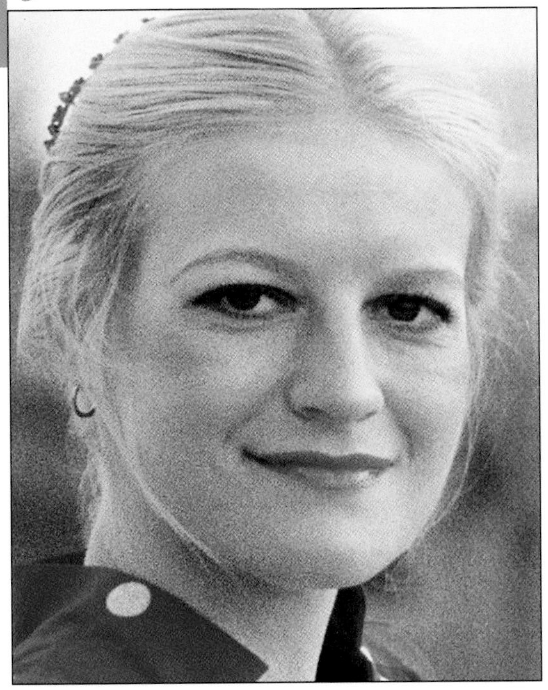

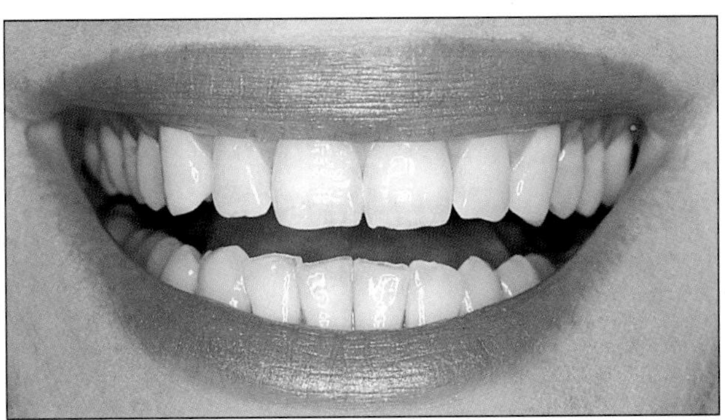

Although multiple plastic surgery procedures over several years resulted in a more youthful and attractive facial appearance, her teeth remained an obvious flaw.

CHIPPED, CROOKED AND WORN TEETH

This forty-year-old media personality was unhappy with her appearance.

After

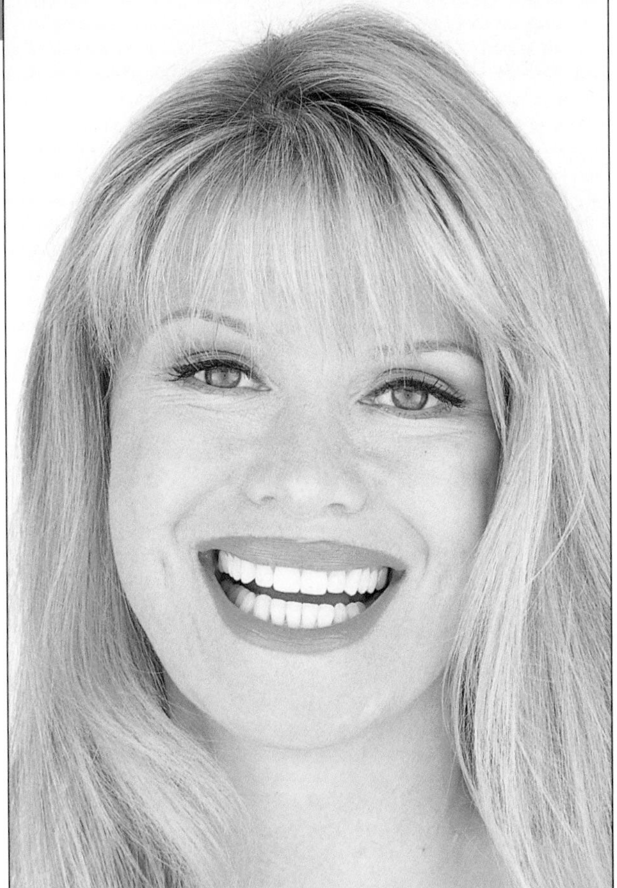

COSMETIC CONTOURING

Cosmetic contouring made her teeth appear straighter and younger looking. The new smileline helped complete a total esthetic result.

Now That You've Changed It, Use It!

Many people who've had corrective dental treatment forget that their smile looks better. If, for example, you've spent years hiding your mouth with your hand whenever you laughed or smiled because you were embarrassed by your teeth, it will probably take conscious effort to break yourself of the habit.

When you complete your cosmetic dental treatment, practice smiling in front of a large mirror. Ease into a broad grin. Think of something funny so that you really reveal your teeth. Repeat this until you get used to smiling again.

Then remember to smile often. It increases your face value.

Before

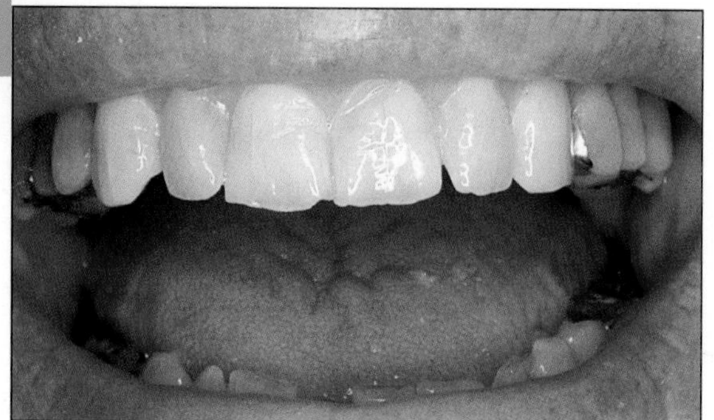

Discolored, Chipped, Worn and Eroded Anterior Teeth

This internationally known entertainer wanted bright, white teeth to enhance her tremendous smile and laugh.

After

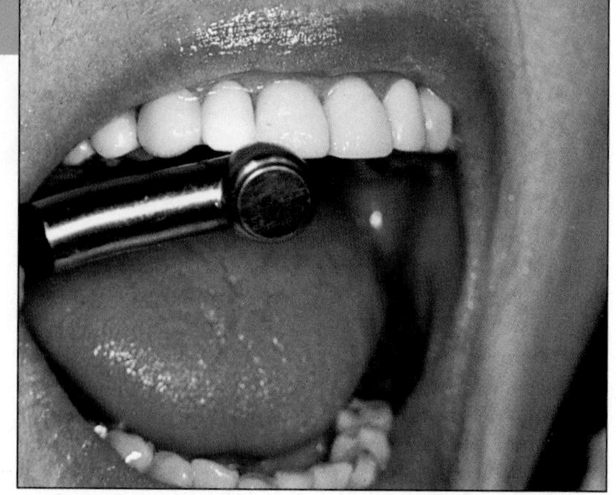

Composite Resin Bonding and Cosmetic Contouring

It took one ten-hour appointment to transform this lady's smile. Here cosmetic contouring is done to make the shapes of the teeth appear more feminine.

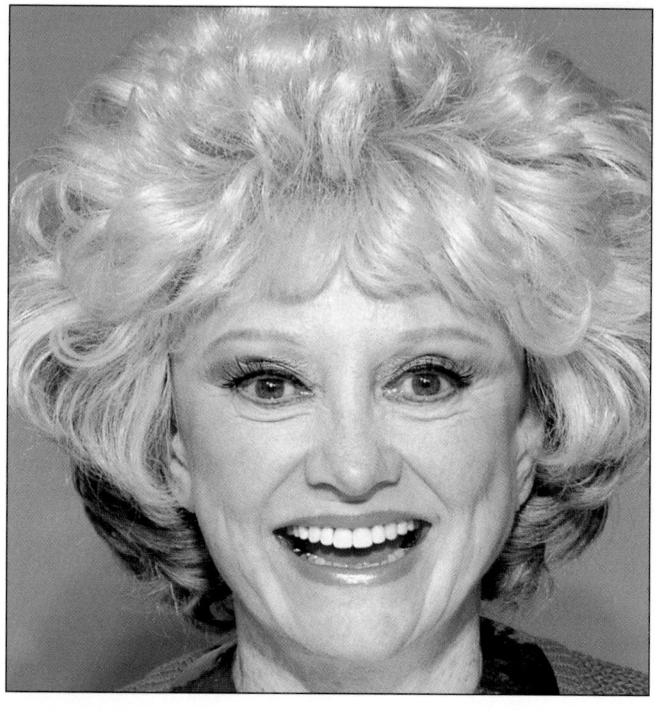

A more youthful and flattering smile resulted immediately.

APPENDIX

How Technology Can Change Your Smile

Esthetic dentistry is entering its most exciting era. Many procedures that were once uncomfortable and time-consuming can now be performed quickly and comfortably using state-of-the-art techniques and equipment. New technology allows you to participate actively in your diagnosis and treatment and even preview end results!

Dentists are incorporating the following high-tech tools into their practices:

Extraoral Video Camera

The extraoral video camera provides an audiovisual record of your ideas, preferences, expectations and complaints as well as your dentist's suggestions and explanations of various treatment options. It also allows your dentist to have a detailed record of your face while you move and talk—a much more helpful tool than a still photograph.

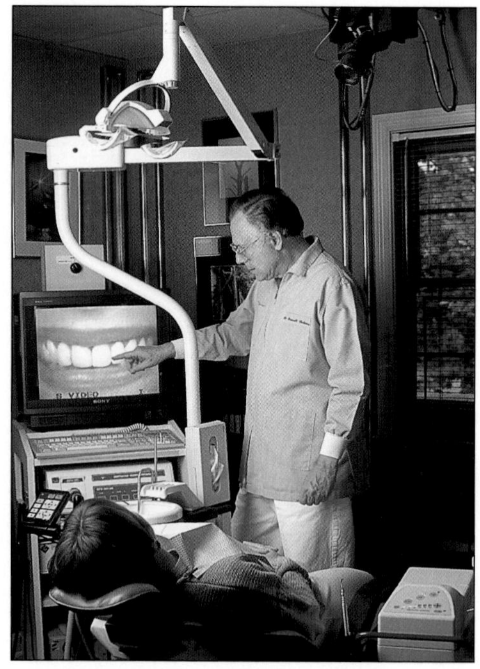

Seeing yourself on a close-up TV screen gives both you and your dentist a valuable look at what needs to be done to give you a great new smile. Additionally, you can analyze your smile much better in this way than you can when you look at yourself in the mirror. (Photo © Bill Lisenby)

Intraoral Video Camera

The intraoral video camera allows you to get a real "inside" view of your mouth. Most intraoral cameras are no bigger than a thumbnail yet provide unparalleled diagnostic capabilities. With it your dentist can explain certain conditions and treatment options much more accurately than with sketches, mirrors and X-rays.

Computer or Voice-Activated Data Entry

Using voice-activated technology, dentists and hygienists can document their findings by speaking into a microphone that is connected to a computer which has been "trained" to recognize a limited vocabulary. The computer then stores the information and even displays graphics on a monitor so that you and your dentist can discuss various procedures.

T-Scan

The T-Scan allows your dentist to determine the force of your occlusion, or bite. When you bite down on the horseshoe-shaped sensor, the information is transmitted to a computer that provides a three-dimensional representation of your chewing contacts.

Digital Radiography

An alternative to traditional X-rays, digital radiography is a filmless technique that uses up to 90 percent less radiation. It also provides high-quality, digitally encoded information that can be adjusted electronically to alter contrast density or to magnify specific areas.

CAD/CAM

With CAD/CAM (computer-assisted design/computer-assisted manufacture) technology, dentists can design and make inlays, onlays, veneers and crowns while you wait! Information for fabricating the restorations is supplied to a computer via optical imaging or by tracing the tooth with a device that records its dimensions. The restoration is then milled by the computer instead of a laboratory and is fitted by the dentist in one easy appointment.

Lasers

The dental laser uses a beam of light in place of a scalpel to perform delicate gum surgery. Benefits of the laser include less discomfort after surgery, virtually no bleeding and reduced risk of infection. Some minor procedures can actually be performed without anesthesia. Among other uses, laser surgery offers a patient-friendly approach to enhancing a smile by reshaping the gum lines. Lasers are also being used to speed up the bonding process.

Computer Imaging

This exciting state-of-the-art technology allows you to "see" various looks before deciding on treatment. For example, if you want to know how you would look with whiter, straighter teeth, your dentist or the imaging technician can show you by electronically altering a video image of your smile. Computer imaging improves communication between you and your dentist by allowing both of you to visualize, evaluate and agree on treatment before you invest your time or money.

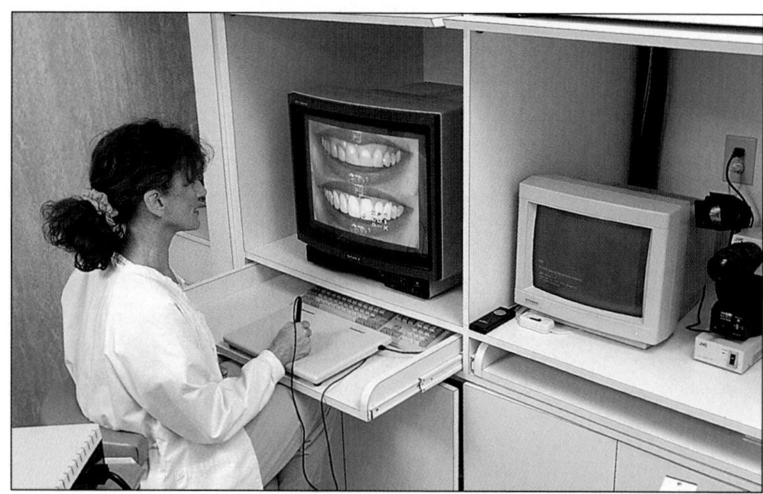

Computer imaging can provide you with a preview of how your new smile will look. It also helps you make certain that your dentist's ideas for improvement coincide with your own vision. (Photo © Bill Lisenby)

Abrasive Technology

Although abrasive technology doesn't replace the dental drill for filling teeth, it often provides an alternative. Working much like a precise miniature sandblaster, this instrument gently sprays away decayed tooth structure using a microscopically fine powder called *alpha alumina*, a nontoxic ingredient that is also used in whitening toothpastes. Because abrasive technology produces virtually no heat or vibration, it can usually be used without anesthetic injections.

Although abrasive technology cannot remove metal (amalgam) fillings or prepare teeth for crowning, it offers a rapid and comfortable way to remove stain and early decay. In fact, abrasive technology frequently uncovers "veins of decay" that are hidden beneath the "stain pockets" of active tooth destruction that sometimes cannot even be detected by X-rays. Thanks to this breakthrough, dentists now have an effective way to not only completely free the mouth of decay but also eliminate all of the stained areas that are potential breeding grounds for decay-causing bacteria.

This technology is also useful during repairs to existing composite or porcelain restorations because it roughens these surfaces, allowing the reparative materials to bond to them more readily. Thanks to abrasive technology, precision and lack of vibration, veneers can be repaired without risk of damaging the porcelain. While nearly all patients find abrasive technology to be a welcome advance, it is especially helpful in the treatment of children and in patients whose medical conditions restrict the use of anesthesia.

These high-tech tools open up a whole new world of possibilities and allow you to achieve the smile you have always wanted. Although few dentists will have every high-tech tool available, find out which dentists in your area offer state-of-the-art cosmetic treatment. They are most likely the ones who will also provide you with the best dental care.

Glossary

Abrasion Loss of tooth structure from mechanical wear other than chewing.

Abrasive technology Working like a miniature "sandblaster," an instrument using abrasive technology gently sprays away dental decay using a fine nontoxic powder; anesthetic injections are not usually required with abrasive technology.

Abutment A tooth or root used to anchor a fixed or removable bridge.

Amalgam A silver-colored metal filling material usually made up of silver, zinc, tin, copper and mercury.

Arches Horseshoe-shaped ridges that support the upper and lower teeth. Usually distinguished as *upper* and *lower* arches.

Attrition Gradual wearing away of the biting surfaces of the teeth.

Bleaching Treating the teeth with a strong oxidizing or bleaching agent to reduce or eliminate stains.

Bonding (Composite resin bonding) Mildly etching a tooth surface to create microscopic voids for receiving a plastic material that will change the tooth's shape or improve its appearance, or to help attach another material to the tooth.

Bridge A dental appliance (fixed or removable) replacing lost teeth.

Bruxism Excessive grinding of the teeth that can cause unnatural wear of the chewing surfaces.

CAD/CAM Computer-assisted design/computer-assisted manufacture technology. Information is supplied to the computer through imaging or by tracing the tooth, which allows the dentist to make inlays, onlays, veneers and crowns while the patient waits.

Cement A material used to attach a restoration to a tooth.

Closed bite Insufficient distance between the upper and lower arches, generally leading to partial collapse of the lower facial tissue.

Composite resin A plastic filling material to which filler has been added for strength.

Computer imaging Computer enhancement of a video image of your smile or face, which allows you to "see" various looks before deciding on treatment.

Cosmetic contouring Reshaping or reducing the natural teeth to make them appear straighter.

Crossbite A bad bite where the lower teeth overlap the upper teeth when the mouth is in a closed position.

Crown A cap, cover or restoration replacing the portion of the tooth exposed in the mouth.

Acrylic Entire surface made of plastic.

Aluminous porcelain Made of reinforced or stronger porcelain. An esthetic all-glass tooth replacement.

Ceramo-metal (porcelain fused to metal) Made of porcelain and metal. The entire undersurface usually is metal.

Gold Entire visible surface of tooth made of gold.

Gold veneer Under and chewing surfaces of tooth made of gold. Front made of either porcelain or acrylic.

Porcelain All-ceramic.

Stainless steel Entire tooth surface made of stainless steel.

Telescopic An outer crown that is attached to a metal thimble inserted on the remaining prepared tooth.

Crowning Making a crown (cap) for a tooth.

Cuspid (canine) The "corner" teeth in the arch so named because of correspondence to a dog's long teeth. The third tooth on each side of the midline.

Decay Tooth destruction caused by bacteria and their by-products.

Deep overbite Almost complete overlapping of the upper front teeth over the lower front teeth.

Dentin The layer of the tooth under the enamel or cementum.

Dentin tubules Minute channels in the dentin that extend from the pulp to the enamel or the cementum.

Diastema A space between two teeth.

Digital radiography A computerized alternative to conventional X-rays. A filmless X-ray technique that uses up to 90 percent less radiation.

Enamel The visible, hard, white part of the tooth that covers and protects the dentin.

Erosion Loss of tooth structure due to chemical rather than bacterial action.

Fixed bridge A fixed appliance used to replace a missing tooth or teeth, cemented in the mouth on adjacent teeth that have been reduced to provide anchor support.

Full denture An appliance that replaces all of the natural teeth.

Gingiva Gum tissue.

High lipline When the widest smile reveals gum tissue above the upper teeth.

Incisal Refers to the biting or cutting edges of the front teeth.

Incisal embrasure Slight opening between the teeth at the biting edges, helping to make the teeth look individual rather than like a unit.

Incisor The central or lateral teeth with cutting edges. The four front teeth, two upper and two lower.

Inlay Porcelain or gold filling that helps restore the tooth, made to fit a prepared cavity and cemented into place.

Interdental tissue Gum tissue between the teeth.

Intraoral camera A small video camera that can enlarge the image of a tooth twenty to thirty times, enabling detection of tooth defects at their earliest onset.

Invisible braces Orthodontic brackets attached to the inside surface of the teeth so that they are not visible from the front view.

Laminate veneer Thin porcelain or plastic shell bonded to the enamel of the front teeth.

Laminating Applying a thin veneer of porcelain, composite resin or preformed plastic to the tooth.

Laser Technology that uses a beam of light in place of a scalpel to perform delicate surgery.

Low lipline When the widest smile barely reveals the bottom edges of the upper teeth and no gum or interdental tissue shows.

Malocclusion A bad bite caused by incorrect positions of the upper or lower teeth.

Margin Junction between tooth and crown or filling material.

Medium lipline When the widest smile reveals the interdental gum tissue but not the gum tissue above the upper teeth.

Microabrasion A method of removing dental stains that consists of mildly abrading the tooth with acid.

Microcrack Microscopic cracks in teeth usually visible when stained or in intense light.

Midline An imaginary vertical line that divides the face into two equal parts.

Occlusal equilibration The reshaping process of refining and perfecting the occlusion or bite, usually by adjusting the natural teeth.

Onlay Porcelain or gold filling that protects a tooth by covering the chewing surface.

Open bite A bad bite where the front teeth remain open when the lower teeth return to the closed chewing position.

Overdenture A removable bridge that completely covers the teeth and ridges and is attached to the remaining roots.

Partial denture An appliance that replaces some of the natural teeth.

Pin A thin metal support that is either tapped, cemented or screwed into the dentin to help retain filling material.

Plaque A sticky, colorless film containing bacteria that is constantly forming on the teeth.

Pontic An artificial tooth that replaces a missing tooth by being suspended on a fixed bridge anchored to adjacent teeth.

Porcelain A fine, tooth-colored material consisting mainly of feldspar, kaolin and flux. It fuses at high temperatures to form a hard, enamel-like substance.

Porcelain laminate Thin porcelain shell that is etched from the inside, enabling it to be bonded to tooth structure.

Post A thick metal or ceramic reinforcement inserted into a tooth (that has undergone a root canal) to help strengthen it.

Posterior bonded resin composite A tooth-colored filling in the back teeth.

Precision attachment A specially machined part used in some bridges to hide the attachment of the removable appliance to the anchor teeth.
Prophylaxis Tooth cleaning to remove stains and calculus (tartar).
Protrusion A bad bite in which teeth protrude.
Pulp Nerves, arteries, veins and connective tissue in the pulp chamber inside the tooth.

Resin-bonded bridge An acid-etched, thin, usually metal-reinforced bridge requiring only slight or no reduction of the anchor teeth.
Restoration A filling, laminate, crown, bridge or other means used to repair or replace part or all of a tooth.
Ridge augmentation A surgical buildup of missing bone and tissue.
Root The part of the tooth that is usually anchored in the jawbone.
Rubber dam A thin piece of rubber that can isolate teeth to control moisture during treatment.

Shade A degree or intensity of color usually referring to the descriptive color of a tooth.
Splint An appliance of metal, acrylic or composite resin usually used to hold and stabilize loose teeth.

T-Scan A computerized method of measuring the bite (occlusion).
Tartar (calculus) A cement-like substance that forms when plaque is not removed from teeth.
Temporary crown A protective interim covering placed after a tooth is prepared for a final crown. It can also give the patient a good idea of what the final crown will look like.
Temporomandibular joint (TMJ) The joint that connects the upper and lower jaws.
Tetracycline An antibiotic that can discolor the teeth if taken before the age of eight or in people whose mothers took it during pregnancy.
Try-in Checking the fit and appearance of a laminate, crown, bridge or other dental restoration or appliance.

Vital bleaching Bleaching live teeth.

Walking bleach Temporarily sealing a bleaching agent in a tooth that has undergone a root canal.

REFERENCES

No book is an island unto itself. Other works influence and spark ideas that may take other forms. The major references for this book are listed below. The reader who desires additional information is encouraged to consult the following sources:

Berns JM. Understanding Periodontal Diseases. Chicago: Quintessence, 1993.

Berns JM. Why Replace a Missing Back Tooth? Chicago: Quintessence, 1994.

Berscheid E, Walster E, Bohrnstedt G. The happy American body: a survey report. Psych Today 7:119, 1973.

Christensen GJ. A Consumer's Guide to Dentistry. St. Louis: Mosby Year Book, Inc, 1994.

Collins DA. Your Teeth—A Handbook of Dental Care for the Whole Family. Garden City, New York: Doubleday & Co, 1967.

Denholtz M, Denholtz E. The Dental Facelift. New York: Van Nostrand Reinhold, 1981.

Garfield S. Teeth, Teeth, Teeth. Beverly Hills, California: Valient Books, 1969.

Gibson RM. The Miracle of Smilepower. Honolulu: The Smilepower Institute, 1977.

Goldstein RE, Garber DA. Complete Dental Bleaching. Chicago: Quintessence, 1995.

Goldstein RE. Esthetics in Dentistry. Philadelphia: JH Lippincott Co, 1976.

Jablonski S. Illustrated Dictionary of Dentistry. Philadelphia: WB Saunders, 1982.

Liggett J. The Human Face. New York: Stein & Day, 1974.

McGuire T. The Tooth Trip. New York: Random House, 1972.

McKeown J. Everybody's Tooth Book. Santa Cruz, California: Happy Valley Apple Press, 1977.

Moss SJ. Growing Up Cavity Free: A Patient's Guide to Prevention. Chicago: Quintessence, 1993.

Rosenthal S. Cosmetic Surgery: A Consumer's Guide. New York: Tree Communications, 1977.

Sawchenko T. Cosmetic Dentistry. Phoenix, Arizona: Sims Printing, 1974.

Shelby DS. Anterior Restoration, Fixed Bridgework, and Esthetics. Springfield, IL: Charles C. Thomas, 1976.

Smigel I. Dental Health, Dental Beauty. New York: M Evans, 1979.

Taylor TD, Laney WR. Dental Implants: Are They For Me? Chicago: Quintessence, 1993.

Consultants

Dr. Leonard Abrams, Philadelphia, Pennsylvania
Dr. Morton Amsterdam, Philadelphia, Pennsylvania
Ms. Suzanne Boswell, Dallas, Texas
Dr. Michael Burns, Atlanta, Georgia
Dr. Frank Celenza, New York, New York
Dr. Gerard J. Chiche, New Orleans, Louisiana
Dr. Rella P. Christensen, Provo, Utah
Dr. Gordon Christensen, Provo, Utah
Dr. Walter Cohen, Philadelphia, Pennsylvania
Mr. Richard Davis, Atlanta, Georgia
Dr. Peter Dawson, St. Petersburg, Florida
Dr. Norman Feigenbaum, Tamarac, Florida
Dr. Mark Friedman, Encino, California
Dr. Michael Fritz, Atlanta, Georgia
Dr. Phillipe G. Gallon, Paris, France
Dr. David Garber, Atlanta, Georgia
Ms. Lynn Garber, Philadelphia, Pennsylvania
Dr. Cary Goldstein, Atlanta, Georgia
Dr. Cathy Goldstein-Schwartz, Atlanta, Georgia
Dr. Marvin Goldstein, Atlanta, Georgia
Dr. Ken Goldstein, Atlanta, Georgia
Dr. Joseph Greenberg, Ardmore, Pennyslvania
Dr. Pierre N. Guilbert, Paris, France
Dr. Van Haywood, Augusta, Georgia
Dr. Harald Heymann, Chapel Hill, North Carolina
Dr. Sumiya Hobo, Tokyo, Japan
Dr. Abraham Ingher, Bethesda, Maryland
Dr. Stuart L. Isler, Denville, New Jersey
Ms. Cathy Jameson, Davis, Oklahoma
Dr. Vincent Kokich, Tacoma, Washington
Dr. Fritz R. Kopp, Zurich, Switzerland
Mr. Masahiro Kuwata, Tokyo, Japan
Dr. Alan Lackey, Pacific Grove, California
Dr. Roger Levine, Baltimore, Maryland
Dr. Theodore Levitas, Atlanta, Georgia
Mr. Bob Levoy, Rosyln, New York
Dr. Tom Limoli, Atlanta, Georgia
Dr. Ronald L. Maitland, New York, New York
Dr. Kenneth A. Malament, Boston, Massachusetts
Dr. John W. McLean, London, England
Mrs. Linda Miles, Virginia Beach, Virginia
Dr. Lloyd L. Miller, Weston, Massachusetts
Dr. Marilyn Miller, Princeton, New Jersey
Dr. Charles Miller, Pittsburgh, Pennsylvania
Dr. William Mopper, Winnetka, Illinois
Dr. Stephen Moss, New York, New York
Dr. Dan Nathanson, Boston, Massachusetts
Dr. Linda Niessen, Dallas, Texas
Dr. Ralph O'Connor, Tacoma, Washington
Dr. Jack Preston, Los Angeles, California
Dr. James Pride, Greenbrae, California
Mrs. Naomi Rhode, Phoenix, Arizona
Mr. James Rhode, Phoenix, Arizona
Dr. Giano Ricci, Firenze, Italy
Dr. Robert M. Ricketts, Scottsdale, Arizona
Dr. Carl Rieder, Newport Beach, California
Dr. Louis F. Rose, Philadelphia, Pennsylvania
Dr. Ed Rosenberg, Philadelphia, Pennsylvania
Dr. Serge Rozanes, Paris, France
Dr. Maurice Salama, Atlanta, Georgia
Dr. Peter Scharer, Zurich, Switzerland
Dr. Cherilyn G. Sheets, Newport Beach, California
Dr. David Shelby, New York, New York
Dr. Richard Simonsen, Maplewood, Minnesota
Dr. R. Sheldon Stein, Boston, Massachusetts
Dr. Frank Spear, Seattle, Washington
Ms. Jennifer De St. Georges, Los Gatos, California
Dr. Richard Sugarman, Atlanta, Georgia
Dr. Bernard Touati, Paris, France
Dr. Arnold Weisgold, Philadelphia, Pennsylvania
Dr. John D. West, Tacoma, Washington
Dr. Paul Yurfest, Atlanta, Georgia

INDEX

Boldface indicates pages on which treatment summaries appear.

A

B

D

E

F

G

H

I

J

L

M

N

O

P

T

V

W